Advances in Robotic-Assisted Urologic Surgery

Editor

ASHOK K. HEMAL

UROLOGIC CLINICS OF NORTH AMERICA

www.urologic.theclinics.com

Consulting Editor
SAMIR S. TANEJA

November 2014 • Volume 41 • Number 4

ELSEVIER

1600 John F. Kennedy Boulevard • Suite 1800 • Philadelphia, Pennsylvania, 19103-2899

http://www.theclinics.com

UROLOGIC CLINICS OF NORTH AMERICA Volume 41, Number 4
November 2014 ISSN 0094-0143, ISBN-13: 978-0-323-32391-8

Editor: Kerry Holland
Developmental Editor: Susan Showalter

Urologic Clinics of North America (ISSN 0094-0143) is published quarterly by Elsevier Inc., 360 Park Avenue South, New York, NY 10010-1710. Months of issue are February, May, August, and November. Business and Editorial Offices: 1600 John F. Kennedy Blvd., Suite 1800, Philadelphia, PA 19103-2899. Periodicals postage paid at New York, NY and additional mailing offices. Subscription prices are $355.00 per year (US individuals), $602.00 per year (US institutions), $415.00 per year (Canadian individuals), $752.00 per year (Canadian institutions), $515.00 per year (foreign individuals), and $752.00 per year (foreign institutions). Foreign air speed delivery is included in all *Clinics* subscription prices. All prices are subject to change without notice. **POSTMASTER:** Send address changes to *Urologic Clinics of North America*, Elsevier Health Sciences Division, Subscription Customer Service, 3251 Riverport Lane, Maryland Heights, MO 63043. Customer Service: 1-800-654-2452 (US). From outside the United States, call 1-314-447-8871. Fax: 1-314-447-8029. E-mail: JournalsCustomerServiceusa@elsevier.com (for print support) and JournalsOnlineSupport-usa@elsevier.com (for online support).

Reprints. For copies of 100 or more, of articles in this publication, please contact the Commercial Reprints Department, Elsevier Inc., 360 Park Avenue South, New York, New York 10010-1710. Tel.: 212-633-3874; Fax: 212-633-3820; E-mail: reprints@elsevier.com.

Urologic Clinics of North America is covered in MEDLINE/PubMed (*Index Medicus*), *Excerpta Medica, Current Contents/Clinical Medicine, Science Citation Index,* and *ISI/BIOMED*.

PROGRAM OBJECTIVE

The goal of *Urologic Clinics of North America* is to keep practicing urologists and urology residents up to date with current clinical practice in urology by providing timely articles reviewing the state of the art in patient care.

TARGET AUDIENCE

Practicing urologists, urology residents and other health care professionals practicing in the discipline of urology.

LEARNING OBJECTIVES

Upon completion of this activity, participants will be able to:

1. Recognize the economics of robotic urologic surgery.
2. Review robot-assisted adrealectomy, robot-assisted partial nephrectomy, and robot-assisted adrenalectomy.
3. Discuss simulators, surgery and credentialing with respect to training in robotic surgery.

ACCREDITATION

The Elsevier Office of Continuing Medical Education (EOCME) is accredited by the Accreditation Council for Continuing Medical Education (ACCME) to provide continuing medical education for physicians.

The EOCME designates this enduring material for a maximum of 15 *AMA PRA Category 1 Credit*(s)™. Physicians should claim only the credit commensurate with the extent of their participation in the activity.

All other health care professionals requesting continuing education credit for this enduring material will be issued a certificate of participation.

DISCLOSURE OF CONFLICTS OF INTEREST

The EOCME assesses conflict of interest with its instructors, faculty, planners, and other individuals who are in a position to control the content of CME activities. All relevant conflicts of interest that are identified are thoroughly vetted by EOCME for fair balance, scientific objectivity, and patient care recommendations. EOCME is committed to providing its learners with CME activities that promote improvements or quality in healthcare and not a specific proprietary business or a commercial interest.

The planning committee, staff, authors and editors listed below have identified no financial relationships or relationships to products or devices they or their spouse/life partner have with commercial interest related to the content of this CME activity:

Ali AL-Daghmin; Mohamad E. Allaf, MD; Clinton D. Bahler, MD; Mark W. Ball, MD; Jamin V. Brahmbhatt; Michael S. Cookson, MD; John B. Eifler, MD; Robert F. Elder, MD; Farzeen Firoozi; Giorgio Gandaglia, MD; Ahmet Gudeloglu, MD; Khurshid A. Guru; Kristen Helm; Ashok K. Hemal, MD; Kerry Holland; Jim C. Hu; Brynne Hunter; Wooju Jeong, MD; L Spencer Krane, MD; Indu Kumari; Sandy Lavery; Susan Marshall; Jill McNair; Mani Menon, MD; Christopher R. Mitchell; Sijo J. Parekattil, MD; Lindsay Parnell; Manish N. Patel, MD; James O. Peabody, MD; Ryan B. Pickens, MD; Kristopher Prado; Johar Raza Syed, MD, MRCS, FCPS (Urol); Akshay Sood, MD; Chandru P. Sundaram, MD; Mohammed Tawfeeq; Stephen B. Williams, MD.

The planning committee, staff, authors and editors listed below have identified financial relationships or relationships to products or devices they or their spouse/life partner have with commercial interest related to the content of this CME activity:

S. Duke Herrell, MD is a consultant/advisor for and has a research grant from Galil Medical.

Michael Stifelman is on speakers bureau and has stock ownership with Intuitive Surgical, Inc.; is a consultant/advisor for Vascular Technology, Inc. and Surgiquest, Inc.

Samir S. Taneja, MD is a consultant/advisor for Eigen Pharma LLC, GTx, Inc., Bayer Healthcare Pharmaceuticals, Healthtronics, Inc. and Hitachi, Ltd.

Quoc-Dien Trinh, MD is on speakers bureau for Intuitive Surgical.

Wesley M. White, MD is a consultant/advisor for Coloplast.

UNAPPROVED/OFF-LABEL USE DISCLOSURE

The EOCME requires CME faculty to disclose to the participants:

1. When products or procedures being discussed are off-label, unlabelled, experimental, and/or investigational (not US Food and Drug Administration [FDA] approved); and
2. Any limitations on the information presented, such as data that are preliminary or that represent ongoing research, interim analyses, and/or unsupported opinions. Faculty may discuss information about pharmaceutical agents that is outside of FDA-approved labelling. This information is intended solely for CME and is not intended to promote off-label use of these medications. If you have any questions, contact the medical affairs department of the manufacturer for the most recent prescribing information.

TO ENROLL

To enroll in the *Urologic Clinics of North America* Continuing Medical Education program, call customer service at 1-800-654-2452 or sign up online at http://www.theclinics.com/home/cme. The CME program is available to subscribers for an additional annual fee of $270 USD.

METHOD OF PARTICIPATION

In order to claim credit, participants must complete the following:

1. Complete enrolment as indicated above.
2. Read the activity.
3. Complete the CME Test and Evaluation. Participants must achieve a score of 70% on the test. All CME Tests and Evaluations must be completed online.

CME INQUIRIES/SPECIAL NEEDS

For all CME inquiries or special needs, please contact elsevierCME@elsevier.com.

Contributors

CONSULTING EDITOR

SAMIR S. TANEJA, MD
The James M. Neissa and Janet Riha Neissa Professor of Urologic Oncology; Professor of Urology and Radiology; Director, Division of Urologic Oncology; Co-Director, Smilow Comprehensive Prostate Cancer Center, Department of Urology, NYU Langone Medical Center, New York, New York

EDITOR

ASHOK K. HEMAL, MD, MCh, FAMS, FACS, FRCS(Glasg)
Professor, Department of Urology, Comprehensive Cancer Center; Professor, Wake Forest Institute for Regenerative Medicine; Director, Robotics and Minimally Invasive Surgery, Wake Forest Baptist Medical Center, School of Medicine, Wake Forest University, Winston-Salem, North Carolina

AUTHORS

ALI AL-DAGHMIN, MD
Roswell Park Cancer Institute, Buffalo, New York

MOHAMAD E. ALLAF, MD
Department of Urology, The James Buchanan Brady Urological Institute, The Johns Hopkins University School of Medicine, Baltimore, Maryland

CLINTON D. BAHLER, MD
Fellow, Department of Urology, Indiana University, Indianapolis, Indiana

MARK W. BALL, MD
Department of Urology, The James Buchanan Brady Urological Institute, The Johns Hopkins University School of Medicine, Baltimore, Maryland

JAMIN V. BRAHMBHATT, MD
Co-Director, The PUR Clinic (Personalized Urology and Robotics), South Lake Hospital, Clermont, Florida

MICHAEL S. COOKSON, MD, MMHC
Chairman and Professor, Department of Urology, University of Oklahoma College of Medicine, Oklahoma City, Oklahoma

JOHN B. EIFLER, MD
Clinical Instructor, Department of Urologic Surgery, Vanderbilt University Medical Center, Nashville, Tennessee

ROBERT F. ELDER, MD
Department of Obstetrics and Gynecology, The University of Tennessee Medical Center, Knoxville, Tennessee

FARZEEN FIROOZI, MD
Center for Female Pelvic Health and Reconstructive Surgery, The Arthur Smith Institute for Urology, Hofstra North Shore-LIJ School of Medicine, New Hyde Park, New York

GIORGIO GANDAGLIA, MD
Division of Oncology, Unit of Urology, Urological Research Institute, San Raffaele Scientific Institute, IRCCS Ospedale San Raffaele, Vita-Salute San Raffaele University, Milan, Italy

AHMET GUDELOGLU, MD
Department of Urology, Memorial Ankara Hospital, Ankara, Turkey; European Regional Director, The PUR Clinic (Personalized Urology and Robotics), Clermont, Florida

KHURSHID A. GURU, MD
Director, Robotic Surgery and ATLAS (Applied Technology Laboratory for Advanced Surgery), Robert P. Huben Endowed Professor of Urologic Oncology, Roswell Park Cancer Institute, Buffalo, New York

ASHOK K. HEMAL, MD, MCh, FAMS, FACS, FRCS(Glasg)
Professor, Department of Urology, Comprehensive Cancer Center; Professor, Wake Forest Institute for Regenerative Medicine; Director, Robotics and Minimally Invasive Surgery, Wake Forest Baptist Medical Center, School of Medicine, Wake Forest University, Winston-Salem, North Carolina

S. DUKE HERRELL, MD
Professor of Urology, Department of Urologic Surgery, Vanderbilt University Medical Center, Nashville, Tennessee

JIM C. HU, MD, MPH
Department of Urology, David Geffen School of Medicine at UCLA, Los Angeles, California

WOOJU JEONG, MD
Senior Staff, Vattikuti Urology Institute, Henry Ford Health System, Detroit, Michigan

L. SPENCER KRANE, MD
Department of Urology, Wake Forest University School of Medicine, Winston-Salem, North Carolina

SUSAN MARSHALL, MD
Clinical Instructor, Department of Urology, NYU Langone Medical Center, New York, New York

MANI MENON, MD
The Raj and Padma Vattikuti Distinguished Chair; Director, Vattikuti Urology Institute, Henry Ford Health System, Detroit, Michigan

CHRISTOPHER R. MITCHELL, MD
Instructor of Urology, Department of Urologic Surgery, Vanderbilt University Medical Center, Nashville, Tennessee

SIJO J. PAREKATTIL, MD
Co-Director, The PUR Clinic (Personalized Urology and Robotics), South Lake Hospital, Clermont, Florida

MANISH N. PATEL, MD
Chief Resident, Wake Forest Medical School and Baptist Medical, Winston-Salem, North Carolina

JAMES O. PEABODY, MD
Senior Staff, Fellowship Director, Vattikuti Urology Institute, Henry Ford Health System, Detroit, Michigan

RYAN B. PICKENS, MD
Department of Urology, The University of Tennessee Medical Center, Knoxville, Tennessee

KRIS PRADO, MD
Department of Urology, David Geffen School of Medicine at UCLA, Los Angeles, California

SYED JOHAR RAZA, MD, FCPS (Urol)
Roswell Park Cancer Institute, Buffalo, New York

AKSHAY SOOD, MD
Resident PGY-1, Vattikuti Urology Institute, Henry Ford Health System, Detroit, Michigan

MICHAEL STIFELMAN, MD
Professor of Urology, NYU School of Medicine, Director, NYU Robotic Surgery Center, Chief of Service, Tisch Hospital, New York, New York

CHANDRU P. SUNDARAM, MD
Professor, Director of Residency Program and Minimally Invasive Surgery Fellowship, Department of Urology, Indiana University, Indianapolis, Indiana

MOHAMMED TAWFEEQ, MD
Roswell Park Cancer Institute, Buffalo, New York

QUOC-DIEN TRINH, MD
Division of Urologic Surgery and Center for Surgery and Public Health, Brigham and Women's Hospital, Dana-Farber Cancer Institute, Harvard Medical School, Boston, Massachusetts

WESLEY M. WHITE, MD
Director of Laparoscopic and Robotic Urologic Surgery, Department of Urology, The University of Tennessee Medical Center, Knoxville, Tennessee

STEPHEN B. WILLIAMS, MD
Department of Urology, The University of Texas MD Anderson Cancer Center, Houston, Texas

Contents

Foreword: Advances in Robotic-Assisted Urologic Surgery xv

Samir S. Taneja

Preface: Urology Robotic Surgery: 15-year Path xvii

Ashok K. Hemal

Robot-Assisted Radical Prostatectomy: Inching Toward Gold Standard 473

Akshay Sood, Wooju Jeong, James O. Peabody, Ashok K. Hemal, and Mani Menon

Robot-assisted radical prostatectomy (RARP) offers excellent and lasting oncologic control. Technical refinements in apical dissection, such as the retroapical approach of synchronous urethral transection, and adoption of real-time frozen section analysis of the excised prostate during RARP have substantially reduced positive surgical margin rates, particularly in high-risk disease patients. Furthermore, precision offered by the robotic platform and technical evolution of radical prostatectomy, including enhanced nerve sparing (veil), have led to improved potency and continence outcomes as well as better safety profile in patients undergoing surgical therapy for prostate cancer.

Robot-Assisted Laparoscopic Simple Anatomic Prostatectomy 485

Manish N. Patel and Ashok K. Hemal

Management options for men with symptomatic benign prostatic hyperplasia have increased in recent years. Surgery is recommended for patients who have renal insufficiency secondary to benign prostatic hyperplasia (BPH), who have recurrent urinary tract infections, bladder stones or gross hematuria caused by BPH, and those who have lower urinary tract symptoms refractory to other therapies. Technology is improving, and the use of endoscopic techniques with lasers has gained popularity. The use of robotics overcomes the limitations of pure laparoscopy. Robotic assistance helps in quicker skills acquisition. This article describes techniques for robotic-assisted laparoscopic simple anatomic prostatectomy in a step-by-step manner.

Best Evidence Regarding the Superiority or Inferiority of Robot-Assisted Radical Prostatectomy 493

John B. Eifler and Michael S. Cookson

Robotic-assisted laparoscopic radical prostatectomy (RALP) has enjoyed rapid adoption over the past decade without rigorous clinical studies demonstrating superior clinical outcomes over radical retropubic prostatectomy (RRP). This article reviews the literature comparing RALP and RRP with regard to oncologic, perioperative, and functional outcomes, summarizing evidence for and against the superiority of RALP.

Robot-assisted Intracorporeal Urinary Diversion: Where Do We Stand in 2014? 503

Syed Johar Raza, Mohammed Tawfeeq, Ali Al-Daghmin, and Khurshid A. Guru

Radical cystectomy can only be considered as minimally invasive when both extirpative and reconstructive part of the procedure are performed with an intracorporeal approach. Robot-assisted radical cystectomy makes it possible to achieve this task, which seemed difficult with conventional laparoscopy. Intracorporeal urinary diversion (ICUD) is associated with better perioperative outcomes. Quality-of-life assessments and functional outcomes from continent ICUD are encouraging. Working in high-volumes center with mentored training can help robotic surgeons to learn the techniques of ICUD in conjunction with robot-assisted radical cystectomy. This article discusses the perioperative and functional outcomes of ICUD with a review of literature.

Emerging Technologies to Improve Techniques and Outcomes of Robotic Partial Nephrectomy: Striving Toward the Pentafecta **511**

L. Spencer Krane and Ashok K. Hemal

The technique of robotic partial nephrectomy continues to evolve, but the goals remain the same. Achievement of pentafecta outcomes is difficult to obtain; however, surgeons should continue to strive for this standard of excellence. The future continues to be bright for patients and surgeons alike in continuing to perform robot-assisted partial nephrectomy.

Robot-Assisted Surgery for the Treatment of Upper Urinary Tract Urothelial Carcinoma **521**

Susan Marshall and Michael Stifelman

Robot-assisted laparoscopic surgery is increasingly used in urologic oncologic surgery. Robotic nephroureterectomy is still a relatively new technique. As upper tract urothelial carcinoma is a rare disease, intermediate- and long-term outcome data are scarce. However, robotic nephroureterectomy does seem to offer advantages to open and laparoscopic counterparts, with comparable short-term oncologic and functional outcomes. Here the authors review the robotic surgical management of upper tract urothelial carcinoma, with a review of the steps and tips on making this approach more widely adoptable.

Robot-Assisted Adrenalectomy (Total, Partial, & Metastasectomy) **539**

Mark W. Ball and Mohamad E. Allaf

Robotic-assisted adrenalectomy is an increasingly used intervention for patients with a variety of surgical adrenal lesions, including adenomas, aldosteronomas, pheochromocytomas, and metastases to the adrenal gland. Compared with traditional laparoscopy, robotic adrenalectomy has comparable perioperative outcomes and is associated with improved hospital length of stay and blood loss, though it does come at a cost premium. Emerging literature also supports a role for robotics in partial adrenalectomy and metastasectomy. Ultimately, well-conducted prospective trials are needed to fully define the role of robotics in the surgical management of adrenal disease.

Robotic-assisted Sacrocolpopexy for Pelvic Organ Prolapse **549**

Wesley M. White, Ryan B. Pickens, Robert F. Elder, and Farzeen Firoozi

The demand for surgical correction of pelvic organ prolapse is expected to grow as the aging population remains active and focused on quality of life. Definitive correction of pelvic organ prolapse can be accomplished through both vaginal and abdominal approaches. This article provides a contemporary reference source that specifically addresses the historical framework, diagnostic algorithm, and therapeutic options for the treatment of female pelvic organ prolapse. Particular emphasis is placed on the role and technique of abdominal-based reconstruction using robotic technology and the evolving controversy regarding the use of synthetic vaginal mesh.

Robot-Assisted Microsurgery in Male Infertility and Andrology **559**

Ahmet Gudeloglu, Jamin V. Brahmbhatt, and Sijo J. Parekattil

Use of the operative microscope marked a new era for microsurgery in male infertility and andrology in the 1970s. More than a decade has passed since the initial description of the first robotic-assisted microsurgical vasovasostomy. Large single-center series have recently been published on robotic-assisted microsurgery for vasectomy reversal, especially in the past few years. Multicenter studies are also beginning to be reported, and the potential for this new platform for microsurgery is starting to become more apparent. This article describes the basic technical details of robotic-assisted microsurgery in male infertility and andrology, and reviews the latest literature.

Image-Guided Surgery and Emerging Molecular Imaging: Advances to Complement Minimally Invasive Surgery **567**

Christopher R. Mitchell and S. Duke Herrell

Recent technologic advances have ushered in an era of surgery with a focus on development of minimally invasive surgical techniques. Specifically, robotic platforms, with robotic-assisted instrumentation, have helped overcome previous barriers to widespread adoption of laparoscopic surgery. Along these lines, image guidance will soon be incorporated into many laparoscopic/robotic procedures to improve surgeon ease, accuracy, and comfort with these complex operations. Thus, we explore recent advances in image-guided surgery and emerging molecular imaging technologies for minimally invasive urologic surgery.

Training in Robotic Surgery: Simulators, Surgery, and Credentialing **581**

Clinton D. Bahler and Chandru P. Sundaram

The use of robot-assisted laparoscopic surgery has increased rapidly and with it, the need to better define a structured curriculum and credentialing process. Numerous efforts have been made by surgical societies to define the requisite skills for robotic surgeons, but individual institutions have the responsibility for granting privileges. Recently, efforts have focused on creating a standardized curriculum with competency-based assessments. A competency-based approach offers a better hope of honoring the principle of "above all, do no harm" and obtaining continued acceptance of new operative technologies such as robot-assisted surgery.

Economics of Robotic Surgery: Does It Make Sense and for Whom? **591**

Stephen B. Williams, Kris Prado, and Jim C. Hu

The authors performed a literature review to identify cost-effectiveness research as it pertains to robotic surgery. There is increased utilization of robotic surgery in urology with limited comparative effectiveness research demonstrating superiority over conventional, less costly treatment options. Further research into identifying determinants for optimal utilization of robotics and newer technology is needed.

Models of Assessment of Comparative Outcomes of Robot-Assisted Surgery: Best Evidence Regarding the Superiority or Inferiority of Robot-Assisted Radical Prostatectomy **597**

Giorgio Gandaglia and Quoc-Dien Trinh

The widespread dissemination of robot-assisted radical prostatectomy (RARP) occurred despite the absence of high-level evidence supporting its safety and efficacy in patients with clinically localized prostate cancer. This study aims at systematically evaluating the models adopted in scientific reports assessing the comparative effectiveness of RARP versus open radical prostatectomy (ORP). Although several retrospective observational studies have assessed the comparative effectiveness of RARP and ORP, currently no published randomized data are available to comprehensively evaluate this issue. Furthermore, well-designed prospective investigations are needed to ultimately assess the benefits of RARP compared with other treatment modalities in patients with clinically localized prostate cancer.

Index **607**

UROLOGIC CLINICS OF NORTH AMERICA

FORTHCOMING ISSUES

February 2015
Minimally Invasive Pediatric Urologic Surgery
Aseem R. Shukla, *Editor*

May 2015
Multimodal Treatment of Urothelial Cancer
Arjun Balar and Matt Milowsky, *Editors*

August 2015
Testicular Cancer
Daniel W. Lin, *Editor*

RECENT ISSUES

August 2014
Urodynamics
Benjamin M. Brucker and Victor W. Nitti, *Editors*

May 2014
Early Stage Prostate Cancer: Screening and Detection
Stacy Loeb and Matthew R. Cooperberg, *Editors*

February 2014
Current Management of Male Infertility
Craig S. Niederberger, *Editor*

RELATED INTEREST

Magnetic Resonance Imaging Clinics of North America May 2014 (Vol. 22)
The Male Pelvis
Mukesh G. Harisinghani, *Editor*

Foreword
Advances in Robotic-Assisted Urologic Surgery

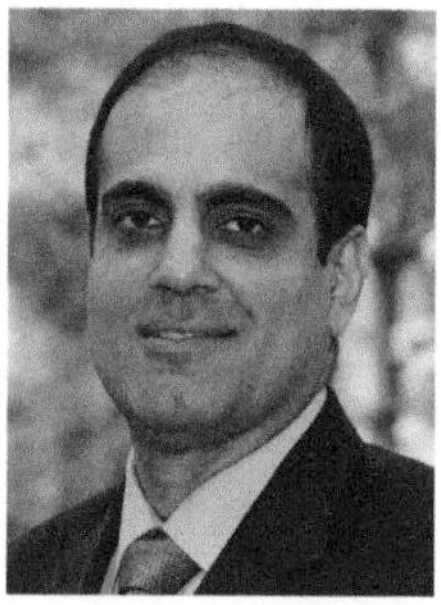

Samir S. Taneja, MD
Consulting Editor

The role of robotics has shifted from the nouveau to standard fare in American urology. In many centers (mine included), the decision-making process, when evaluating patients for planned surgery, starts first with the question of whether surgery can be done with robotic assistance. This shift in paradigm follows a rapid adaptation of most common urologic procedures to fit the robotic-assisted surgical paradigm. As we are truly in the infancy of surgical robotic tools, future adaptation of the majority of surgical procedures, common or uncommon, is very likely. Questions remain regarding candidate selection, measurement of benefit, and balancing benefit against cost.

Although there is ongoing controversy regarding the degree of improvement in surgical outcomes achieved with robotics, I believe there is general consensus that recovery from minimally invasive surgery is easier for patients, that short-term complications related to recovery are fewer, and that robotics, while costly, is a tool that facilitates a surgeon's transition to minimally invasive techniques. In the case of the latter, the current controversies may be misdirected. While measuring outcome improvement on an individual case basis is unlikely to show benefit (after all, a great open surgeon should not be any different than a great robotic surgeon), the true impact of robotic technology may be at a population level. By providing surgeons a comfort level in attempting procedures with which they may not have otherwise been comfortable, robotic assistance has increased access to procedures for which competent surgeons may have not previously been available. This assumes, of course, that surgeons can be trained to perform these procedures safely.

A number of challenges remain in implementation of robotic surgery. The first on everyone's mind is cost. Can the cost of robotics be sustained by a struggling health care economy? If not demonstrable in the direct, measurable, cost of care, the justification of cost could be measured, perhaps, in opportunity cost and improvement in quality of care—difficult, but necessary metrics. Surgeon training and safety of the transition to robotics-assisted surgery are major hurdles for the community. Adaptation of simulators, training programs, and standardized credentialing will be necessary. Finally, maintaining the ability of young surgeons to perform open surgery when needed is a unique challenge created by the introduction of robotics into our field. It is important not only from the perspective of being able to salvage a case not progressing robotically but also for the purpose of ensuring proper candidate selection for robotic procedures. Our ability to solve these challenges, in my opinion, will determine the fate of technological advance in surgery.

In this issue of *Urologic Clinics of North America*, edited by Dr Ashok Hemal, a global leader in the

Urol Clin N Am 41 (2014) xv–xvi
http://dx.doi.org/10.1016/j.ucl.2014.08.002

field of robotic-assisted surgery, we attempt to demonstrate the progress robotic surgeons have made in utilizing the approach across urologic practice. In creating the table of contents, Dr Hemal has included discussion of a number of the aforementioned controversies as well as a critical discussion of the public health impact of robotic surgery. He has invited a number of the most critical minds in the field to offer perspective on robotic surgery, its current practice, its limitations, and future directions. I am extremely indebted to Dr Hemal, and the esteemed article contributors, for what should be a very informative issue of *Urologic Clinics of North America.*

Samir S. Taneja, MD
Division of Urologic Oncology
Smilow Comprehensive Prostate Cancer Center
Department of Urology
NYU Langone Medical Center
150 East 32nd Street, Suite 200
New York, NY 10016, USA

E-mail address:
samir.taneja@nyumc.org

Preface
Urology Robotic Surgery: 15-year Path

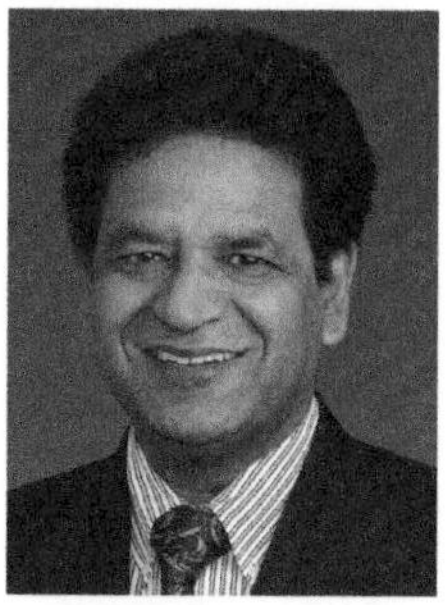

Ashok K. Hemal, MD, MCh, FAMS, FACS, FRCS(Glasg)
Editor

Urologists have always been at the forefront of new developments and have changed the face of open surgery by embracing ever-changing improvements and technological advances. Robotic-assisted laparoscopic urologic surgery is a major evolution in the field and has now become a major subspecialty. Robotic-assisted laparoscopic urologic surgery was first performed in 2000, and the last 15 years have been testimony to its exponential growth and overwhelming adoption by surgeons and patients across the world.

There is an ever-increasing amount of information available on the subject that surgeons need to quickly assimilate. This issue of *Urologic Clinics of North America* aims to provide comprehensive, state-of-the-art information about the recent developments in the areas of Uro-Oncology, Reconstructive Urology, and Female Urology. Topics such as issue of training, evidence-based practice, the economics of robotic surgery, and the impact on public and global health are also covered.

The contributors are truly pioneers and the best experts in the field. I am extremely grateful to all the individual authors and believe the information they have shared will be extremely useful to present and future urologists who have embraced this form of minimally invasive surgery.

It is an honor and privilege for me to write the preface as I have been involved in robotic surgery since its inception and it has been an astounding and eclectic journey.

Ashok K. Hemal, MD, MCh, FAMS, FACS, FRCS(Glasg)
Department of Urology
Comprehensive Cancer Center
Wake Forest Institute for Regenerative Medicine

Robotics and Minimally Invasive Surgery
Wake Forest Baptist Medical Center
Wake Forest School of Medicine
Winston-Salem, NC 27157, USA

E-mail address:
ashokkhemal@gmail.com

Urol Clin N Am 41 (2014) xvii
http://dx.doi.org/10.1016/j.ucl.2014.08.001
0094-0143/14/$ – see front matter

Robot-Assisted Radical Prostatectomy

Inching Toward Gold Standard

Akshay Sood, MD[a,*,1], Wooju Jeong, MD[a,1],
James O. Peabody, MD[a],
Ashok K. Hemal, MD, MCh, FAMS, FACS, FRCS(Glasg)[b],
Mani Menon, MD[a]

KEYWORDS

• Minimally invasive surgery • Robotics • Prostatectomy • Prostate cancer

KEY POINTS

- Surgical management of clinically localized prostate cancer leads to superior survival when compared with observation or radiotherapy.
- Robot-assisted radical prostatectomy (RARP) has become the modality of choice for surgical management of prostate cancer and has evolved dramatically since its inception in the early 2000s.
- RARP offers excellent and lasting oncologic control.
- Technical refinements in apical dissection, such as the retroapical approach of synchronous urethral transection, and adoption of real-time frozen section analysis of the excised prostate during RARP, have substantially reduced positive surgical margin rates, particularly in high-risk disease patients.
- Precision offered by the robotic platform and technical evolution of radical prostatectomy, including enhanced nerve sparing (veil and superveil), have led to improved potency and continence outcomes as well as better safety profile in patients undergoing surgical therapy for prostate cancer.

INTRODUCTION

Prostate cancer (PCa) remains the most common internal organ malignancy and the second leading cause of cancer-related death in men in the United States.[1] Most cases of PCa are clinically localized at the time of diagnosis[2,3] and potentially curable by an array of therapeutic modalities, with the major options being (**Fig. 1**)[4]:

1. Observation (active surveillance and watchful waiting)
2. Radiotherapy (intensity-modulated radiation therapy and external beam radiotherapy)
3. Surgery (radical prostatectomy [RP])

Each modality has its benefits and limitations, although current evidence suggests RP to be the most effective of these modalities. RP leads to better overall and cancer-specific survival when compared with observation[5] or radiotherapy alone[6–8] across all PCa risk groups (D'Amico), with patients with high-risk disease benefitting the most.[6,8]

RP can be performed via an open approach or a laparoscopic approach with or without robotic assistance. In recent years, there has been a remarkable increase in the use of robot-assisted RP (RARP). In 2001, less than 0.3% of all RPs were performed robotically; however, by 2011, 61% to 80% of all RPs in the United States were

Disclosures: none.
Conflicts of interest: none.

[a] Vattikuti Urology Institute, Henry Ford Health System, 2799 West Grand Boulevard, Detroit, MI 48202, USA;
[b] Department of Urology, Wake Forest School of Medicine, Winston-Salem, Medical Center Boulevard, NC 27157-1090, USA
[1] These authors contributed equally to the work.
* Corresponding author.
E-mail address: asood1@hfhs.org

Urol Clin N Am 41 (2014) 473–484
http://dx.doi.org/10.1016/j.ucl.2014.07.002

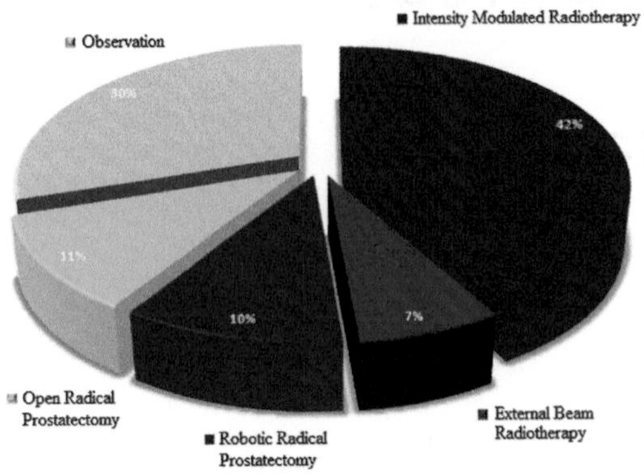

Fig. 1. Major options for treatment of localized PCa. (*Data from* SEER-MEDICARE (2004-2009). Available at: http://seer.cancer.gov/. Accessed July 17, 2014.)

being performed with robotic assistance.[9,10] Recent population-based reports and meta-analyses, constituting level 2a evidence,[9,11–13] have shown that RARP compares favorably with open RP (ORP) in terms of perioperative outcomes, perioperative complications, and functional (continence and potency) results. In terms of oncologic outcomes, whereas the few large retrospective series of RARP have reported equivalent outcomes,[14–16] there is a paucity of long-term definitive data.[17]

In this review, the various technical advances are discussed that have been made in RARP since its inception, leading to increasingly better oncologic, functional, and safety outcomes in patients undergoing RARP for management of PCa.

HISTORICAL PERSPECTIVE

Minimally invasive surgery (MIS) began in 1987 with laparoscopic cholecystectomy.[18] Laparoscopic RP (LRP) was first performed by Schuessler and colleagues[19] in 1991, and further developed and pioneered by Guillonneau and Vallancien,[20] subsequently. The strengths and weaknesses of the MIS approach became apparent quickly. The strengths included smaller incision, less surgical site infection, blood loss, and postoperative pain, shorter hospital stay and convalescence period, and better cosmesis. On the other hand, the weaknesses included loss of haptic feedback, natural hand-eye coordination, and dexterity. These limitations made delicate dissections and anastomoses difficult, if not impossible.[21] Robotic surgery was developed to overcome these limitations of minimally invasive laparoscopic surgery and to enhance the capabilities of surgeons performing open surgery.

RARP was first reported by Abbou and colleagues[22] in 2000. RARP has since been refined and popularized by Menon and colleagues[19] as a minimally invasive technique, with vastly improved ergonomics, superior outcomes, and shorter learning curve relative to LRP. Robotics has since permeated and found its application in many oncologic,[23,24] nononcologic,[25,26] and pediatric[27–29] urologic procedures, and, more recently, in kidney transplantation.[30–33]

INDICATIONS AND CONTRAINDICATIONS

Indications are same as those for ORP. Patients with locally advanced disease (T3–T4 disease) with or without nodal metastasis (N1) may be considered as part of a multimodal/multidisciplinary management strategy and constitute a highly selected group. Relative contraindications include chronic obstructive pulmonary disease and abnormalities of cardiac function caused by difficulties in ventilation, which may occur in patients undergoing RARP as a result of exposure to pneumoperitoneum and steep Trendelenberg position. Previous abdominal/pelvic surgery may also present difficulties but is not a contraindication; a careful laparoscopic review and adhesiolysis at the time of port placement are helpful in avoiding delays and complications later during the procedure. Patient factors, such as morbid obesity, narrow pelvis, large prostate, large median lobe, or surgery in the salvage setting, increase the complexity of RARP, and hence, should be reserved for experienced surgeons.[34]

TECHNICAL ADVANCEMENTS IN CANCER CONTROL

The most important outcome to assess in patients undergoing RP is cancer control. Survival statistics and biochemical recurrence rates are the critical indicators of oncologic control, but all of these require long-term follow-up to assess and can be subject to significant reporting and interpretational biases.[13] Positive surgical margin (PSM) rate thus remains an early oncologic outcome measure of importance when evaluating surgical therapy.

In mature RARP series, overall PSM rates have ranged between 9% and 19%, depending on the patient and surgeon characteristics. In our patients, undergoing the Vattikuti Institute Prostatectomy (VIP) technique[35–37] of RARP, we have previously shown a PSM rate of 13% and 35% in patients with pT2 and pT3 disease, respectively.[38] The most common locations for PSMs during RARP are posterolateral and apical, but location and number do not seem to affect survival.[39] However, an extensive PSM does seem to affect the prognosis adversely.[40] Various technical modifications and tailoring the nerve sparing according to the disease severity have been shown to improve cancer control during RARP. The major technical modifications are listed in **Fig. 2** and are discussed later.

Apical Dissection

Meticulous dissection of the prostatic apex is one of the most challenging steps of RP, for multiple reasons. First, the apex is in a relatively inaccessible location, deep beneath the pubic arch and surrounded with vital structures such as the dorsal venous complex (DVC), converging erectile neurovascular bundles, rectum, and urethral sphincter.[39] Second, the apex lacks the distinct prostatic capsule and periprostatic tissue that surrounds the posterolateral prostate, making the accurate planes of dissection in this area difficult to find. Third, the anatomy of the apex is highly variable from individual to individual, with some glands harboring a distal beak of apical tissue protruding posterior to the urethra (also known as a posterior apical notch). This hidden posterior extension might be violated during surgery, especially if the dissection is carried out in a plane perpendicular to the longitudinal axis of the urethra.[39]

Therefore, to optimize the cancer control (as well as urinary and potency outcomes), surgeons have sought ways to optimally dissect the apical tissue. For example, to prevent the DVC or puboprostatic ligaments from obstructing the view, Tewari and colleagues[41] used a 30° upward-looking lens combined with cephalad retraction of the prostate (by an assistant) to approach the transition of the apex into the membranous urethra from the posterior undersurface of the prostate rather than the conventional anterior approach.[39] This novel retroapical technique decreased the investigators' PSM rates from 4.4% to 1.4%. Other proposed modifications include upfront cold transection of the DVC facilitated by increased pneumoperitoneum and its subsequent ligation.[42,43]

Degree of Nerve Sparing Versus Cancer Control

Before deciding how wide to dissect the neurovascular bundles, the surgeon must take into consideration the clinical patient data, including prostate biopsy findings, prostate-specific antigen levels, digital rectal examination findings, patient age, preoperative sexual function, and patient expectations, because different levels of nerve sparing can be considered based on these factors, and accordingly, different planes of dissection can be entered. Nerve sparing is not an all or none phenomenon, as it was believed to be.

Tewari and colleagues[44] suggested using the periprostatic veins as an anatomic landmark to differentiate among the various fascial compartments. Depending on the preoperative clinical characteristics and how the extent of the tumor at base is appreciated, the surgeon may choose to carry out the dissection in 1 of the 3 periprostatic anatomic planes: in an intrafascial plane (complete nerve sparing as ascertained by the view of glistening prostate), an interfascial plane (partial nerve sparing confirmed by a whitish coloration of the prostate), or an extrafascial plane (non–nerve sparing determined by fatty tissue seen on the prostate).[39] These investigators showed a decline in PSM rate from 2.1% to 1% by adoption of

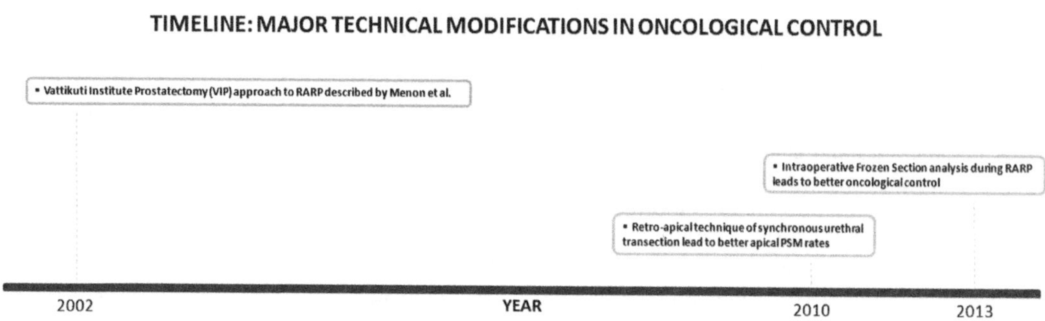

MODIFICATION	YEAR	GROUP	OUTCOME
Retro-apical technique of synchronous urethral transection	2010	Tewari et al.	Decrease in apical positive surgical margin (PSM) rates from 4.4% to 1.4%, without any compromise in potency and continence outcomes.
Intraoperative Frozen Section analysis during RARP	2013	Jeong et al.	In high-risk disease (pT3) patients, the PSM rates decreased from 43% to 17% (P = .05), without any compromise in potency and continence outcomes. No increase in operative time.
	2013	Beyer et al.	In all comers, the PSM rates decreased from 24% to 16% (P = .003). Significant improvement in nerve sparing rates was also noted, increasing from 81% to 97% (P = .001). No increase in operative time.

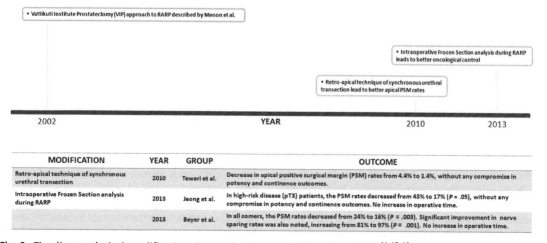

Fig. 2. Timeline: technical modifications in oncologic control. (*Data from* Refs.[41,45,46])

these visual cues, despite an increase in risk categorization of the patients operated.

Intraoperative Frozen Section Analysis

Techniques for extracting prostate intraoperatively during RARP have recently been described by our group and Beyer and colleagues[45,46] These techniques are aimed at increasing the certainty of adequate excision of the tumor by allowing performance of real-time bimanual examination and frozen section histopathology of the excised prostate specimen, especially in patients with aggressive high-risk disease.

In our technique a GelPOINT device (Applied Medical, Rancho Santa Margarita, CA) is used, which allows for rapid specimen extraction without compromising the pneumoperitoneum. The GelPOINT access port is inserted in the periumbilical region through a 4-cm to 5-cm vertical incision. The GelSeal cap, prepared with a 12-mm camera port and a 10-mm assistant port preplaced through it, is secured on top of the access port. Cruciate stab incisions around the 10-mm port on the GelSeal cap are made to facilitate the retrieval of the specimen. Other ports are placed and the patient is put in a 30° Trendelenberg, as previously described.[35] After excision of the prostate, the specimen is retrieved through the stab incision in the GelSeal cap without dedocking the robot, and a bimanual examination is performed on table by the surgeon. Frozen section biopsies are obtained from areas suspicious for PSM and after being carefully marked for anatomic orientation are sent for pathology. Biopsies positive or suspicious for cancer result in more tissue being removed from the corresponding pelvic bed region, which is labeled and sent for permanent sections. Beyer and colleagues, developing on their technique of NeuroSAFE for ORP,[47] also recently described a similar technique for RARP.[45] In contrast with our technique, in the NeuroSAFE technique, the prostate is systematically sectioned in a circumferential manner (rather than targeted biopsies as we do) and the sections are sent for frozen section analysis. Both these studies showed a dramatic reduction in PSMs by performing intraoperative frozen biopsies, without an increase in the operative time or blood loss. Beyer and colleagues found that the overall PSM rate decreased from 24% to 16% ($P = .003$) by adopting the NeuroSAFE technique, and we found that the PSM rates (in patients with pT3 disease) decreased from 43% to 17% ($P = .05$). Beyer and colleagues also showed that in addition to decreasing the PSM rates, the NeuroSAFE technique also improved the nerve sparing rates in the setting of both organ-confined and locally advanced disease.

TECHNICAL ADVANCEMENTS IN URINARY CONTINENCE

Oncologic outcomes achieved with RARP and ORP have been excellent and equivalent, and hence, the focus of innovation has increasingly been on the preservation of quality of life (QOL). Urinary control after RP has the greatest impact on a patient's QOL[48,49] and accordingly, maintaining optimal urinary function after RP takes precedence among outcomes, given ideal control of cancer. As a result, several surgical modifications in technique have been attempted to achieve early return and improve overall continence rates.

Fig. 3 summarizes the various technical modifications and advances that have been made in this regard, and their impact on continence outcomes. Many of these modifications were developed in the ORP model, but because the surgical principles underlying continence preservation are consistent irrespective of the approach, these modifications were readily adapted for robotic surgery. These modifications are detailed later.

Bladder Neck Preservation

As understanding of the continence anatomy and mechanism evolved, the usefulness of bladder neck preservation was shown.[50] Gaker and Steel[51] and Deliveliotis and colleagues[52] both reported that precise dissection of the prostatovesical junction and preservation of the circular muscle fibers of the bladder neck lead to early return of continence, although overall continence rates remained unchanged. Similar results have been reported by other groups as well.[53,54]

Periurethral Suspension

Many investigators have shown the usefulness of periurethral suspension after DVC ligation. Different approaches have been described. Patel and colleagues,[55] using their technique of DVC suspension, showed earlier return of continence as well as higher continence rates at 3 months. Similarly, Campenni and colleagues,[56] using their technique of pubourethral suspension, Noguchi and colleagues,[57] using their approach of vesicourethral anastomosis suspension, and Jorion,[58] using their technique of fascial sling suspension, also reported significantly improvement in continence outcomes. However, the latter modification also increased the risk of urinary retention. We do not perform this step routinely, because we have noted no additional improvement in urinary control by performing periurethral suspension in addition to our routine nerve sparing VIP technique.

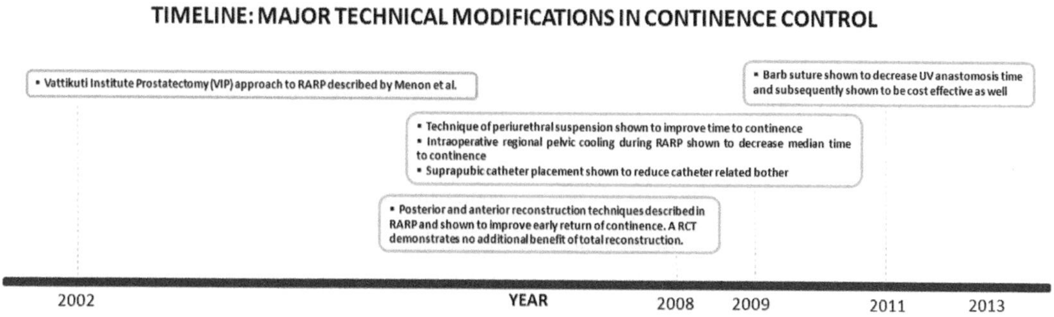

MODIFICATION	YEAR	GROUP	OUTCOME
Periurethral suspension	2009	Patel et al.	Suspension stitch during RARP leads to improved continence at 3 months.
Retzius-sparing approach of RARP	2013	Galfano et al.	This completely intrafascial technique of RARP yielded high continence rates – 96% at 1 year. Further studies needed to establish non-inferiority/superiority of this technique over conventional RARP techniques.
Periurethral reconstruction			
Posterior reconstruction	2008	Nguyen et al.	Improvement in rates of early continence (56% vs. 17% at 6 weeks)
	2011	Coelho et al.	Improvement in rates of early continence (43% vs. 51% at 4 weeks), but no difference in 3/6 month continence rates.
	2011	Sutherland et al.	In this Phase-II RCT, the authors found no difference in continence rates at 3 months in patients with and without posterior reconstruction. Limitation of this study was small sample size.
Anterior reconstruction	2007	Tewari et al.	Decrease in median time to continence.
Total reconstruction	2008	Menon et al.	In this 2-group RCT, the authors found no difference in continence rates in patients with and without total reconstruction (both anterior and posterior).
	2010	Sammon et al.	Single or double layer anastomosis did not correlate to urinary outcomes at 2 years.
Intraoperative regional cooling during RARP	2009	Finley et al.	Regional pelvic cooling during RRP was associated with early return of continence. Longer and deeper cooling improved continence.
Barbed suture utilization for UV anastomosis	2011	Sammon et al.	UV anastomosis using V-loc suture showed a decrease in anastomotic time without change in outcomes.
Suprapubic catheter placement	2009	Krane et al.	Significant decrease in catheter related patient discomfort and utilization of anti-cholinergic medication.
	2012	Orikasa et al.	Improved early quality of life in patients undergoing suprapubic catheter placement.
	2014	Prasad et al.	In this RCT, the authors found no difference in pain and catheter related bother in patients who underwent suprapubic vs. Foley catheter placement.

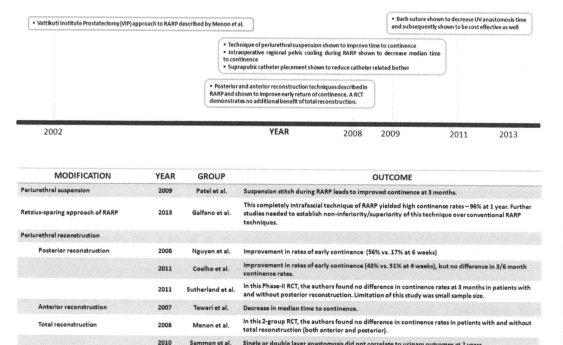

Fig. 3. Technical modifications in continence control. (*Data from* Refs.[55,63,68–70,72,83,84,87–89,110,111])

Puboprostatic Ligament Sparing

It has been hypothesized that preservation of the puboprostatic fibromuscular tissue would provide anterior support to the urethra, leading to better urinary control.[59] Studies by Poore and colleagues[60] and Avant and colleagues[61] reported that preservation of pupoprostatic ligaments facilitated an earlier median return to continence when compared with standard ORP. On the contrary, Deliveliotis and colleagues[52] showed that there was no short-term continence benefit in adding pupoprostatic ligaments preservation to bladder neck sparing. This concept has been translated into Retzius-sparing RARP by Galfano and colleagues[62,63] and Rha and colleagues[64] Conventional RARP technique for bladder neck dissection, nerve sparing, and apical dissection use an anterior approach, but these investigators have suggested a posterior approach without the need for dropping down the bladder. Galfano and colleagues claimed that this technique showed better outcomes in early continence rate, compared with the published data. However, this technique is still in its infancy, and there is lack of high-level evidence to support the superiority of this technique over the conventional approaches.

Periurethral Reconstruction Techniques

Great interest has been paid to periurethral reconstructive techniques: both posterior musculofascial plate and anterior puboprostatic collar repair. The posterior repair technique, using a 2-stitch posterior rhabdosphincter reconstruction before urethrovesical anastomosis, was first proposed by Klein[65] and Rocco and colleagues[66,67] and reported dramatic success in improving early continence in both ORP and LRP settings. Continence rates at 1 month improved from 30% to 79% for ORP and from 32% to 84% for LRP. These results have been replicated in the setting of RARP by Nguyen and colleagues,[68] who showed that the continence rates improved from 17% to 56% at 6 weeks. Coelho and colleagues[69] also reported early return of continence in patients undergoing posterior reconstruction during RARP (42.7% vs 51.6% at 4 weeks), but no difference in continence rates was observed at 3 and 6 months. Tewari and colleagues[70] developed a technique for preservation of the anterior puboprostatic collar, with 1-week and 6-week continence rates of 29% and 62%, respectively; subsequently, a complete vesicourethral repair technique was developed, yielding 1-week and 6-week continence rates of 38% and 83%.[71] Our own experience, in a randomized control trial setting,[72] showed that reconstruction of periprostatic tissue (both anterior and posterior) provided no added benefit in early return to continence (80% vs 74% at 30 days; *P*>.1). The lack of improvement noted in the patients undergoing complete periurethral repair was probably because of the excellent continence outcomes already achieved by the patients in the control group secondary to precise nerve sparing, urethral length preservation, and bladder neck sparing. Despite this finding, we do continue to perform a posterior musculofascial repair before ultraviolet anastomosis.

Preservation of Urethral Length

Multiple studies have reported the importance of preserving membranous urethral length for optimal urinary continence.[73,74] Coakley and colleagues[75] and Nguyen and colleagues,[76] using preoperative magnetic resonance imaging, reported that the membranous urethral length was directly related with continence outcomes after RP. However, the challenge lies in precisely identifying the junction between the prostatic apex and the proximal membranous urethra.[77] The improved visualization of the robotic interface is implicitly beneficial in pursuit of this goal. van Randenborgh and colleagues[78] suggested a technique of craniodorsal retraction of prostate for maximal preservation of urethral length. They reported significant improvement in continence (89% vs 76%; *P*<.05).

Creating a Watertight Anastomosis

Urine extravasation secondary to poor vesicourethral anastomosis has been shown to lead to local inflammation followed by fibrosis and scarring of the vesicourethral junction.[79,80] Van Velthoven described a simple, running, laparoscopic technique for accomplishing a watertight vesicourethral anastomosis. This technique is easily transferrable and reproducible in the robotic environment and has been described by our group in detail previously.[35]

Locoregional Pelvic Hypothermia

Controlled hypothermia is a well-established technique that has been used to limit the inflammatory cascade common to all surgical procedures.[81–83] Finley and colleagues[84] were the first to use, and show the benefits of, regional cooling during RARP. These investigators used an endorectal cooling balloon system, which was continuously irrigated with ice-cold saline at 4°C to maintain effective regional hypothermia throughout the procedure. With this technical modification, the investigators noted a significant decrease in the time to continence (median 39 days vs median 59 days; *P* = .002) as well as improved overall continence rates at 3 months (86.8% vs 68.6%). This technique might aid in improving the potency outcomes as well, because the underlying physiologic principles used are consistent with the athermal technique of cavernosal nerve sparing (see later discussion).

Barbed Suture

Sammon and colleagues[85] performed a randomized control trial showing the usefulness of barbed sutures in decreasing the time for urethrovesical anastomosis (26.8% reduction) and posterior reconstruction (23.3% reduction). V-Loc (Covidien, Mansfield, MA, USA) barbed sutures were used, and knots were not required because of the autolocking properties of the suture. These investigators found no difference in leaks, bladder neck contractures, patient symptoms, or other outcome measures.[86] Subsequently, it has been shown to be a cost-effective approach as well.[85]

Suprapubic Catheter

Traditionally with ORP, the bladder had been drained via urethral catheter for a finite period (2–3 weeks) to maintain urethral patency.[87] Despite this precaution, bladder neck contracture rates ranged from 5% to 32%.[88] With the advent of running anastomosis and the improved visualization of mucosal suturing offered by the robotic platform, postoperative bladder neck contracture rates were reduced to 0% to 3%, questioning the role of urethral catheter in urethral patency after RARP.[88] Further, the desire by both patient and surgeon for early catheter removal, or perhaps to obviate urethral stenting altogether, led us to introduce the suprapubic catheter as an alternative to the urethral catheter. We found that the continence and stricture rates were similar between this group and historical controls, with significant reduction in catheter-related discomfort postoperatively.[86,89] Results from other groups have been mixed, with some mirroring our results,[90] whereas others have reported no benefit.[91] In a subsequent study, we showed that the use of a suprapubic catheter (instead of the urethral catheter) was also associated with an early return of urinary continence.[92] Tewari and colleagues[93] looked at a custom suprapubic catheter with a small bladder neck anastomotic splint, which could be retracted. This pilot study also reported earlier return of continence and decreased patient discomfort.

TECHNICAL ADVANCEMENTS IN POTENCY PRESERVATION

Before the description of the nerve sparing technique of RP by Walsh in 1983,[94] as in the case of urinary control, patients undergoing RP fared poorly in terms of sexual function preservation as well.

Building on the nerve sparing technique described by Walsh and contemporary advances in understanding of the neuroanatomy of the prostatic plexus, coupled with the inherent precision of the robotic platform, various technical modifications in RARP over the years have led to dramatic improvement in potency outcomes. The major technical modifications are summarized in **Fig. 4** and are discussed later.

Hammock Concept and the Veil of Aphrodite

The VIP approach of RARP was first described in 2002 by Menon and colleagues,[95] followed by several refinements and technical modifications, leading to its present description.[35–37] Among these refinements are the development and preservation of the lateral prostatic fascia (ie, veil of Aphrodite).[86] This refinement involves high anterior release of the curtain of cavernosal neural tissue extending along the posterolateral aspects of the prostate bilaterally, up to the fibrous stroma of the dorsal vein complex (ie, sparing of the neural tissue between 1'o clock and 11'o clock).[35,86] More recently, we have described a superveil modification, which was developed for select patients with favorable anatomy and clinical characteristics, allowing for further extension anteriorly of the dissection to preserve the pubovesical ligaments and dorsal vein complex.[36,86] With these techniques, we reported erectile function recovery rates of 93% and 94%, respectively, in the most favorable patient groups. Similarly, Srivastava and colleagues[96] recently published a review of their current technique of neurovascular bundle preservation. Building on basic tenets of RARP, their approach included avoiding unnecessary thermal and traction injury to the neurovascular bundle during the dissection of the trizonal region (see later discussion). Through a medial to lateral dissection approach, beginning with the seminal vesicles and extending along the posterolateral aspect of the prostate, the investigators used sharp, athermal dissection and small pedicle clipping to facilitate intrafascial dissection.[86] In their retrospective analysis of 2317 consecutive men with PCa undergoing RARP,[97] 91% reported the ability to engage in sexual intercourse. For men aged 60 years and younger, rates of erectile function recovery beyond 12 months were approximately 95% when undergoing grade 1 neurovascular bundle preservation. These rates deteriorated incrementally with progressively wider planes of dissection (ie, a greater degree of neurovascular bundle resection [ie, grades 2–4]).

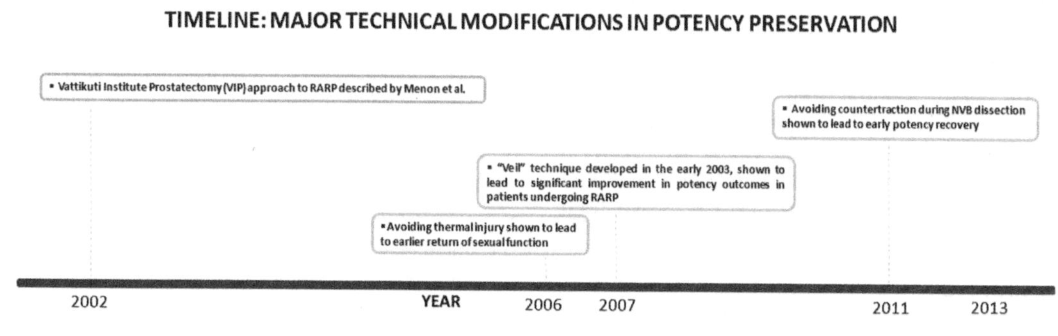

MODIFICATION	YEAR	GROUP	OUTCOME
"Veil" nerve sparing technique	2007 2009	Menon et al. Menon et al.	Significant improvement in potency rates in patients undergoing "Veil" nerve sparing.
Athermal dissection	2006	Ahlering et al.	Avoiding thermal injury leads to earlier return of sexual function.
Traction free dissection	2011	Kowalczyk et al.	Avoidance of countertraction on the NVB leads to earlier return of erectile function.

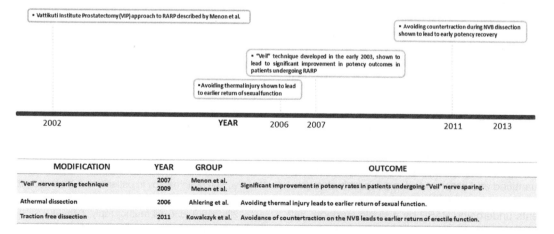

Fig. 4. Technical modifications in potency preservation. (*Data from* Refs.[35,36,105,107])

The rationale for these modifications was based on cadaveric dissections performed by our group and others previously, suggesting that smaller nerves comprising the pelvic neurovascular plexus run along the prostatic and Denonvilliers fascia.[98] Further studies have supported the concept of a neural hammock extending from the posterior surface of the seminal vesicles down along the posterolateral aspect (bilaterally) of the midprostate, and diverging anterolaterally near the membranous urethra.[86,99,100] These studies proposed the concept of a trizonal neural hammock, including the proximal neurovascular bundle posterior to the seminal vesicles, the predominant neurovascular bundle running bilaterally along the posterolateral aspect of the prostate, and the accessory neural pathway.[101]

Athermal Dissection

The use of thermal energy on or near neural tissues can cause neuropraxia, axonotmesis, and subsequently, neurotmesis. Mandhani and colleagues[102] and Ong and colleagues[103] both reported that the use of monopolar cautery, bipolar cautery, or harmonic shears, all resulted in significant thermal tissue insult and lead to cavernosal injury, compared with athermal dissection. This finding was supported by histologic evidence of inflammation and cellular death in the group who underwent nonathermal dissection. As a result of these findings, transection of the pedicles should ideally be accomplished without thermal energy. When cautery must be used, it should be used at the lowest effective power (ie, around 10 W for endopelvic fascia). Ahlering and colleagues[104,105] have reported extensively on improvement in potency outcomes with their athermal technique of RARP using bulldog clamps on the hypogastric vessels. The potency rates at 3, 9, and 24 months in patients with and without thermal utilization (all underwent similar nerve sparing) were 8.3%, 14.7%, and 63.2% and 38.1%, 69.8%, and 92%, respectively. Gill and Ukimura[106] have reported similar results in the LRP model. Hence, great care should be taken to avoid electrocautery use and excessive heat application in the vicinity of cavernosal nerves.

Traction Free

The impact of countertraction (either by the surgeon or by the assistant) on neurovascular injury and secondary neuropraxia has been recently quantified and emphasized in a report by Kowalczyk and colleagues[107] In their report, of 610 patients undergoing RARP by a single surgeon, 342 patients underwent countertraction-free dissection of the neurovascular bundle during nerve sparing RARP. This dissection was accomplished by placing traction on the prostate itself (ie, medial motion of the instruments while performing blunt dissection, rather than lateral) and dissecting it away from the neurovascular bundle. These patients experienced earlier potency recovery (45% vs 28% potent at 5 months), but overall potency rates at 1 year were similar between the groups. These results are in agreement with the findings that have been previously reported in ORP and other RARP series using similar techniques.[108,109]

SUMMARY

RARP has evolved dramatically since its inception in the early 2000s. RARP offers excellent and lasting oncologic control, which is at least equivalent to that achieved with ORP. Technical refinements in apical dissection, such as the retroapical approach of synchronous urethral transection, and adoption of real-time frozen section analysis of the excised prostate during RARP, have further substantially reduced PSM rates, particularly in high-risk disease patients. Furthermore, precision offered by the robotic platform and technical evolution of RP, including enhanced nerve sparing (veil), have led to improved potency and continence outcomes as well as better safety profile in patients undergoing surgical therapy for PCa.

REFERENCES

1. Siegel R, Naishadham D, Jemal A. Cancer statistics, 2012. CA Cancer J Clin 2012;62(1):10–29.
2. Cooperberg MR, Lubeck DP, Mehta SS, et al. Time trends in clinical risk stratification for prostate cancer: implications for outcomes (data from CaPSURE). J Urol 2003;170(6 Pt 2):S21–5 [discussion: S26–7].
3. Gallina A, Chun FK, Suardi N, et al. Comparison of stage migration patterns between Europe and the USA: an analysis of 11 350 men treated with radical prostatectomy for prostate cancer. BJU Int 2008; 101(12):1513–8.
4. Jacobs BL, Zhang Y, Schroeck FR, et al. Use of advanced treatment technologies among men at low risk of dying from prostate cancer. JAMA 2013; 309(24):2587–95.
5. Bill-Axelson A, Holmberg L, Garmo H, et al. Radical prostatectomy or watchful waiting in early prostate cancer. N Engl J Med 2014;370(10):932–42.
6. Abdollah F, Schmitges J, Sun M, et al. Comparison of mortality outcomes after radical prostatectomy versus radiotherapy in patients with localized prostate cancer: a population-based analysis. Int J Urol 2012;19(9):836–44 [author reply: 844–5].
7. Hoffman RM, Koyama T, Fan KH, et al. Mortality after radical prostatectomy or external beam

radiotherapy for localized prostate cancer. J Natl Cancer Inst 2013;105(10):711–8.
8. Sooriakumaran P, Nyberg T, Akre O, et al. Comparative effectiveness of radical prostatectomy and radiotherapy in prostate cancer: observational study of mortality outcomes. BMJ 2014;348:g1502.
9. Trinh QD, Sammon J, Sun M, et al. Perioperative outcomes of robot-assisted radical prostatectomy compared with open radical prostatectomy: results from the nationwide inpatient sample. Eur Urol 2012;61(4):679–85.
10. Tsui C, Klein R, Garabrant M. Minimally invasive surgery: national trends in adoption and future directions for hospital strategy. Surg Endosc 2013;27(7):2253–7.
11. Kowalczyk KJ, Levy JM, Caplan CF, et al. Temporal national trends of minimally invasive and retropubic radical prostatectomy outcomes from 2003 to 2007: results from the 100% Medicare sample. Eur Urol 2012;61(4):803–9.
12. Ficarra V, Novara G, Ahlering TE, et al. Systematic review and meta-analysis of studies reporting potency rates after robot-assisted radical prostatectomy. Eur Urol 2012;62(3):418–30.
13. Tewari A, Sooriakumaran P, Bloch DA, et al. Positive surgical margin and perioperative complication rates of primary surgical treatments for prostate cancer: a systematic review and meta-analysis comparing retropubic, laparoscopic, and robotic prostatectomy. Eur Urol 2012;62(1):1–15.
14. Menon M, Bhandari M, Gupta N, et al. Biochemical recurrence following robot-assisted radical prostatectomy: analysis of 1384 patients with a median 5-year follow-up. Eur Urol 2010;58(6):838–46.
15. Suardi N, Ficarra V, Willemsen P, et al. Long-term biochemical recurrence rates after robot-assisted radical prostatectomy: analysis of a single-center series of patients with a minimum follow-up of 5 years. Urology 2012;79(1):133–8.
16. Sukumar S, Rogers CG, Trinh QD, et al. Oncological outcomes after robot-assisted radical prostatectomy: long term follow-up in 4,803 patients. BJU Int 2013. [Epub ahead of print].
17. Novara G, Ficarra V, Mocellin S, et al. Systematic review and meta-analysis of studies reporting oncologic outcome after robot-assisted radical prostatectomy. Eur Urol 2012;62(3):382–404.
18. Polychronidis A, Laftsidis P, Bounovas A, et al. Twenty years of laparoscopic cholecystectomy: Philippe Mouret–March 17, 1987. JSLS 2008;12(1):109–11.
19. Carlucci JR, Nabizada-Pace F, Samadi DB. Robot-assisted laparoscopic radical prostatectomy: technique and outcomes of 700 cases. Int J Biomed Sci 2009;5(3):201–8.
20. Guillonneau B, Vallancien G. Laparoscopic radical prostatectomy: the Montsouris technique. J Urol 2000;163(6):1643–9.
21. Lanfranco AR, Castellanos AE, Desai JP, et al. Robotic surgery: a current perspective. Ann Surg 2004;239(1):14–21.
22. Abbou CC, Hoznek A, Salomon L, et al. Laparoscopic radical prostatectomy with a remote controlled robot. J Urol 2001;165(6 Pt 1):1964–6.
23. Hayn MH, Hussain A, Mansour AM, et al. The learning curve of robot-assisted radical cystectomy: results from the International Robotic Cystectomy Consortium. Eur Urol 2010;58(2):197–202.
24. Sukumar S, Rogers CG. Robotic partial nephrectomy: surgical technique. BJU Int 2011;108(6 Pt 2):942–7.
25. Ghani KR, Rogers CG, Sood A, et al. Robot-assisted anatrophic nephrolithotomy with renal hypothermia for managing staghorn calculi. J Endourol 2013;27(11):1393–8.
26. Mufarrij PW, Shah OD, Berger AD, et al. Robotic reconstruction of the upper urinary tract. J Urol 2007;178(5):2002–5.
27. Peters CA. Robotically assisted surgery in pediatric urology. Urol Clin North Am 2004;31(4):743–52.
28. Sammon JD, Zhu G, Sood A, et al. Pediatric nephrectomy: incidence, indications and use of minimally invasive techniques. J Urol 2014;191(3):764–70.
29. Sukumar S, Roghmann F, Sood A, et al. Correction of ureteropelvic junction obstruction in children: national trends and comparative effectiveness in operative outcomes. J Endourol 2014;28(5):592–8.
30. Oberholzer J, Giulianotti P, Danielson KK, et al. Minimally invasive robotic kidney transplantation for obese patients previously denied access to transplantation. Am J Transplant 2013;13(3):721–8.
31. Menon M, Abaza R, Sood A, et al. Robotic kidney transplantation with regional hypothermia: evolution of a novel procedure utilizing the IDEAL guidelines (IDEAL phase 0 and 1). Eur Urol 2014;65(5):1001–9.
32. Menon M, Sood A, Bhandari M, et al. Robotic kidney transplantation with regional hypothermia: a step-by-step description of the Vattikuti Urology Institute-Medanta Technique (IDEAL Phase 2a). Eur Urol 2014;65(5):991–1000.
33. Sood A, Ghani KR, Ahlawat R, et al. Application of the statistical process control method for prospective patient safety monitoring during the learning phase: robotic kidney transplantation with regional hypothermia (IDEAL Phase 2a-b). Eur Urol 2014;66(2):371–8.
34. Montorsi F, Wilson TG, Rosen RC, et al. Best practices in robot-assisted radical prostatectomy: recommendations of the Pasadena Consensus Panel. Eur Urol 2012;62(3):368–81.
35. Menon M, Shrivastava A, Kaul S, et al. Vattikuti Institute prostatectomy: contemporary technique and analysis of results. Eur Urol 2007;51(3):648–57 [discussion: 657–8].

36. Menon M, Shrivastava A, Bhandari M, et al. Vattikuti Institute prostatectomy: technical modifications in 2009. Eur Urol 2009;56(1):89–96.
37. Ghani KR, Trinh QD, Menon M. Vattikuti Institute prostatectomy–technique in 2012. J Endourol 2012;26(12):1558–65.
38. Badani KK, Kaul S, Menon M. Evolution of robotic radical prostatectomy: assessment after 2766 procedures. Cancer 2007;110(9):1951–8.
39. Yossepowitch O, Briganti A, Eastham JA, et al. Positive surgical margins after radical prostatectomy: a systematic review and contemporary update. Eur Urol 2014;65(2):303–13.
40. Sammon JD, Trinh QD, Sukumar S, et al. Risk factors for biochemical recurrence following radical perineal prostatectomy in a large contemporary series: a detailed assessment of margin extent and location. Urol Oncol 2013;31(8):1470–6.
41. Tewari AK, Srivastava A, Mudaliar K, et al. Anatomical retro-apical technique of synchronous (posterior and anterior) urethral transection: a novel approach for ameliorating apical margin positivity during robotic radical prostatectomy. BJU Int 2010;106(9):1364–73.
42. Guru KA, Perlmutter AE, Sheldon MJ, et al. Apical margins after robot-assisted radical prostatectomy: does technique matter? J Endourol 2009;23(1):123–7.
43. Sasaki H, Miki J, Kimura T, et al. Upfront transection and subsequent ligation of the dorsal vein complex during laparoscopic radical prostatectomy. Int J Urol 2010;17(11):960–1.
44. Tewari AK, Patel ND, Leung RA, et al. Visual cues as a surrogate for tactile feedback during robotic-assisted laparoscopic prostatectomy: posterolateral margin rates in 1340 consecutive patients. BJU Int 2010;106(4):528–36.
45. Beyer B, Schlomm T, Tennstedt P, et al. A feasible and time-efficient adaptation of NeuroSAFE for da Vinci robot-assisted radical prostatectomy. Eur Urol 2014;66(1):138–44.
46. Jeong W, Sood A, Ghani KR, et al. Bimanual examination of the retrieved specimen and regional hypothermia during robot-assisted radical prostatectomy: a novel technique for reducing positive surgical margin and achieving pelvic cooling. BJU Int 2013. [Epub ahead of print].
47. Schlomm T, Tennstedt P, Huxhold C, et al. Neurovascular structure-adjacent frozen-section examination (NeuroSAFE) increases nerve-sparing frequency and reduces positive surgical margins in open and robot-assisted laparoscopic radical prostatectomy: experience after 11,069 consecutive patients. Eur Urol 2012;62(2):333–40.
48. Jonler M, Nielsen OS, Wolf H. Urinary symptoms, potency, and quality of life in patients with localized prostate cancer followed up with deferred treatment. Urology 1998;52(6):1055–62 [discussion: 1063].
49. Katz G, Rodriguez R. Changes in continence and health-related quality of life after curative treatment and watchful waiting of prostate cancer. Urology 2007;69(6):1157–60.
50. Myers RP. Male urethral sphincteric anatomy and radical prostatectomy. Urol Clin North Am 1991; 18(2):211–27.
51. Gaker DL, Steel BL. Radical prostatectomy with preservation of urinary continence: pathology and long-term results. J Urol 2004;172(6 Pt 2):2549–52.
52. Deliveliotis C, Protogerou V, Alargof E, et al. Radical prostatectomy: bladder neck preservation and puboprostatic ligament sparing–effects on continence and positive margins. Urology 2002; 60(5):855–8.
53. Sakai I, Harada K, Hara I, et al. Intussusception of the bladder neck does not promote early restoration to urinary continence after non-nerve-sparing radical retropubic prostatectomy. Int J Urol 2005;12(3):275–9.
54. Selli C, De Antoni P, Moro U, et al. Role of bladder neck preservation in urinary continence following radical retropubic prostatectomy. Scand J Urol Nephrol 2004;38(1):32–7.
55. Patel VR, Coelho RF, Palmer KJ, et al. Periurethral suspension stitch during robot-assisted laparoscopic radical prostatectomy: description of the technique and continence outcomes. Eur Urol 2009;56(3):472–8.
56. Campenni MA, Harmon JD, Ginsberg PC, et al. Improved continence after radical retropubic prostatectomy using 2 pubo-urethral suspension stitches. Urol Int 2002;68(2):109–12.
57. Noguchi M, Kakuma T, Suekane S, et al. A randomized clinical trial of suspension technique for improving early recovery of urinary continence after radical retropubic prostatectomy. BJU Int 2008; 102(8):958–63.
58. Jorion JL. Rectus fascial sling suspension of the vesicourethral anastomosis after radical prostatectomy. J Urol 1997;157(3):926–8.
59. Jarow JP. Puboprostatic ligament sparing radical retropubic prostatectomy. Semin Urol Oncol 2000; 18(1):28–32.
60. Poore RE, McCullough DL, Jarow JP. Puboprostatic ligament sparing improves urinary continence after radical retropubic prostatectomy. Urology 1998; 51(1):67–72.
61. Avant OL, Jones JA, Beck H, et al. New method to improve treatment outcomes for radical prostatectomy. Urology 2000;56(4):658–62.
62. Galfano A, Ascione A, Grimaldi S, et al. A new anatomic approach for robot-assisted laparoscopic prostatectomy: a feasibility study for completely intrafascial surgery. Eur Urol 2010;58(3):457–61.
63. Galfano A, Di Trapani D, Sozzi F, et al. Beyond the learning curve of the Retzius-sparing approach for robot-assisted laparoscopic radical prostatectomy: oncologic and functional results of the first 200

patients with ± 1 year of follow-up. Eur Urol 2013; 64(6):974–80.
64. Lim SK, Kim KH, Shin TY, et al. Retzius-sparing robot-assisted laparoscopic radical prostatectomy–combining the best of retropubic and perineal approaches. BJU Int 2014;114(2):236–44.
65. Klein EA. Early continence after radical prostatectomy. J Urol 1992;148(1):92–5.
66. Rocco B, Gregori A, Stener S, et al. Posterior reconstruction of the rhabdosphincter allows a rapid recovery of continence after transperitoneal videolaparoscopic radical prostatectomy. Eur Urol 2007;51(4):996–1003.
67. Rocco F, Carmignani L, Acquati P, et al. Restoration of posterior aspect of rhabdosphincter shortens continence time after radical retropubic prostatectomy. J Urol 2006;175(6):2201–6.
68. Nguyen MM, Kamoi K, Stein RJ, et al. Early continence outcomes of posterior musculofascial plate reconstruction during robotic and laparoscopic prostatectomy. BJU Int 2008;101(9):1135–9.
69. Coelho RF, Chauhan S, Orvieto MA, et al. Influence of modified posterior reconstruction of the rhabdosphincter on early recovery of continence and anastomotic leakage rates after robot-assisted radical prostatectomy. Eur Urol 2011;59(1):72–80.
70. Tewari AK, Bigelow K, Rao S, et al. Anatomic restoration technique of continence mechanism and preservation of puboprostatic collar: a novel modification to achieve early urinary continence in men undergoing robotic prostatectomy. Urology 2007; 69(4):726–31.
71. Tewari A, Jhaveri J, Rao S, et al. Total reconstruction of the vesico-urethral junction. BJU Int 2008; 101(7):871–7.
72. Menon M, Muhletaler F, Campos M, et al. Assessment of early continence after reconstruction of the periprostatic tissues in patients undergoing computer assisted (robotic) prostatectomy: results of a 2 group parallel randomized controlled trial. J Urol 2008;180(3):1018–23.
73. Majoros A, Bach D, Keszthelyi A, et al. Analysis of risk factors for urinary incontinence after radical prostatectomy. Urol Int 2007;78(3):202–7.
74. Paparel P, Akin O, Sandhu JS, et al. Recovery of urinary continence after radical prostatectomy: association with urethral length and urethral fibrosis measured by preoperative and postoperative endorectal magnetic resonance imaging. Eur Urol 2009;55(3):629–37.
75. Coakley FV, Eberhardt S, Kattan MW, et al. Urinary continence after radical retropubic prostatectomy: relationship with membranous urethral length on preoperative endorectal magnetic resonance imaging. J Urol 2002;168(3):1032–5.
76. Nguyen L, Jhaveri J, Tewari A. Surgical technique to overcome anatomical shortcoming: balancing post-prostatectomy continence outcomes of urethral sphincter lengths on preoperative magnetic resonance imaging. J Urol 2008;179(5):1907–11.
77. Kojima Y, Takahashi N, Haga N. Urinary incontinence after robot-assisted radical prostatectomy: pathophysiology and intraoperative techniques to improve surgical outcome. Int J Urol 2013;20(11): 1052–63.
78. van Randenborgh H, Paul R, Kubler H, et al. Improved urinary continence after radical retropubic prostatectomy with preparation of a long, partially intraprostatic portion of the membraneous urethra: an analysis of 1013 consecutive cases. Prostate Cancer Prostatic Dis 2004;7(3):253–7.
79. Popken G, Sommerkamp H, Schultze-Seemann W, et al. Anastomotic stricture after radical prostatectomy. Incidence, findings and treatment. Eur Urol 1998;33(4):382–6.
80. Surya BV, Provet J, Johanson KE, et al. Anastomotic strictures following radical prostatectomy: risk factors and management. J Urol 1990;143(4): 755–8.
81. Cambria RP, Davison JK, Zannetti S, et al. Clinical experience with epidural cooling for spinal cord protection during thoracic and thoracoabdominal aneurysm repair. J Vasc Surg 1997;25(2):234–41 [discussion: 241–3].
82. Polderman KH. Induced hypothermia and fever control for prevention and treatment of neurological injuries. Lancet 2008;371(9628):1955–69.
83. Westermann S, Vollmar B, Thorlacius H, et al. Surface cooling inhibits tumor necrosis factor-alpha-induced microvascular perfusion failure, leukocyte adhesion, and apoptosis in the striated muscle. Surgery 1999;126(5):881–9.
84. Finley DS, Osann K, Skarecky D, et al. Hypothermic nerve-sparing radical prostatectomy: rationale, feasibility, and effect on early continence. Urology 2009;73(4):691–6.
85. Sammon J, Kim TK, Trinh QD, et al. Anastomosis during robot-assisted radical prostatectomy: randomized controlled trial comparing barbed and standard monofilament suture. Urology 2011; 78(3):572–9.
86. Jacobs EF, Boris R, Masterson TA. Advances in Robotic-Assisted Radical Prostatectomy over Time. Prostate Cancer 2013;2013:902686.
87. Walsh PC. Anatomic radical prostatectomy: evolution of the surgical technique. J Urol 1998;160(6 Pt 2):2418–24.
88. Msezane LP, Reynolds WS, Gofrit ON, et al. Bladder neck contracture after robot-assisted laparoscopic radical prostatectomy: evaluation of incidence and risk factors and impact on urinary function. J Endourol 2008;22(2):377–83.
89. Krane LS, Bhandari M, Peabody JO, et al. Impact of percutaneous suprapubic tube drainage on

patient discomfort after radical prostatectomy. Eur Urol 2009;56(2):325–30.

90. Orikasa S, Kanbe K, Shirai S, et al. Suprapubic versus transurethral bladder drainage after radical prostatectomy: impact on patient discomfort. Int J Urol 2012;19(6):587–90.
91. Prasad SM, Large MC, Patel AR, et al. Randomized, controlled trial of early removal of urethral catheter with suprapubic tube drainage versus urethral catheter drainage alone following robot-assisted laparoscopic radical prostatectomy. J Urol 2014;192(1):89–96.
92. Sammon JD, Sharma P, Trinh QD, et al. Predictors of immediate continence following robot-assisted radical prostatectomy. J Endourol 2013;27(4): 442–6.
93. Tewari A, Rao S, Mandhani A. Catheter-less robotic radical prostatectomy using a custom-made synchronous anastomotic splint and vesical urinary diversion device: report of the initial series and perioperative outcomes. BJU Int 2008;102(8): 1000–4.
94. Walsh PC, Lepor H, Eggleston JC. Radical prostatectomy with preservation of sexual function: anatomical and pathological considerations. Prostate 1983;4(5):473–85.
95. Menon M, Tewari A, Peabody J. Vattikuti Institute prostatectomy: technique. J Urol 2003;169(6): 2289–92.
96. Srivastava A, Grover S, Sooriakumaran P, et al. Neuroanatomic basis for traction-free preservation of the neural hammock during athermal robotic radical prostatectomy. Curr Opin Urol 2011;21(1): 49–59.
97. Tewari AK, Srivastava A, Huang MW, et al. Anatomical grades of nerve sparing: a risk-stratified approach to neural-hammock sparing during robot-assisted radical prostatectomy (RARP). BJU Int 2011;108(6 Pt 2):984–92.
98. Tewari A, Peabody JO, Fischer M, et al. An operative and anatomic study to help in nerve sparing during laparoscopic and robotic radical prostatectomy. Eur Urol 2003;43(5):444–54.
99. Costello AJ, Brooks M, Cole OJ. Anatomical studies of the neurovascular bundle and cavernosal nerves. BJU Int 2004;94(7):1071–6.
100. Eichelberg C, Erbersdobler A, Michl U, et al. Nerve distribution along the prostatic capsule. Eur Urol 2007;51(1):105–10 [discussion: 110–1].
101. Tewari A, Takenaka A, Mtui E, et al. The proximal neurovascular plate and the tri-zonal neural architecture around the prostate gland: importance in the athermal robotic technique of nerve-sparing prostatectomy. BJU Int 2006;98(2):314–23.
102. Mandhani A, Dorsey PJ Jr, Ramanathan R, et al. Real time monitoring of temperature changes in neurovascular bundles during robotic radical prostatectomy: thermal map for nerve-sparing radical prostatectomy. J Endourol 2008;22(10): 2313–7.
103. Ong AM, Su LM, Varkarakis I, et al. Nerve sparing radical prostatectomy: effects of hemostatic energy sources on the recovery of cavernous nerve function in a canine model. J Urol 2004;172(4 Pt 1):1318–22.
104. Ahlering TE, Eichel L, Skarecky D. Evaluation of long-term thermal injury using cautery during nerve sparing robotic prostatectomy. Urology 2008;72(6): 1371–4.
105. Ahlering TE, Skarecky D, Borin J. Impact of cautery versus cautery-free preservation of neurovascular bundles on early return of potency. J Endourol 2006;20(8):586–9.
106. Gill IS, Ukimura O. Thermal energy-free laparoscopic nerve-sparing radical prostatectomy: one-year potency outcomes. Urology 2007;70(2): 309–14.
107. Kowalczyk KJ, Huang AC, Hevelone ND, et al. Stepwise approach for nerve sparing without countertraction during robot-assisted radical prostatectomy: technique and outcomes. Eur Urol 2011; 60(3):536–47.
108. Masterson TA, Serio AM, Mulhall JP, et al. Modified technique for neurovascular bundle preservation during radical prostatectomy: association between technique and recovery of erectile function. BJU Int 2008;101(10):1217–22.
109. Mattei A, Naspro R, Annino F, et al. Tension and energy-free robotic-assisted laparoscopic radical prostatectomy with interfascial dissection of the neurovascular bundles. Eur Urol 2007;52(3):687–94.
110. Sutherland DE, Linder B, Guzman AM, et al. Posterior rhabdosphincter reconstruction during robotic assisted radical prostatectomy: results from a phase II randomized clinical trial. J Urol 2011; 185(4):1262–7.
111. Sammon JD, Muhletaler F, Peabody JO, et al. Long-term functional urinary outcomes comparing single- vs double-layer urethrovesical anastomosis: two-year follow-up of a two-group parallel randomized controlled trial. Urology 2010;76(5): 1102–7.

Robot-Assisted Laparoscopic Simple Anatomic Prostatectomy

Manish N. Patel, MD,
Ashok K. Hemal, MD, MCh, FAMS, FACS, FRCS(Glasg)*

KEYWORDS

• Robotic • Laparoscopy • Simple prostatectomy • Benign prostatic hypertrophy
• Bladder outlet obstruction • Lower urinary tract symptoms

KEY POINTS

- This article demonstrates multiple surgical approaches for robot-assisted simple prostatectomy (RALSP) in patients suffering from lower urinary tract symptoms from large prostatic adenomas.
- RALSP is a technically feasible and viable treatment option that also allows management of other pathologies concomitantly.
- RALSP with complete urethrovesical reconstruction is a minimally invasive technique for a large prostatic adenoma that provides excellent outcomes.
- RALSP can also be performed with other modified techniques as described.
- Larger studies with longer follow-up are needed to assess the long-term results of this procedure on alleviation of voiding symptoms.

INTRODUCTION

Management options for men with symptomatic benign prostatic hyperplasia have increased over the past few decades. For most men with small glands and lower urinary tract symptoms, the standard therapy includes alpha blockers as a first-line treatment. In previous studies of 1-year duration or less, combination with a 5-alpha reductase inhibitor proved equal to alpha-blocker therapy in efficacy and safety, but superior to 5-alpha reducatase inhibitor (ARI) therapy alone. However, the Medical Therapy of Prostate Symptoms (MTOPS) study[1] demonstrated that in the long term, among men with larger prostates, combination therapy is superior to either alpha-blocker or 5-ARI therapy in preventing progression and improving symptoms.

According to the American Urological Association (AUA) guidelines, surgery is recommended for patients who have renal insufficiency secondary to benign prostatic hyperplasia (BPH), who have recurrent urinary tract infections (UTIs), bladder stones or gross hematuria due to BPH, and those who have lower urinary tract symptoms (LUTS) refractory to other therapies. Minimally invasive interventions are the standard therapy for this group of patients.

Technology is rapidly improving, and the use of various endoscopic techniques along with lasers has gained popularity because of the lower morbidity and mortality compared with the traditional gold standard of transurethral resection of the prostate (TURP).[2] Other approved technologies for treatment of outlet obstruction include visual laser ablation of the prostate (VLAP), transurethral needle ablation of the prostate (TUNA), transurethral electrovaporization of the prostate (TUEVP), microwave ablation of the prostate, Greenlight photovaprorization of the prostate using a KTP laser, and holmium enucleation of the prostate. The AUA guidelines state that in men with larger prostates who would likely require

Department of Urology, Wake Forest University School of Medicine, Medical Center Boulevard, Winston-Salem, NC 27157, USA
* Corresponding author.
E-mail address: ahemal@wakehealth.edu

Urol Clin N Am 41 (2014) 485–492
http://dx.doi.org/10.1016/j.ucl.2014.07.003
0094-0143/14/$ – see front matter

a staged procedure, open prostatectomy is an appropriate and effective treatment alternative for men with moderate-to-severe LUTS who are significantly bothered by their symptoms.

Open simple prostatectomy is recommended by the European Association of Urology guidelines for men with large glands (>80–100 mL). Although the guidelines last updated in 2010 did not give a formal recommendation to minimally invasive approaches to simple prostatectomy, techniques been developed and are now commonly being performed to help men suffering from significant lower urinary tract symptoms who would otherwise undergo a difficult transurethral procedure.

The first laparoscopic simple prostatectomy was performed in 2006,[3] and numerous subsequent series have demonstrated function outcomes similar to the open technique.[4,5] Although these series demonstrated the equivalence of performing simple prostatectomy using a minimally invasive approach, this technique is difficult to master and disseminate. The authors first started developing a technique of robot-assisted laparoscopic simple prostatectomy (RALSP) in 2009 at Wake Forest based on experience of the senior author, who has previously performed laparoscopic and robot-assisted simple prostatectomy.[6,7]

The use of robotics overcomes the limitations of pure laparoscopy by providing stereoscopic 3-dimensional vision, wristed instruments with 7° of freedom, and tremor control. Robotic assistance helps in quicker skills acquisition, and the learning curve for RALSP is actually steeper than for laparoscopic simple prostatectomy, as learning is longer and shallower with the latter. This article describes multiple techniques for RALSP in a step-by-step manner presents the authors' results.

Indications for RALSP include

1. Large prostate over 75 to 100 g
2. Acute urinary retention
3. Bladder outlet obstruction recalcitrant to medical therapy
4. Bladder outlet obstruction with diverticulum
5. Recurrent hematuria due to BPH
6. Upper tract changes
7. Bladder calculi

METHODS AND PATIENTS

Twenty consecutive cases of RALSP for BPH-related LUTS were performed by a single surgeon. Some of these procedures were performed as a live demonstration for educational purposes.

Initial workup included a complete history and physical examination, International Prostrate Symptom Score (IPSS) (if applicable, ie, not with an indwelling Foley urethral catheter for urinary retention), office uroflowmetry, urine analysis, urine culture, serum electrolytes including creatinine, prostate-specific antigen, and axial imaging (**Fig. 1**). All patients who were younger than 70 with an elevated prostrate-specific antigen (PSA) test underwent transrectal ultrasound-guided prostate biopsy to exclude prostate cancer prior to surgery before their referral to the authors. All patients had failed medical therapy prior to intervention. Patients were counseled regarding treatment options including continuing medical therapy, prostatectomy (both open and minimally invasive), TURP, laser prostatectomy, and photovaporization of the prostate. After appropriate workup and counseling, informed consent was obtained.

Multiple techniques can be employed to perform RALSP. Each approach recapitulated the open technique with few modifications.

Technique I—RALSP Transperitoneal Anatomic Approach

The step-by-step video of this technique can be seen on the *Urologic Clinics of North America* Web site.

Positioning

The patient is placed in the dorsal lithotomy position with all pressure points padded. The patient

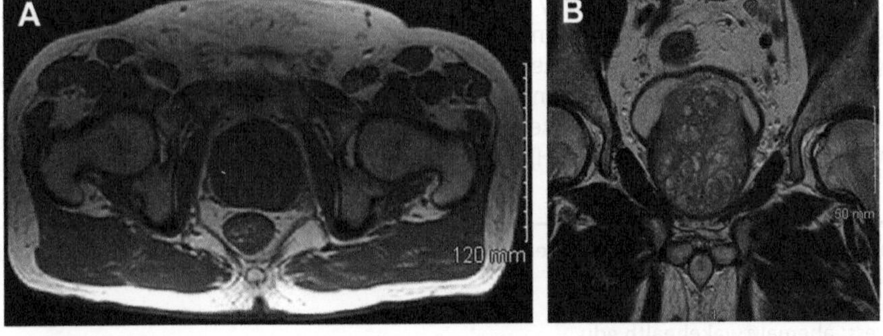

Fig. 1. (*A*) Magnetic resonance imaging (MRI) axial images of large prostatic adenoma. (*B*) MRI coronal images demonstrating significant intravesical prostatic protrusion of prostatic adenoma.

is secured to the table with straps or pads across the chest or shoulders. The patient is prepared and draped with a 20 F Foley catheter in place. The patient is then placed in the Trendelenberg position at about 30° or more as needed.

Placement of ports

A Veress needle is inserted periumbilically, and the abdomen is insufflated to a pressure of 15 mm of Hg. A 12 mm camera port is then placed in the midline just below or above the umbilicus based on body habitus of the patient by making a longitudinal incision. The abdomen is inspected to assess for adhesions or any bowel injury during Veress needle or port placement. Two 8 mm robotic ports are placed about 8 cm lateral and an inch caudal to the camera port on either side of the rectus muscle. A third 8 mm robotic port is placed on the left side at the same level as the other working ports in the anterior axillary line above the anterior superior iliac spine. A 12 mm assistant port is placed on the right about 3 cm above the right anterior–superior iliac spine. A 5 mm assistant port is placed about 3 cm lateral to the midline on the right just cranial to the camera port (**Fig. 2**).

Bladder mobilization

The bladder is filled with water or saline to easily identify it. The anterior peritoneum is incised medial to the medial umbilical ligaments to the level of the vasa deferentia bilaterally (**Fig. 3**). In case of very large prostates, over 150 g, or in patients with a small or narrow pelvis, it is better to excise lateral-to-medial umbilical ligaments to give wide exposure for dissection and manipulation of the gland. The bladder is dropped off anterior to the abdominal wall to reach into the space of retzius. The bladder is then drained.

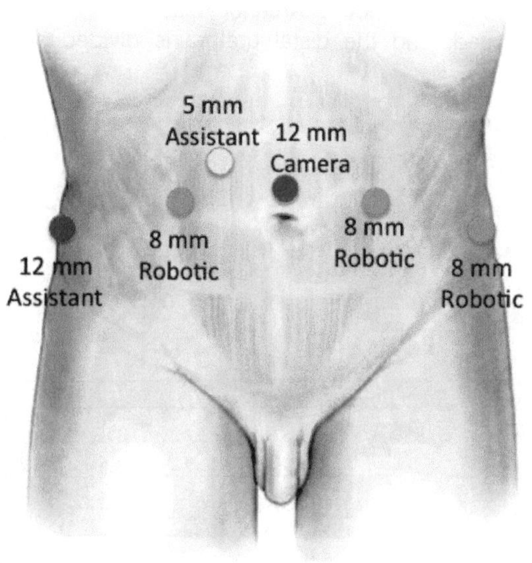

Fig. 2. Port placement.

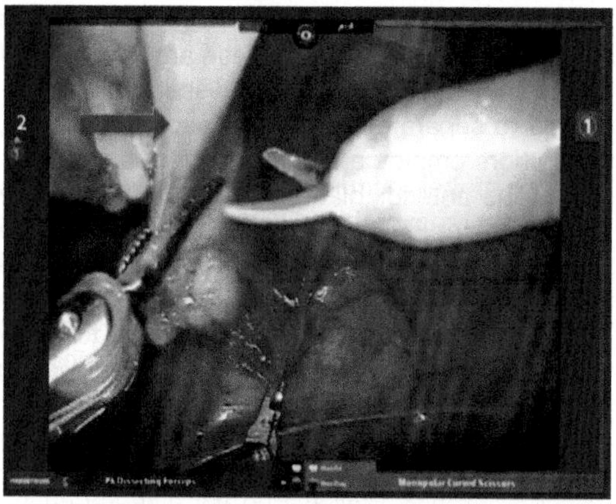

Fig. 3. Incision of the medial umbilical ligament, which is identified by the red arrow.

Apical dissection

Once retropubic space is entered, the fat over the prostate and prostato–vesical junction is dissected to expose the bladder neck (**Fig. 4**). The superficial branch is fulgurated and divided at the apex and at the level of bladder neck. In most cases, unlike radical prostatectomy, the authors do not dissect endopelvic fascia (EPF), perform apical dissection, or control dorsal vascular complex (DVC) with the suture at the apex. However, if there is concern, or if the surgeon feels it is not optimal, then endopelvic fascia is incised laterally; however, spare puboprostatic ligament and DVC is controlled with 0 monocryl on computed tomography (CT) 1 needle.

Bladder neck dissection and division

The prostate is visualized and the bladder neck identified by pulling the catheter in and out. There

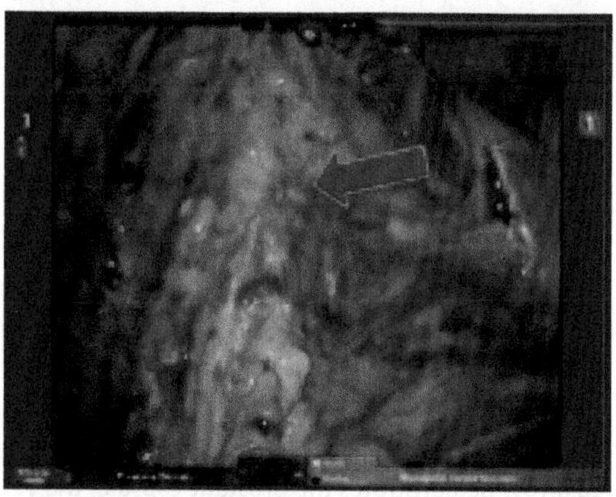

Fig. 4. Prostate dissected free (*red arrow*) showing the location of the bladder neck.

are sometimes superficial dorsal veins that run over the bladder neck, and these are fulgurated if present. Gentle and careful dissection is performed to separate the bladder neck. If possible, the authors employ a bladder neck-sparing technique. The anterior bladder neck is divided. The Foley catheter is removed (**Fig. 5**). If the prostate is very large, and median lobes are going inside the bladder, a polydioxanone (PDS) or Monocryl stay suture is placed into the prostate to allow for retraction, which is helpful while enucleating the prostatic adenoma (**Fig. 6**).

In patients who have bladder stones or bladder diverticuli, a wide bladder neck incision is made to ensure good visualization. In the authors' series, 3 patients had secondary bladder stones related to their outlet obstruction, which were removed prior to proceeding. One patient had a bladder diverticulum, which was excised by transvesical diverticulectomy.

Dissection of prostate adenoma

An incision is made between the anterior prostatic capsule and adenoma at the level of the bladder neck. This plane is advanced between the prostate capsule and adenoma in order to avoid dorsal vascular complex. Posterior dissection is started at the level of the anatomic capsule with blunt and sharp dissection. Traction sutures are used to retract and assist with dissection. By staying close to adenoma, there is less chances of bleeding (**Fig. 7**).

When nearing completion of the posterior dissection, anterolateral dissection is carried out to mobilize the lateral lobes. Most of the time, because of the large size of the gland, it can be difficult to perform sequential dissection of the

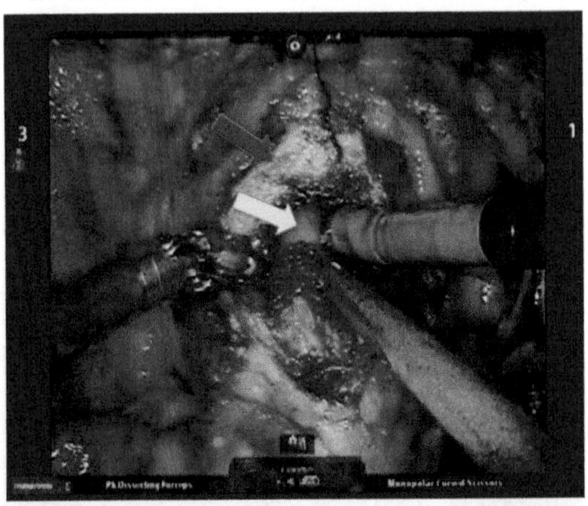

Fig. 5. Bladder neck incision and Foley removal. The red arrow demonstrates the prostatic capsule; the yellow arrow demonstrates the Foley catheter in the urethra.

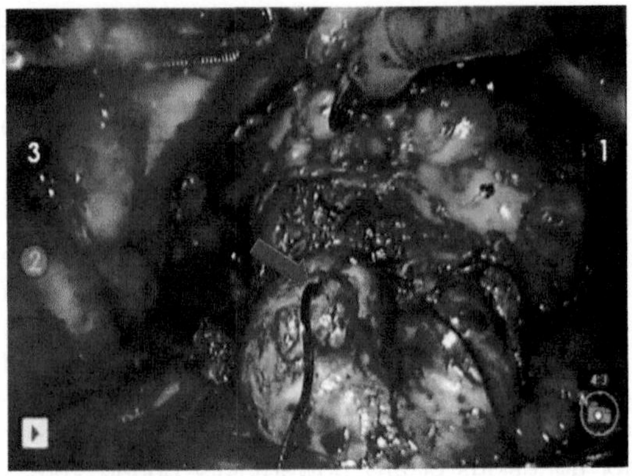

Fig. 6. Stay suture in prostate for retraction as shown by the red arrow.

gland. In these situations, one can toggle between anterior, posterior, and lateral dissection as needed in order to continue to progress. The goal is to shell out entire prostatic adenoma between anatomic and surgical capsule.

Of course, endowristed instruments are helpful in following various angles of the capsular plane. It also helps in hemostasis and meticulous dissection by allowing focal coagulation of bleeders. If the patient has a history of recurrent UTIs or prior surgery, these planes may be difficult to dissect and may lead to avulsion of the prostatic capsule.

Dissection and division of the distal prostatic urethra

Before starting dissection, make sure the Foley catheter is advanced. The 3-dimensional vision coupled with magnification allows for a precise apical dissection underneath the anterior capsule of the prostate, thereby avoiding injury to the external sphincter. Anterior dissection is performed, and the distal urethra is divided after

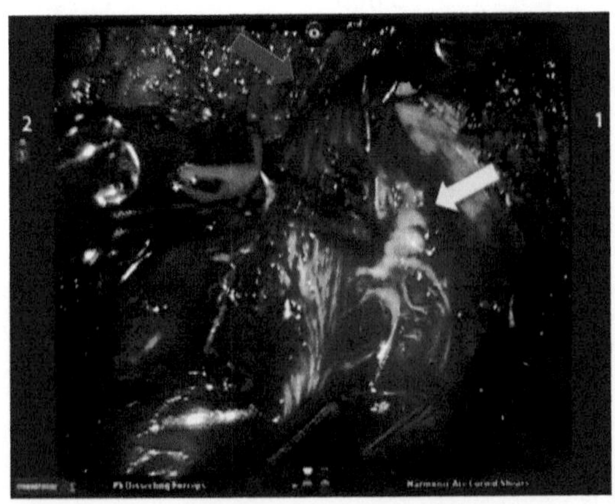

Fig. 7. Dissection of the lateral lobes (*yellow arrow*) away from the prostatic capsule (*red arrow*).

circumferential dissection. It is lifted with a left arm instrument. The urethra is then divided sharply at the apex, freeing the specimen from the prostatic capsule. Once the specimen is free, it is bagged in to a specimen bag (sometimes the larger 15 mm specimen bag is needed depending on the size of the prostate).

Control of hemostasis

At this point, hemostasis is ensured using bipolar cautery. If there are small bleeders, they can be controlled with the plasmakinetic or fenestrated bipolar forceps or 3-0 Monocryl suture. Alternatively, an ultrasonic device can be used for dissection.

Vesico-urethral anastomosis

Unlike the standard description, the authors perform a complete anatomic reconstruction.[7] A single 3-0 Monocryl suture is used to reapproximate the posterior prostatic capsule, which can help in hemostasis. Then, the vesicourethral anastomosis is performed using a 3-0 barbed suture in a running fashion; alternatively, a Monocryl suture can be used to save on cost.[8] When performing the posterior portion of the anastomosis, care is taken to identify and avoid the ureteral orifices (**Fig. 8**). Finally, the anterior capsule is reapproximated to the outer surface of the bladder with a 3-0 Monocryl suture. If suture is not used, the capsule will spontaneously cover the anastomosis (**Fig. 9**).

Closure

A new 20 F 2-way Foley catheter is placed, and the balloon is inflated with 15 cc of water inside the bladder lumen. A Jackson Pratt drain is placed is placed into the rectovesical pouch. The assistant 12 mm port is closed with a 1-0 vicryl suture using a reusable Carter-Thompson closure device. The

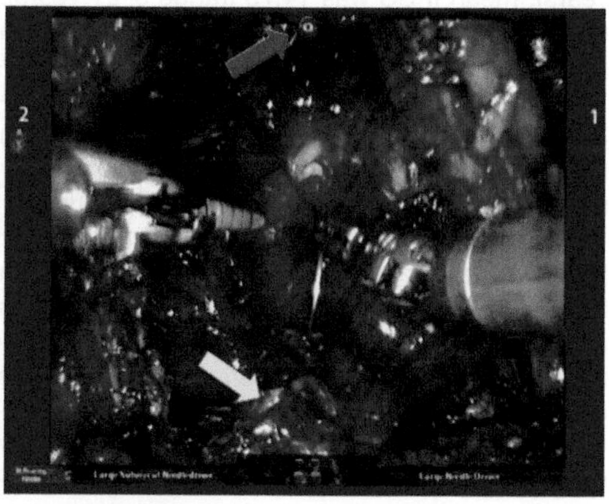

Fig. 8. Vesicourethral anastomosis. Red arrow demonstrates the urethra and the yellow arrow demonstrates the bladder neck.

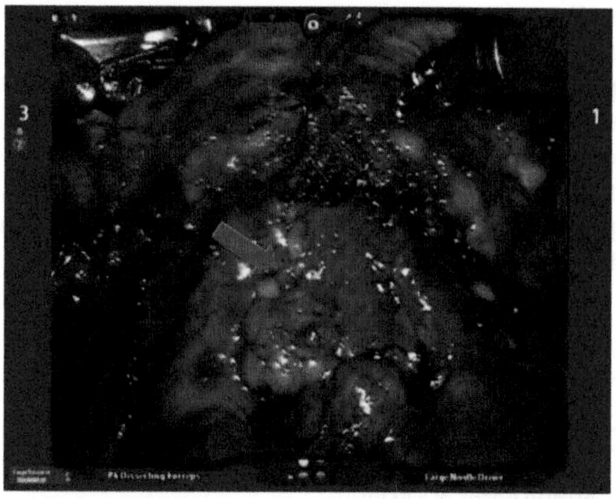

Fig. 9. Approximation of the anterior prostatic capsule (*red arrow*).

specimen is extracted by extending the midline camera port. The fascia is closed using a 0-PDS suture, and the skin is closed using a 4-0 Monocryl subcuticular suture. The 8 mm robotic trocars sites and the 5 mm assistant port sites are closed using a subcuticular 4-0 Monocryl suture.

Technique II—RALSP with Extraperitoneal Approach

Initial access

The initial access is obtained via a 2 to 3 cm infraumbilical incision to expose the anterior rectus sheath. A vertical incision is made in the anterior sheath so as to expose the rectus muscles. The muscles are split in the midline to delineate posterior sheath. Once visualized, a PDB 1000 balloon dilator (Covidien, Dublin, Ireland) is inserted over the posterior sheath, slowly advancing down toward the space of Retzius. It allows the laparoscope to pass through the balloon port, which helps in creating an extraperitoneal space under direct vision. The epigastric vessels can be visualized, with care taken not to dissect them off of the lower aspect of the rectus muscles. Once the space has been created satisfactorily, this balloon is replaced with blunt tip balloon trocar. Then under endoscopic vision. secondary ports are placed.

One should be careful to avoid in inadvertent rent in the peritoneum, because a small peritoneal rent may lead to loss or decreases in the extraperitoneal space. Although the procedure can still be undertaken, considerable experience may be required if this occurs.

Port placement

Four to 5 additional ports are placed under direct endoscopic vision, with enough space left in between the robotic trocars to avoid instrument collision, and the assistant port should not be too lateral. All of these ports are below the camera port. The advantage of this technique is that once the extraperitoneal space is developed, access to the prostate is immediate. With the exception of the creation of the extraperitoneal space, port placement and technique are similar to the transperitoneal approach.

Technique III—Robot-Assisted Laparoscopic Simple Retropubic Prostatectomy (Millin Technique)

This can also be done by transperitoneal and extraperitoneal approach.

Initial steps

Positioning, port placement, and bladder mobilization are done as with the previously described approach for transperitoneal and extraperitoneal access.

Prostate capsule incision

The Foley catheter balloon is pulled in and out to determine the location of the bladder neck. Stay sutures are taken distally, proximally, and laterally on both sides of the lateral edge of the prostate. A transverse incision is made in the prostatic capsule and followed down into the prostatic adenoma. The adenoma is mobilized on the anterior and lateral sides from the capsule. A 0-vicryl stay suture can be used for countertraction of the prostate adenoma during mobilization of posterior part of adenoma. The urethra is identified and transected sharply at the apex of the prostate.

Capsular closure

Hemostasis is achieved with bipolar or plasmakinetic forceps. If bleeding continues to be an issue, large figure-of-eight sutures can be taken at the 5 o'clock and 7 o'clock positions at the bladder neck, or any obvious bleeders can be ligated. In addition, a single 3-0 monocryl suture is used to reapproximate the posterior plate. A 20 F Foley catheter is replaced with the balloon deflated. Then anterior capsule is sewn closed. The Foley balloon is inflated inside the bladder, and mild traction is given.

Technique IV—Robot-Assisted Laparoscopic Simple Transvesical Prostatectomy (Frayer Technique)

This can also be done by transperitoneal and extraperitoneal approach.

Preparation

Positioning, port placement, and bladder mobilization are done as with the previous techniques.

Bladder incision

The Foley balloon is pulled to determine the location of the bladder neck. A longitudinal incision is made in the anterior wall of the bladder proximal to the bladder neck, and the Foley balloon is visualized. The Foley balloon is taken down, and the Foley catheter is retracted. The mucosa around the adenoma is scored, taking care to avoid the ureteral orifices. Using a combination of blunt and sharp dissections, the adenoma is mobilized away from the prostatic capsule. This is begun at the posterior surface, then on the lateral aspects of the adenoma, and then continued anteriorly. A 0-vicryl stay suture can be placed to help retract the prostate during mobilization. The urethra is identified and transected sharply. The adenoma is pulled anteriorly, and the posterior aspect is then mobilized. The adenoma is then removed and placed into a specimen bag.

Hemostasis is achieved with cautery. If hemostasis continues to be an issue, large figure-of-eight sutures can be taken at the 5 o'clock and 7 o'clock positions at the bladder neck to ligate any branches from the prostatic pedicles. Obvious bleeders were also tied.

At this point, a single 3-0 monocryl suture is used to reapproximate the posterior plate. A 20 F Foley catheter is replaced with the balloon deflated. Then the bladder closure is performed using a 3-0 vicryl single barbed suture in a running fashion. Finally, the anterior capsule is reapproximated with a 3-0 monocryl suture to aid with hemostasis.

RESULTS

Robot-assisted simple prostatectomy was successfully performed by a single surgeon in 20 patients using different surgical approaches. The mean patient age was 70.8 years (range 61–87 years); mean IPSS was 14.75 (range 9–21 years); mean PSA was 7.6 (range 1.5–18.9). Mean postvoid residual urine was 414 cc (range 123–750 cc). Four patients who underwent simple prostatectomy were in urinary retention with indwelling Foley urethral catheter. Two patients had bladder stones, and 1 patient had a large diverticulum.

All patients had failed medical therapy (either 5-alpha reeducates inhibitors and/or alpha blockers), and 2 patients had undergone previous interventions for BPH including transurethral resection of the prostate. All patients under 70 years of age underwent preoperative evaluation for prostate cancer and had a negative prostate biopsy prior to surgery. All patients underwent preoperative cystoscopy to evaluate for intravesical prostatic protrusion, with 5 of 9 patients having a prominent median lobe.

Six patients had concomitant procedures, including inguinal hernia repairs in 2 patients, cystolithotomy in 3 patients, and bladder diverticulectomy in 1 patient. Mean length of stay was 1.7 days (range 1–5 days). There were 2 complications. Despite administration of second-generation cephalosporin, 1 patient developed a UTI requiring prolonged treatment with oral antibiotics (Clavien grade 2). One patient developed an ileus postoperatively, which was treated with conservative management but necessitated a prolonged hospital stay (Clavien grade 1).

A complete urethrovesical anastomosis performed with a 3-0 barbed or monocryl suture allowed the authors to leave the catheter postoperatively for 3 to 5 days and remove it without a voiding cystourethrogram except for initial cases. Postoperatively, all patients were able to void with minimal postvoid residual after catheter removal. On pathologic review, mean excised prostate adenoma weight was 134.7 g (range 74–384 g). Two patients were diagnosed with Gleason 3 + 3 = 6 adenocarcinoma, pathologic stage T1a. Both of those patients continue to have regular PSA to monitor their disease.

DISCUSSION

This series demonstrates the multiple approaches to robot-assisted simple prostatectomy that recapitulate the open technique. Transurethral resection and open simple prostatectomy have traditionally been the standard methods of treatment for men with BPH with significant bother. As technology has advanced, the use of lasers has entered the treatment arena with the introduction of photovaporization of the prostate and holmium enucleation of the prostate. Randomized control trials have shown equivalent short-tem outcomes for photovaporization of the prostate[9] and intermediate-term outcomes for holmium enucleation of the prostate[10] in regards to IPSS scores and QMax compared with open simple prostatectomy.

One of the major reasons endoscopic treatments for BPH were created was the concern for high complication rates related to open simple prostatectomy. Bleeding is a major concern, with a large-volume center reporting a 12.7% rate of blood transfusions, a 12.3% infection rate, and 3.2% bladder neck contracture rate.[11] In 1 prospective study of 56 patients, the mean estimated blood loss was 1181.3 mL, with a 36% rate of blood transfusion.[12]

The first published series of a minimally invasive approach to simple prostatectomy was published by Mariano and colleagues,[3] which demonstrated improved pain and shorter recovery compared with the open approach. However, blood loss was still a major issue, with nearly 10.2% of the laparoscopic group requiring blood transfusions. The laparoscopic approach to simple prostatectomy remains a challenge for most surgeons because of the limited ergonomics of the instruments and the narrow confines of the pelvis and difficulty of performing intracorporeal suture.

The use of robotics has overcome the challenges of performing minimally invasive laparoscopic procedures, making the procedure technically easier for the surgeon. Using the techniques they developed beginning in 2009, the authors have successfully performed 20 procedures.[6,7]

The authors' series demonstrated no blood transfusions, which is consistent with published reports of robot-assisted simple prostatectomy.[13–15] Factors that may be significant for this discrepancy between blood loss using the robotic approach and the traditional open approach may be the pneumoperitoneum contributing to a taponade of small vessels, better hemostatic control using laparoclip (Covidien, Dublin, Ireland) under 3-dimensional magnified stereoscopic vision, and articulated instruments. In addition, the authors perform a complete anatomic reconstruction of vesicourethral junction and inflation of balloon inside the bladder. This maneuver completely obliterates the prostatic cavity and has the potential for better hemostasis and early catheter removal.

Another advantage of the robotic approach is the ease of treating additional coexisting pathologies as done in the present series. Using the robotic approach, these concomitant procedures were very quick to perform and minimize the morbidity for the patient in need of an additional anesthetic or prolonged operative time.

In the authors' opinion, RALSP is a viable option for patients with large glands, preferably over 100 g, that would not be amenable to single-stage transurethral resection or patients would otherwise be candidates for an open procedure. This technique also helps in treating concomitant pelvic pathology. The robotic approach is a recapitulation of the open approach with modifications as described. It demonstrates decreased blood loss, shorter convalescence, minimal catheter duration, no suprapubic catheterization, no continuous bladder irrigation, and lower complication rates. This series is limited by the small sample size and single surgeon experience, as the authors do not believe in operating on a small-sized prostate with RALSP, which can be handled with alternative less costly approaches. A larger cohort of patients would allow greater reproducibility. Additionally, long-term follow-up is necessary to evaluate outcomes.

SUMMARY

This article demonstrated multiple surgical approaches for robot-assisted simple prostatectomy in patients suffering from LUTS from large prostatic adenomas. Robot-assisted simple prostatectomy is a technically feasible and viable treatment option that also allows management of other pathologies concomitantly. RALSP with complete urethrovescial reconstruction is a minimally invasive technique for a large prostatic adenoma that provides excellent outcomes. RALSP can also be performed with other modified techniques as described. Larger studies with longer follow-up are needed to assess the long-term results of this procedure on alleviation of voiding symptoms.

REFERENCES

1. McConnell JD, Roehrborn CG, Bautista OM, et al. The long-term effect of doxazosin, finasteride, and combination therapy on the clinical progression of benign prostatic hyperplasia. N Engl J Med 2003; 349(25):2387–98.
2. Reich O, Gratzke C, Bachmann A, et al. Morbidity, mortality and early outcome of transurethral resection of the prostate: a prospective multicenter evaluation of 10,654 patients. J Urol 2008;180(1):246–9.
3. Mariano MB, Graziottin TM, Tefilli MV. Laparoscopic prostatectomy with vascular control for benign prostatic hyperplasia. J Urol 2002;167(6):2528–9.
4. Baumert H, Ballaro A, Dugardin F, et al. Laparoscopic versus open simple prostatectomy: a comparative study. J Urol 2006;175(5):1691–4.
5. McCullough TC, Heldwein FL, Soon SJ, et al. Laparoscopic versus open simple prostatectomy: an evaluation of morbidity. J Endourol 2009;23(1):129–33.
6. Singh I, Hudson JE, Hemal AK. Robot-assisted laparoscopic prostatectomy for a giant prostate with retrieval of vesical stones. Int Urol Nephrol 2010; 42(3):615–9.
7. Dubey D, Hemal AK. Robotic-assisted simple prostatectomy with complete urethrovesical reconstruction. Indian J Urol 2012;28(2):231–2.
8. Hemal AK, Agarwal MM, Babbar P. Impact of newer unidirectional and bidirectional barbed suture on vesicourethral anastomosis during robot-assisted radical prostatectomy and its comparison with polyglecaprone-25 suture: an initial experience. Int Urol Nephrol 2012;44(1):125–32.
9. Alivizatos G, Skolarikos A, Chalikopoulos D, et al. Transurethral photoselective vaporization versus transvesical open enucleation for prostatic adenomas >80 ml: 12-mo results of a randomized prospective study. Eur Urol 2008;54(2):427–37.
10. Kuntz RM, Lehrich K, Ahyai SA. Holmium laser enucleation of the prostate versus open prostatectomy for prostates greater than 100 grams: 5-year follow-up results of a randomised clinical trial. Eur Urol 2008;53(1):160–6.
11. Suer E, Gokce I, Yaman O, et al. Open prostatectomy is still a valid option for large prostates: a high-volume, single-center experience. Urology 2008;72(1):90–4.
12. Helfand B, Mouli S, Dedhia R, et al. Management of lower urinary tract symptoms secondary to benign prostatic hyperplasia with open prostatectomy: results of a contemporary series. J Urol 2006;176(6 Pt 1):2557–61 [discussion: 2561].
13. Leslie S, de Castro Abreu AL, Chopra S, et al. Transvesical robotic simple prostatectomy: initial clinical experience. Eur Urol 2014. pii:S0302-2838(13) 01381-X.
14. John H, Bucher C, Engel N, et al. Preperitoneal robotic prostate adenomectomy. Urology 2009; 73(4):811–5.
15. Sotelo R, Clavijo R, Carmona O, et al. Robotic simple prostatectomy. J Urol 2008;179(2):513–5.

Best Evidence Regarding the Superiority or Inferiority of Robot-Assisted Radical Prostatectomy

John B. Eifler, MD[a,*], Michael S. Cookson, MD, MMHC[b]

KEYWORDS

• Prostate cancer • Radical prostatectomy • Robotic surgery • Comparative effectiveness

KEY POINTS

- Oncologic outcomes are generally excellent for both robotic-assisted laparoscopic radical prostatectomy (RALP) and radical retropubic prostatectomy (RRP), with no consistent oncologic outcome difference.
- Studies consistently report significantly lesser blood loss with RALP than RRP, and many report lower prolonged duration of stay and bladder neck contracture rates.
- In expert hands, urinary incontinence and potency outcomes are similar between RALP and RRP.
- Ultimately, the skill and experience of the surgeon remain the greatest determinant of surgical outcomes after RALP and RRP.

INTRODUCTION

Since the first robotic-assisted laparoscopic radical prostatectomy (RALP) in 2000, a tectonic shift has occurred in the operative management of prostate cancer.[1] With the rapid diffusion of this innovation, estimates now suggests more than 60% of all radical prostatectomies were performed robotically by the end of the decade and this percentage may increase to greater than 75% in the near future. Proponents of robotic surgery tout the 3-dimensional visualization, wristed instrumentation, and comfortable seated position.[2] When combined with the lower blood loss, robotic systems may allow better visualization of the apex and greater magnification when dissecting surgical planes, both of which may lead to improved surgical outcomes.[3] Detractors note that the widespread adoption was a result of aggressive marketing rather than proven benefits, and that claims for the superiority of the robotic technique remain unproven.[4] Furthermore, the anatomic considerations that allow improved hemostasis and visualization of the prostatic apex were pioneered by Walsh and are common to both open and robotic techniques.[5]

Available evidence regarding outcomes from RALP and RRP arise from retrospective reviews of single-center experience, metaanalyses, and results from administrative datasets. To date, no prospective, randomized trials exist to guide clinical decisions. In addition, given the strong preferences patients harbor coupled with surgeon biases, a randomized trial in the United States would be difficult, if not impossible, to perform in the current health care environment.[6,7] Thus, we

[a] Department of Urologic Surgery, Vanderbilt University Medical Center, A1302/Medical Center North, 1161 21st Avenue, South, Nashville, TN 37232, USA; [b] Department of Urology, University of Oklahoma College of Medicine, 920 Stanton L. Young Boulevard, Oklahoma City, OK 73104, USA
* Corresponding author.
E-mail address: john.b.eifler@vanderbilt.edu

Urol Clin N Am 41 (2014) 493–502
http://dx.doi.org/10.1016/j.ucl.2014.07.004
0094-0143/14/$ – see front matter

are faced with existing retrospective data comparing the 2 modalities, which has significant limitations. First, given the impact of the robotic learning curve, outcomes early in the robotic experience are inferior to the mature outcomes achieved after more than 300 cases.[8,9] Second, in centers that have transitioned predominantly to robotic prostatectomy, patients who undergo RRP may be poorer operative candidates,[1,10] biasing statistical analyses of surgical outcomes. Furthermore, continued stage migration between 2000 (when RRP was predominant) and current times (when RALP is more common than RRP) may bias oncologic outcomes in favor of RALP. Administrative datasets traditionally have lacked of a modifier distinguishing RALP from laparoscopic radical prostatectomy (LRP), limiting the ability to compare robotic and open surgery directly. With these limitations in consideration, the objective of the current review is to weigh the available evidence for superiority, inferiority, or equivalence of RALP compared with RRP.

ONCOLOGIC OUTCOMES

Although no randomized, controlled trials comparing oncologic outcomes for RALP and RRP currently exist, observational studies of administrative datasets and retrospective analyses from high-volume centers allow limited comparisons of RALP and RRP. Retrospective analyses of data from single institutions benefit from granular data collection, centralized pathology review, and often from a uniform surgical pathway. However, selection bias and lack of power to detect small differences remain legitimate concerns. Early comparisons of oncologic outcomes between RRP and RALP were based on analyses of single institutions.

Several groups have assessed the risk of positive surgical margin (PSM) between the 2 techniques, with some studies reporting lower PSM after RALP,[11] and others reporting no difference[12,13] or higher PSM rates.[14,15] To reduce potential biases that result from including multiple surgeons who may utilize different surgical techniques, Masterson and colleagues[12] evaluated the experience from a single, high-volume surgeon and a single pathologist to determine whether the robotic technique was associated with decreased surgical margins. The study included 357 men who underwent RRP and 669 who underwent RALP, finding no difference in surgical margin rate after stratifying by TNM stage. No multivariable analysis was included in this study. Of course, the results are limited by potential selection bias in choosing patients for each modality. Magheli and colleagues[14] compared PSM rates after RRP, RALP, or LRP, controlling for selection bias by propensity score matching based on preoperative characteristics. PSM rates were lower in men undergoing RRP (14.4%) and LRP (13.0%) compared with RALP (19.5%) after adjusting based on propensity score (hazard ratio [HR] 1.64 for RALP vs radical prostatectomy [RP] for PSM; $P = .026$). Barocas and colleagues,[16] on the contrary, found a lower PSM rate among men who underwent RALP in their institution (19.9% vs 30.1%; $P<.01$). The authors evaluated 2132 men and found no association between 3-year biochemical recurrence (BCR) and surgical modality after adjusting for pathologic stage, surgical margin status, and pathologic Gleason score, with an HR of 1.01 ($P = .93$).[16] The lack of difference in BCR has been confirmed in other populations.[17]

Single-institution series rely on the experience of 1 or a few surgeons, and the results may not be generalizable. Population studies comparing RALP and RRP have the advantage of diluting the impact of any individual surgeon and allowing an assessment of the collective impact of robotic surgery on oncologic outcomes. Hu and colleagues[18] sought to evaluate oncologic outcomes of RALP and RRP in a propensity-matched analysis of the Surveillance, Epidemiology, and End Results (SEER)-Medicare database. The investigators assessed the rate of PSMs as well as need for additional therapies after surgery in 13,004 men who underwent either RALP or RRP between 2004 and 2010. After propensity matching using data on socioeconomic background, comorbidities, and disease characteristics, the rate of PSM decreased among men who underwent RALP compared with RRP (13.6% vs 18.3%, respectively; HR, 0.70; $P<.001$), particularly in men with intermediate (15.0% vs 21.0%) or high-risk disease (15.1% vs 20.6%). The use of adjuvant therapies was decreased at 6, 12, and 24 months as well (odds ratio [OR], 0.75; $P<.001$) in a multivariable model. The results may have been influenced by differing practice patterns among open and robotic surgeons (eg, propensity for adjuvant therapy utilization), lack of centralized pathology review, and misclassification resulting from unreliable use of the Current Procedural Terminology code for minimally invasive RP (MIRP) during the study period. Unfortunately, SEER does not capture post-prostatectomy prostate-specific antigen (PSA) values, and BCR data were not available. In the Victorian Prostate Cancer Registry, Evans and colleagues[19] found improved oncologic outcomes with RALP. In multivariable models including hospital volume, National Comprehensive Cancer Network risk criteria, hospital type (public vs private), and surgical modality, RALP was significantly less likely than RRP to result in a PSM (OR, 0.69; $P = .002$), and in a separate analysis also including pathologic stage and margin status, RALP was associated with fewer secondary treatments (OR, 0.59; $P = .010$). In a separate population-based comparative effectiveness study of the Health Professionals Follow-up Study, Alemozaffar and colleagues[20] noted no difference in PSM between RALP and RRP (24.4% vs 23.1%; $P = .51$) among the 903 men in the study population. No difference was found in 3- or 5-year BCR rates between RALP and RRP.

Similar conclusions regarding decreased PSM with RALP compared with RRP were reached in a large, multiinstitutional study of 14 high-volume centers in Europe, the United States, and Australia. Sooriakumaran and colleagues[21] compared PSM rates in 22,393 patients, adjusting for differences in age, PSA, Gleason score, pathologic stage, and year of surgery. PSM rates were lowest for RALP (13.8%) compared with LRP (16.3%) and RRP (22.8%), although a greater proportion of men undergoing RRP had high-risk disease and were treated at a significantly earlier time point. After adjustment using either logistic regression analysis or propensity score matching, the HR for PSM was 0.76 when comparing either RALP to RRP or LRP to RRP ($P<.001$ for all analyses). No difference was found between RALP and LRP. It should be noted that surgeon volume could not be controlled for in the analysis and may have contributed to the results. Of note, a similar HR for PSM was seen between the study of Sooriakumaran and colleagues[21] (HR, 0.76) as the PSM rate seen in the analysis of SEER-Medicare data (HR, 0.70).

Early in the robotic experience, it was postulated that RRP would be superior for high-risk prostate cancer (HRCaP) because tactile feedback would allow wider excision in palpably suspicious areas and the open approach would allow wider lymphadenectomy. However, in studies limited to HRCaP, the rates of PSM and BCR are comparable for each modality. Pierorazio and colleagues[22] compared PSM, BCR, and lymphadenectomy data from 913 patients with HRCaP at a single high-volume institution who underwent RRP or MIRP (encompassing both RALP and LRP). PSM rates were similar for RRP and MIRP overall (29.4% vs 31.8%; $P = .53$) and for pT2 disease (1.9% vs 2.9%; $P = .6$). In a multivariable logistic regression controlling for age, PSA, Gleason score, and clinical and pathologic stage, RALP was not associated with BCR ($P = .359$). Of note, a greater number of lymph nodes were removed via the open approach (median of 8 vs 6; $P<.001$). Although the cohort was well matched, the authors acknowledge the possibility of selection bias, given that 92% of patients had only 1 high-risk feature and a greater number of HRCaP in RRP patients was based on Gleason score (40.3% for RRP vs 33.0% for RALP). Other single-institution studies of HRCaP have found no difference in the PSM rate for RRP and RALP.[23,24] Of note, Punnen and colleagues[24] report that 37% of high-risk patients undergoing RALP did not receive pelvic lymphadenectomy, compared with 5% in the RRP cohort, whereas Harty and colleagues[23] report that 44% of RALP patients and 62% of LRP patients with high-risk disease did not undergo lymphadenectomy.

Oncologic outcomes are generally excellent for both RALP and RRP. Single-institution studies, typically from expert RP surgeons, have not consistently demonstrated a clear oncologic outcome difference between RALP and RRP. On the other hand, available data from SEER-Medicare[18] and the Victorian Prostate Cancer Registry[19] have suggested lower rates of PSM and adjuvant therapies among men undergoing RALP than those undergoing RRP. A likely explanation for the lack of consistency is that PSM is surgeon dependent rather than modality dependent. Critical to oncologic and functional outcomes is developing the optimal plane between the neurovascular bundles and prostatic capsule. Err too close to the capsule and PSM will increase; stay too far from the capsule and functional outcomes will suffer. The surgical robot is a tool that can assist a surgeon with exposure and visibility, but the greatest determinants of oncologic and functional outcomes are likely the skill and experience of the surgeon. Some believe that, for young surgeons without extensive experience in either robotic or open surgery, oncologic outcomes for RALP are superior to RRP, as has been reported by Di Pierro and colleagues.[25] The authors report the results of 150 consecutive patients (75 RRP, 75 RALP) who underwent surgery early in the robotic experience at a single institution between 2007 and 2009, finding men who underwent RALP to have lower rate of PSM than those who underwent RRP (16% vs 32%, respectively; $P = .0016$), especially for patients with pT2 disease (8.3% vs 24.1%; $P = .0107$). If other studies reproduce this improvement in the learning curve, it could be the greatest contribution of RALP to surgery for prostate cancer.

LYMPH NODE DISSECTION

In the early RALP experience, robotic pelvic lymphadenectomy (PLND) was limited in its extent[26] and underutilized[27,28] compared with open PLND. Hu and colleagues[28] analyzed SEER-Medicare linked data for men undergoing RP between 2004 and 2006, finding that 87.6% of men undergoing RRP had PLND compared with 38.3% for men undergoing RALP or LRP ($P<.001$). Most studies assessing lymph node yields have documented higher yields from RRP than RALP.[25,29–31] As Silberstein and associates note, the extent of lymph node dissection is at the discretion of the surgeon, and variation in nodal yields likely reflect differences in surgeon preferences and pathologic processing rather than limitations characteristic of the robotic approach.[31] Recent reports from experienced robotic surgeons suggest that the extent of robotic PLND is comparable with open PLND in experienced hands.[32–34]

Complications associated with PLND, such as lymphocele,[35] thromboembolism,[36] or intraoperative complications (eg, obturator nerve injury), are germane to both modalities.[34,37] No study has directly compared complication rates of PLND between modalities, and comparison between the 2 modalities would be difficult because the most common complication of PLND—lymphocele—has been reported in more than 50% of patients undergoing PLND.[35] Thus, differences in rates of lymphocele primarily depend on the willingness of the surgeon to search for them rather than operative technique. One may conclude that complications with PLND are uncommon after both RALP and RRP with little, if any, difference in complication rates between the two.

PERIOPERATIVE OUTCOMES

With the advent of robotic technology, investigators studied whether complication rates decreased after RALP. Single-institution case series, metaanalyses, and population-based studies of administrative datasets have been undertaken to determine how RALP compares with RRP regarding perioperative outcomes. Trinh and colleagues[1] compared the rates of blood transfusions, perioperative complications (based on International Classification of Diseases, 9th edition, diagnostic codes), prolonged length of stay (pLOS), and in-hospital mortality between men undergoing RALP and RRP in the Nationwide Inpatient Sample, which includes hospital discharge data for more than 8 million hospital discharges since 2009. After adjusting for patient characteristics (age, race, Charlson Comorbidity Index, year of surgery, insurance status) and hospital characteristics (volume, academic vs private hospital, location) using propensity score matching, men who underwent RALP had a lower transfusion rate (OR, 0.34; 95% CI, 0.28–0.40), were less likely to experience an intraoperative complication (OR, 0.47; 95% CI, 0.31–0.71), postoperative complication (OR, 0.86; 95% CI, 0.77–0.96), or a pLOS (OR, 0.28; 95% CI, 0.26–0.30) than men undergoing RRP. No difference was seen in in-hospital mortality (OR, 0.21 for RALP vs RRP; $P = .168$) In 2 previous studies of SEER-Medicare data,[38,39] no difference was seen between MIRP and RRP (OR, 0.95; 95% CI, 0.77–1.16), a fact that Trinh and colleagues attribute to the lack of the robotic-assisted modifier code in the former study and the earlier time of the study, before the full maturation of the robotic experience. Recently, an updated analysis of perioperative complications between RALP and RRP in SEER-Medicare data was reported. The authors reported similar rates of overall complications and readmissions for each modality, and similar to Trinh and colleagues, men undergoing RALP had lower transfusion rates and a lesser likelihood of pLOS.[40]

Results from administrative datasets represent accumulated results from multiple practice settings, in which the surgeons are often not experts and the hospitals often not high-volume centers. Conversely, Pierorazio and colleagues[41] compared perioperative complication rate and pLOS, defined as length of stay at the 98th percentile or below, among men treated at a single, high-volume center by expert surgeons over a 20-year period, finding that men who underwent RRP were less likely to experience pLOS than men who underwent RALP (1.20% vs 4.01%; $P<.001$). The majority of men experienced pLOS owing to ileus. Interestingly, in this center, patients who underwent RALP were more likely to develop ileus ($P<.001$), experience a urine leak ($P = .009$), and require blood transfusion ($P = .01$). Surgeon experience (HR, 0.98; $P = .02$), African-American race (HR, 1.92; $P = .004$), and RALP (HR, 2.23; $P<.001$) were significantly associated with pLOS in multivariable analysis. These results, when considered in the context of other single-center studies, demonstrate the importance of surgeon and hospital experience in determining complication rates and length of stay after RP, suggesting that experience may matter more than modality. The importance of institutional experience, which has been demonstrated in SEER-Medicare data as an important contributor to mortality rates after cystectomy,[42] likely also contributed to the low complication rates after RRP at this institution.

In studies from centers specialized in RALP, significantly less blood loss and lower transfusion rates have been seen, although overall complication rates are similar in many centers.[25,43–47] Cumulative analyses of single-institution studies demonstrated significantly lower blood loss and transfusion rates for RARP compared with RRP.[43] Of course, patient characteristics such as body mass index, comorbidities, prostate volume, prior surgery, and age were not considered in the cumulative analysis and may have influenced the results. Fewer bladder neck contractures have been reported with RALP than RRP in multiple studies,[48,49] although some authors have not found a difference.[50] The incidence of bladder neck contracture after RALP (0.2%–1.6%) in reported series is lower than historical series of RRP (often >5%),[51] although these results must be interpreted with caution; more recent studies have noted comparable bladder neck contracture rates between RALP and RRP.[49]

FUNCTIONAL OUTCOMES

Urinary Continence

The majority of publications regarding functional outcomes associated with surgical modality are retrospective reviews of single surgeon's or single center's experience. These studies have considerable limitations.[7] As RALP has become the predominant modality for RP in the United States, patients who undergo RRP are poor RALP candidates owing to prior surgeries, aggressive disease characteristics, or body habitus. As a result, studies in these populations are biased in favor of RALP, and many of these biases (prior surgeries, body habitus) are difficult to quantify in comparative studies. Few of these studies used validated questionnaires to assess postoperative return of continence or potency, and patients may overestimate their functional status in interviews with their surgeons.

A few studies of administrative datasets compare the urinary outcomes of men who undergo RP by surgical modality. Barry and colleagues[10] analyzed a survey sent to Medicare enrollees who underwent RP in 2008. A total of 86% of men answered the questionnaire, which were completed between 343 and 558 days after surgery. A surprisingly high proportion of men had bothersome urinary incontinence (31.1% overall), and after controlling for age, education level, and mental and overall health, men who underwent RALP were more likely to report moderate or big problems with urinary incontinence (P = .007). A major limitation of the study is that no preoperative information was available regarding health status or preoperative incontinence or erectile dysfunction, which in other analyses of the SEER database have been lower in patients undergoing MIRP.[38] Also, all men included in the study were Medicare enrollees, who represent a minority of patients undergoing RP, which likely contributed to the high rate of bothersome urinary incontinence. Rather than using postoperative surveys, Hu and colleagues[38] examined the SEER-Medicare claims file data for a diagnosis of urinary incontinence at least 18 months after surgery for men who underwent RP between 2003 and 2007. These patients underwent RP before the robotic modifier was added to the SEER database, meaning that LRP and RALP were indistinguishable in the analysis and called MIRP. Men who underwent MIRP were more likely to be diagnosed with urinary incontinence 18 months after surgery (based on diagnosis codes) than men who underwent RRP (15.9 vs 12.2 per 100 person-years; OR, 1.3; 95% CI, 1.05–1.61) even after adjusting for baseline urinary incontinence. Importantly, no significant increase in rates of incontinence procedures were seen for men undergoing MIRP, and because it was well documented that men in the MIRP group had an higher socioeconomic status, the higher diagnosis rate may be reflective of closer follow-up in this population.[38]

A number of investigators have compared urinary continence outcomes between RRP and RALP in nonrandomized, single-institution series (**Table 1**). Ahlering and colleagues[13] transitioned from RRP to RALP in 2002 and compared their RALP outcomes (after the learning curve matured by case 45) with the last 60 RRP cases. He reported equivalent urinary continence outcomes for both techniques, finding that 76% of men wore no pads after 3 months with RALP and 75% with RRP. Di Pierro and colleagues[25] reported urinary functional outcomes in patients who underwent RRP and RALP at a smaller center. These authors found improved 3-month continence, defined as "no leakage at all," with RALP compared with RRP (95% vs 83%; P = .003), although no difference was present at 1 year (89% vs 80%; P = .092). Ficarra and colleagues[44] used a validated questionnaire (the International Consultation on Incontinence Modular Questionnaire for Urinary Incontinence [ICIQ-UI]) to assess continence, defining patients who reported "no leak" or leaking "about once a week or less" as continent. The authors found that 69% of men after RALP to be continent at the time of catheter removal, compared with 41% after RRP (P<.001). At 12 months after surgery, 88% of men undergoing RRP were continent, compared with 97% of men undergoing RALP (P = .01). Krambeck and colleagues[7] analyzed the early RALP experience at their institution. The authors included as a comparison group men who underwent RRP during the same time period, matched in a 2:1 ratio of

Table 1
Single-institution studies comparing continence after robotic-assisted laparoscopic radical prostatectomy (RALP) and radical retropubic prostatectomy (RRP)

First Author, Year	N	Continence Definition	Continence Instrument	Urinary Continence Rate (%)	
				3 mo	12 mo
Ahlering et al,[13] 2004	RRP, 60 RALP, 60	0 pads	Nonvalidated questionnaire	75 76	
Di Pierro et al,[25] 2011	RRP, 75 RALP, 75	0 pads	Nonvalidated questionnaire	83 95	80 89
Ficarra et al,[44] 2009	RRP, 105 RALP, 103	Leakage <1 per week	Validated questionnaire	41[a] 69[a]	88 97
Krambeck et al,[7] 2009	RRP, 588 RALP, 294	≤1 pad per day	Nonvalidated questionnaire		93.7 91.8
Geraerts et al,[52] 2013	RRP, 116 RALP, 64	0 g	24-h pad test	78 87	96 97
Tewari et al,[2] 2003	RRP, 100 RALP, 200	0 pads	Third-party interview	160 d[b] 44 d[b]	

[a] Immediately upon catheter removal.
[b] Median time to return of continence.
Data from Refs.[2,7,13,25,44,52]

RRP:RALP based on age, preoperative serum PSA, clinical stage, and biopsy Gleason grade. The authors found no difference in urinary continence at 1 year after surgery, but no earlier time point was available to assess early urinary continence return. Tewari and colleagues[2] also found that men who underwent RALP recovered urinary continence more quickly at a median of 44 days, compared with 160 days for RRP ($P<.05$). Geraerts and colleagues[52] performed a more granular analysis of time to continence in men who underwent RP in a prospective study from a Belgian institution and entered a weekly outpatient pelvic floor muscle-training program. The authors suggest that the early return of continence may be related to surgical technique rather than patient selection, because men undergoing RALP regained continence sooner than those undergoing RRP (16 vs 46 days, respectively; $P = .026$), which remained significant in a multivariable analysis (HR, 1.522; $P = .036$) controlling for D'Amico risk group, nerve-sparing status, surgical margin status, preoperative urinary incontinence, and body mass index. The authors also assessed the difference in continence rates at 1, 3, 6, and 12 months, only finding a significant difference at 1 month. At 1 year, 96% and 97% of men were continent after RRP and RALP, respectively.[52]

In a metaanalysis of single-institution series comparing RALP and RRP, Ficarra and colleagues[53] found that the rate of urinary incontinence was 11.3% after RRP and 7.5% after RALP at 12 months (OR, 1.53; $P = .003$). Of course, these results must be considered in the context of each individual series included in the analysis, each of which has its own definition of continence and postoperative data collection method. Furthermore, many of the studies report the experience at institutions with expert RALP surgeons, with only 1 institution reporting the experience from a center well known for RRP expertise.[7]

Potency

Comparing erectile function outcomes is complicated by lack of consensus for the definition of potency, by a large proportion of patients with suboptimal erectile function preoperatively, and by variation in surgical techniques to preserve potency among open and robotic surgeons. Although potency results in men with perfect preoperative erectile function may be excellent after RALP and RRP, only 28% to 58% of men have perfect preoperative function.[54] The series, which assessed potency outcomes, are largely the same as those that assessed continence outcomes, and thus the limitations germane to the single-institution comparisons for urinary incontinence also apply to potency. The majority of studies found a higher potency rate for men undergoing RALP at 12 months (or faster recovery of potency) than those who underwent RRP (**Table 2**).[2,25,44,55,56] Of note, each of the studies

Table 2
Single-institution studies comparing potency after robotic-assisted laparoscopic radical prostatectomy (RALP) and radical retropubic prostatectomy (RRP)

First Author, Year	N	Potency Definition	Potency Instrument	Potency Rate (%) 3 mo	Potency Rate (%) 12 mo
Rocco et al,[55] 2009	RRP, 100 RALP, 200	Sufficient for intercourse	Third-party interview	18 31	41 61
Di Pierro et al,[25] 2011	RRP, 75 RALP, 75	Sufficient for intercourse	Nonvalidated questionnaire	25 68	26 55
Ficarra et al,[44] 2009	RRP, 105 RALP, 103	IIEF-5 > 17	Validated questionnaire		49 81
Krambeck et al,[7] 2009	RRP, 588 RALP, 294	Sufficient for intercourse	Nonvalidated questionnaire		62.8 70.0
Kim et al,[56] 2011	RRP, 235 RALP, 528	Sufficient for intercourse	Interview		28.1 57.1
Tewari et al,[2] 2003	RRP, 100 RALP, 200	Presence of erection	Third-party interview	440 d[a] 180 d[a]	

Abbreviation: IIEF, International Index of Erectile Function.
[a] Median time to return of potency.
Data from Refs.[2,7,25,44,55,56]

included in the analysis only men who were potent preoperatively. Tewari and colleagues[2] found a shorter time to potency recovery after RALP than RRP at their institution (180 vs 440 days, respectively; $P<.05$). In a cumulative analysis of these studies, the 12-month potency was 52.2% after RRP and 75.8% after RALP (OR, 2.84; $P = .002$).[57] When considering these results, one must again consider that the comparison is typically performed at centers with preeminent RALP surgeons but not RRP surgeons. Furthermore, because many studies only include patients with perfect preoperative potency who underwent an ideal, bilateral, nerve-sparing procedure, unbiased comparison with potency rates in historical RRP series (which were typically not limited to these men) becomes difficult. As noted by Eastham, in a comparable series of patients who underwent RRP by a preeminent RRP surgeon, the rate of potency at 12 months was 79%, which is higher than the potency rate after RALP in the majority of reported series.[4,58]

Studies of administrative datasets do not reveal a significant potency advantage to RALP, although methodologic restrictions limit their ability to do so. In the survey of SEER-Medicare patients who underwent RP conducted by Barry and colleagues,[10] there was no difference in the proportion of patients who reported problems with sexual function (89.0% after RRP vs 87.5% after RALP; $P = .57$). Even after adjustment for mental and overall health, age, and education level, no difference in the likelihood of harboring moderate or big problems with sexual function (OR, 0.87; 95% CI, 0.51–1.49). However, in SEER-Medicare data, men treated from 2003 to 2007 were more likely to be diagnosed with erectile dysfunction at least 18 months after surgery if they underwent RALP rather than RRP (26.8 vs 19.2 per 100 person-years, respectively; $P = .009$), although no greater rate of secondary procedures for erectile dysfunction were noted.[38] In the Health Professionals Follow-up Study, 132 men who underwent RALP and 468 who underwent RRP completed the Expanded Prostate Cancer Index Composite (EPIC)-26 questionnaire after surgery.[20] No difference was seen between men undergoing RALP and RRP in patient-reported sexual function outcomes ($P = .66$).

Is there a difference in sexual function outcomes after RALP and RRP? Although single-institution studies from RALP centers suggest that sexual function after RALP is better than after RRP, comparing RALP experts with RRP experts probably yields comparable sexual function outcomes.[4] Results from SEER-Medicare data suggest slightly better outcomes after RRP, although significant methodologic restrictions limit our ability to interpret the data. Furthermore, the dates of treatment from 2003 to 2007 likely represent the early robotic era, and a later analysis may alter the results. In the Health Professionals Follow-up Study, no difference in sexual function was found between the 2 modalities. Thus, one cannot conclude that 1 modality is significantly better than the other, and as has been previously noted,[59] potency outcomes are largely dependent on the expertise of the surgeon.

Although the functional outcomes after RALP are similar to RRP, patients who undergo RALP may expect better results. Schroeck and colleagues[60] surveyed men who had undergone either RRP or RALP at their institution between 2000 and 2007, finding that men who underwent RRP were more satisfied with their functional outcome than those undergoing RALP (OR, 4.45; 95% CI, 1.9–10.4). The study included patients early in the robotic experience, possibly owing to irrational exuberance related to the advertising of RALP by the robotic device manufacturer. Even with the maturation of the robotic experience, long-term functional outcomes after RALP are similar to those of RRP, and patients should be counseled accordingly.

SUMMARY

Are surgical outcomes of RALP superior to those of RRP? Studies consistently report significantly lower blood loss with RALP, and many report a lower pLOS and bladder neck contracture rate. When assessing the trifecta outcomes (urinary incontinence, potency, and oncologic outcomes), the results seem to be highly surgeon dependent. Unfortunately, no prospective, randomized, controlled trials currently exist comparing the 2 modalities directly. However, a well-designed, randomized trial is currently accruing patients in Australia and promises to give some insight on this important question.[61] Yet in the current state, comparative efficacy of these surgical techniques will be limited to data sets as described in this review and subject to the limitations and biases inherent to these studies. In experienced hands, the surgical robot has proven itself to be an effective tool in the performance of RP, although ultimately the skill and experience of the surgeon remain the greatest determinant of surgical outcomes.

REFERENCES

1. Trinh QD, Sammon J, Sun M, et al. Perioperative outcomes of robot-assisted radical prostatectomy compared with open radical prostatectomy: results from the nationwide inpatient sample. Eur Urol 2012;61:679.
2. Tewari A, Srivasatava A, Menon M. A prospective comparison of radical retropubic and robot-assisted prostatectomy: experience in one institution. BJU Int 2003;92:205.
3. Menon M. Robot-assisted radical prostatectomy: is the dust settling? Eur Urol 2011;59:7.
4. Eastham JA. Robotic-assisted prostatectomy: is there truth in advertising? Eur Urol 2008;54:720.
5. Walsh PC. Anatomic radical prostatectomy: evolution of the surgical technique. J Urol 1998;160:2418.
6. Meeks JJ, Eastham JA. Robotic prostatectomy: the rise of the machines or judgment day. Eur Urol 2012;61:686.
7. Krambeck AE, DiMarco DS, Rangel LJ, et al. Radical prostatectomy for prostatic adenocarcinoma: a matched comparison of open retropubic and robot-assisted techniques. BJU Int 2009; 103:448.
8. Herrell SD, Smith JA Jr. Robotic-assisted laparoscopic prostatectomy: what is the learning curve? Urology 2005;66:105.
9. Alemozaffar M, Duclos A, Hevelone ND, et al. Technical refinement and learning curve for attenuating neurapraxia during robotic-assisted radical prostatectomy to improve sexual function. Eur Urol 2012; 61:1222.
10. Barry MJ, Gallagher PM, Skinner JS, et al. Adverse effects of robotic-assisted laparoscopic versus open retropubic radical prostatectomy among a nationwide random sample of Medicare-age men. J Clin Oncol 2012;30:513.
11. Smith JA Jr, Chan RC, Chang SS, et al. A comparison of the incidence and location of positive surgical margins in robotic assisted laparoscopic radical prostatectomy and open retropubic radical prostatectomy. J Urol 2007;178:2385.
12. Masterson TA, Cheng L, Boris RS, et al. Open vs. robotic-assisted radical prostatectomy: a single surgeon and pathologist comparison of pathologic and oncologic outcomes. Urol Oncol 2013;31:1043.
13. Ahlering TE, Woo D, Eichel L, et al. Robot-assisted versus open radical prostatectomy: a comparison of one surgeon's outcomes. Urology 2004;63:819.
14. Magheli A, Gonzalgo ML, Su LM, et al. Impact of surgical technique (open vs laparoscopic vs robotic-assisted) on pathological and biochemical outcomes following radical prostatectomy: an analysis using propensity score matching. BJU Int 1956;107:2010.
15. Touijer K, Kuroiwa K, Eastham JA, et al. Risk-adjusted analysis of positive surgical margins following laparoscopic and retropubic radical prostatectomy. Eur Urol 2007;52:1090.
16. Barocas DA, Salem S, Kordan Y, et al. Robotic assisted laparoscopic prostatectomy versus radical retropubic prostatectomy for clinically localized prostate cancer: comparison of short-term biochemical recurrence-free survival. J Urol 2010;183:990.
17. Choo MS, Cho SY, Ko K, et al. Impact of positive surgical margins and their locations after radical prostatectomy: comparison of biochemical recurrence according to risk stratification and surgical modality. World J Urol 2013. [Epub ahead of print].

18. Hu JC, Gandaglia G, Karakiewicz PI, et al. Comparative effectiveness of robot-assisted versus open radical prostatectomy cancer control. Eur Urol 2014. [Epub ahead of print].
19. Evans SM, Millar JL, Frydenberg M, et al. Positive surgical margins: rate, contributing factors and impact on further treatment: findings from the Prostate Cancer Registry. BJU Int 2013. [Epub ahead of print].
20. Alemozaffar M, Sanda M, Yecies D, et al. Benchmarks for operative outcomes of robotic and open radical prostatectomy: results from the health professionals follow-up study. Eur Urol 2014. [Epub ahead of print].
21. Sooriakumaran P, Srivastava A, Shariat SF, et al. A multinational, multi-institutional study comparing positive surgical margin rates among 22393 open, laparoscopic, and robot-assisted radical prostatectomy patients. Eur Urol 2013. [Epub ahead of print].
22. Pierorazio PM, Mullins JK, Eifler JB, et al. Contemporaneous comparison of open vs minimally-invasive radical prostatectomy for high-risk prostate cancer. BJU Int 2013;112:751.
23. Harty NJ, Kozinn SI, Canes D, et al. Comparison of positive surgical margin rates in high risk prostate cancer: open versus minimally invasive radical prostatectomy. Int Braz J Urol 2013;39:639.
24. Punnen S, Meng MV, Cooperberg MR, et al. How does robot-assisted radical prostatectomy (RARP) compare with open surgery in men with high-risk prostate cancer? BJU Int 2013;112:E314.
25. Di Pierro GB, Baumeister P, Stucki P, et al. A prospective trial comparing consecutive series of open retropubic and robot-assisted laparoscopic radical prostatectomy in a centre with a limited caseload. Eur Urol 2011;59:1.
26. Guazzoni G, Montorsi F, Bergamaschi F, et al. Open surgical revision of laparoscopic pelvic lymphadenectomy for staging of prostate cancer: the impact of laparoscopic learning curve. J Urol 1994;151:930.
27. Prasad SM, Keating NL, Wang Q, et al. Variations in surgeon volume and use of pelvic lymph node dissection with open and minimally invasive radical prostatectomy. Urology 2008;72:647.
28. Hu JC, Prasad SM, Gu X, et al. Determinants of performing radical prostatectomy pelvic lymph node dissection and the number of lymph nodes removed in elderly men. Urology 2011;77:402.
29. Cooperberg MR, Kane CJ, Cowan JE, et al. Adequacy of lymphadenectomy among men undergoing robot-assisted laparoscopic radical prostatectomy. BJU Int 2009;105:88.
30. Yates J, Haleblian G, Stein B, et al. The impact of robotic surgery on pelvic lymph node dissection during radical prostatectomy for localized prostate cancer: the Brown University early robotic experience. Can J Urol 2009;16:4842.
31. Silberstein JL, Vickers AJ, Power NE, et al. Pelvic lymph node dissection for patients with elevated risk of lymph node invasion during radical prostatectomy: comparison of open, laparoscopic and robot-assisted procedures. J Endourol 2012;26:748.
32. Abaza R, Dangle PP, Gong MC, et al. Quality of lymphadenectomy is equivalent with robotic and open cystectomy using an extended template. J Urol 2012;187:1200.
33. Lallas CD, Pe ML, Thumar AB, et al. Comparison of lymph node yield in robot-assisted laparoscopic prostatectomy with that in open radical retropubic prostatectomy. BJU Int 2011;107:1136.
34. Yuh BE, Ruel NH, Mejia R, et al. Standardized comparison of robot-assisted limited and extended pelvic lymphadenectomy for prostate cancer. BJU Int 2013;112:81.
35. Orvieto MA, Coelho RF, Chauhan S, et al. Incidence of lymphoceles after robot-assisted pelvic lymph node dissection. BJU Int 2011;108:1185.
36. Eifler JB, Levinson AW, Hyndman ME, et al. Pelvic lymph node dissection is associated with symptomatic venous thromboembolism risk during laparoscopic radical prostatectomy. J Urol 2011;185:1661.
37. Ploussard G, Briganti A, de la Taille A, et al. Pelvic lymph node dissection during robot-assisted radical prostatectomy: efficacy, limitations, and complications-a systematic review of the literature. Eur Urol 2013;65:7.
38. Hu JC, Gu X, Lipsitz SR, et al. Comparative effectiveness of minimally invasive vs open radical prostatectomy. JAMA 2009;302:1557.
39. Lowrance WT, Elkin EB, Jacks LM, et al. Comparative effectiveness of prostate cancer surgical treatments: a population based analysis of postoperative outcomes. J Urol 2010;183:1366.
40. Gandaglia G, Sammon JD, Chang SL, et al. Comparative effectiveness of robot-assisted and open radical prostatectomy in the postdissemination era. J Clin Oncol 2014;32(14):1419–26.
41. Pierorazio PM, Mullins JK, Ross AE, et al. Trends in immediate perioperative morbidity and delay in discharge after open and minimally invasive radical prostatectomy (RP): a 20-year institutional experience. BJU Int 2013;112:45.
42. Morgan TM, Barocas DA, Keegan KA, et al. Volume outcomes of cystectomy–is it the surgeon or the setting? J Urol 2012;188:2139.
43. Novara G, Ficarra V, Rosen RC, et al. Systematic review and meta-analysis of perioperative outcomes and complications after robot-assisted radical prostatectomy. Eur Urol 2012;62:431.
44. Ficarra V, Novara G, Fracalanza S, et al. A prospective, non-randomized trial comparing robot-assisted laparoscopic and retropubic radical

prostatectomy in one European institution. BJU Int 2009;104:534.
45. Doumerc N, Yuen C, Savdie R, et al. Should experienced open prostatic surgeons convert to robotic surgery? The real learning curve for one surgeon over 3 years. BJU Int 2010;106:378.
46. Kordan Y, Barocas DA, Altamar HO, et al. Comparison of transfusion requirements between open and robotic-assisted laparoscopic radical prostatectomy. BJU Int 2010;106:1036.
47. Ou YC, Yang CR, Wang J, et al. Comparison of robotic-assisted versus retropubic radical prostatectomy performed by a single surgeon. Anticancer Res 2009;29:1637.
48. Carlsson S, Nilsson AE, Schumacher MC, et al. Surgery-related complications in 1253 robot-assisted and 485 open retropubic radical prostatectomies at the Karolinska University Hospital, Sweden. Urology 2010;75:1092.
49. Webb DR, Sethi K, Gee K. An analysis of the causes of bladder neck contracture after open and robot-assisted laparoscopic radical prostatectomy. BJU Int 2009;103:957.
50. Breyer BN, Davis CB, Cowan JE, et al. Incidence of bladder neck contracture after robot-assisted laparoscopic and open radical prostatectomy. BJU Int 2010;106:1734.
51. Parihar JS, Ha YS, Kim IY. Bladder neck contracture-incidence and management following contemporary robot assisted radical prostatectomy technique. Prostate Int 2014;2:12–8.
52. Geraerts I, Van Poppel H, Devoogdt N, et al. Prospective evaluation of urinary incontinence, voiding symptoms and quality of life after open and robot-assisted radical prostatectomy. BJU Int 2013; 112:936.
53. Ficarra V, Novara G, Rosen RC, et al. Systematic review and meta-analysis of studies reporting urinary continence recovery after robot-assisted radical prostatectomy. Eur Urol 2012;62:405.
54. Ficarra V, Sooriakumaran P, Novara G, et al. Systematic review of methods for reporting combined outcomes after radical prostatectomy and proposal of a novel system: the survival, continence, and potency (SCP) classification. Eur Urol 2012;61:541.
55. Rocco B, Matei DV, Melegari S, et al. Robotic vs open prostatectomy in a laparoscopically naive centre: a matched-pair analysis. BJU Int 2009;104:991.
56. Kim SC, Song C, Kim W, et al. Factors determining functional outcomes after radical prostatectomy: robot-assisted versus retropubic. Eur Urol 2011; 60:413.
57. Ficarra V, Novara G, Ahlering TE, et al. Systematic review and meta-analysis of studies reporting potency rates after robot-assisted radical prostatectomy. Eur Urol 2012;62:418.
58. Masterson TA, Serio AM, Mulhall JP, et al. Modified technique for neurovascular bundle preservation during radical prostatectomy: association between technique and recovery of erectile function. BJU Int 2008;101:1217.
59. Schmid M, Gandaglia G, Trinh QD. The controversy that will not go away. Eur Urol 2014. [Epub ahead of print].
60. Schroeck FR, Krupski TL, Sun L, et al. Satisfaction and regret after open retropubic or robot-assisted laparoscopic radical prostatectomy. Eur Urol 2008;54:785.
61. Gardiner RA, Coughlin GD, Yaxley JW, et al. A progress report on a prospective randomised trial of open and robotic prostatectomy. Eur Urol 2014;65:512.

Robot-assisted Intracorporeal Urinary Diversion

Where Do We Stand in 2014?

Syed Johar Raza, MD, FCPS (Urol)[a], Mohammed Tawfeeq, MD[a], Ali Al-Daghmin, MD[a], Khurshid A. Guru, MD[b,*]

KEYWORDS

• Robot-assisted radical cystectomy • Intracorporeal urinary diversion • Outcomes • Robotic surgery

KEY POINTS

- Robot-assisted radical cystectomy with intracorporeal urinary diversion (ICUD) has made considerable progress.
- Long duration of operation was a major limitation when it was first adopted, but results from selective centers are encouraging.
- Reduced complications, readmissions, and mortality rates are key benefits that have been reported for ICUD.
- Sequential case number and mentored training in high-volume centers can help robotic surgeons to incorporate ICUD in their practices.

INTRODUCTION

Nearly a decade ago Menon and colleagues[1] reported the first robot-assisted radical cystectomy (RARC). This development was much anticipated after the success of robotic technology for performing radical prostatectomy. Open radical cystectomy (ORC) remains the gold standard treatment of localized muscle invasive bladder cancer; however, the use of a minimally invasive approach is advocated to reduce the morbidity and mortality associated with the open technique.[2,3] Use of robotic technology allows the surgeon to perform delicate operative steps in the confined pelvic space with precision and accuracy; steps that may be difficult to perform with open or conventional laparoscopic approach.[2] In addition, the 10-times magnification and EndoWrist technology provide an ideal platform to perform an intracorporeal urinary diversion, which would allow the procedure to be performed in a minimally invasive way, and may eventually reduce the complications of a morbid procedure. Soon after RARC, the first robot-assisted intracorporeal neobladder was reported by Beecken and colleagues.[4] Despite an early report of intracorporeal urinary diversion (ICUD), it was selectively performed. Increase in operative time, lack of expertise with the new technology, and the learning curve for the extirpative part of the procedure were the probable reasons for slow adoption of ICUD. With increasing expertise and better results more centers are performing ICUD, which is a logical progression after RARC, to prove its benefit. RARC with ICUD provides better operative outcomes compared to open surgery, with minimal blood loss, fluid shifts, and electrolyte disturbance, and a decrease in perioperative morbidity.[1,5] In addition, ICUD provides

[a] Department of Urology, Roswell Park Cancer Institute, Elm and Carlton streets, Buffalo, NY 14263, USA; [b] Robotic Surgery and ATLAS (Applied Technology Laboratory for Advanced Surgery), Roswell Park Cancer Institute, Elm and Carlton Streets, Buffalo, NY 14263, USA
* Corresponding author.
E-mail address: khurshid.guru@roswellpark.org

Urol Clin N Am 41 (2014) 503–509
http://dx.doi.org/10.1016/j.ucl.2014.07.005
0094-0143/14/$ – see front matter

better cosmesis and improved quality-of-life (QoL) outcomes.[1] Most commonly performed ICUD includes intracorporeal ileal conduit (ICIC) and intracorporeal neobladder (ICNB) of the Studer type. This article presents the current status of ICUD and reviews the literature evaluating the operative and functional outcome parameters related to ICUD.

OPERATIVE CONSIDERATIONS

Intracorporeal Ileal Conduit (ICIC)

Important surgical points of consideration from previously described techniques include:

1. **Port placement**. In order to perform the ICIC, the postplacement for the RARC needs to be slightly higher (cranial) than that commonly used for robot-assisted radical prostatectomy. This placement allows the arms to adequately reach the bowel mesentery. The 6-port configuration includes placement of an additional 12-mm port near the pubic symphysis. This port is used to perform the enteroenteric anastomosis using the GIA stapler.
2. **Marionette stitch**. This stitch is place percutaneously, using 150 cm (60 in) of 1 silk suture with a Keith needle. The needle is passed through the hypogastrium and through the distal end of the bowel segment; it is then brought back through the same location on the anterior abdominal wall. This stitch is kept untied to give free movement of the bowel segment during the creation of the conduit.[6] The marionette stitch is placed lower than the stoma site to improve ease of fourth arm manipulation.[7]

Intracorporeal Neobladder (ICNB)

A large number of ICNB series have been reported by the Karolinska group, highlighting the key steps of the procedure. Similar to the ICIC, the port placement is important to allow access to the bowel mesentery. The following points are of special consideration while performing ICNB:

3. **Reducing the Trendelenburg**. In case of a limitation to perform a tension-free urethroneobladder anastomosis, the Trendelenburg and break in the operating table should be reduced to allow mobilization of the mesentery deep into the pelvis, for a tension-free anastomosis.
4. **Use of traction stitches or loops**. Some investigators recommend performing the urethroneobladder anastomosis before the bowel is configured into a pouch. In order to protect the anastomosis from any traction, it can be held securely on either side by passing a loop around the bowel.

PERIOPERATIVE OUTCOMES AND COMPLICATIONS

RARC with urinary diversion was introduced to decrease postoperative complications and improve convalescence. Despite these benefits ICUD was not popular with robotic surgeons. Factors that may have encouraged the recent attempts to incorporate ICUD in RARC include:

1. Standardization of RARC, promising oncologic outcomes and extended pelvic lymph node dissection (ePLND) technique.
2. The ability of a robotic platform to facilitate the suturing maneuverability inherent in the intracorporeal technique.
3. Most importantly, performing the entire procedure intracorporeal results in decreased insensible fluid losses, early return of bowel function, and less incisional morbidity, because of the decreased bowel manipulation and exposure.[8]

Intra Corporeal Ileal Conduit

The data on perioperative outcomes have the limitation of not reporting the diversion time. Few studies have reported the time for diversion separately from overall operative time. In addition, it is difficult to differentiate complications of the extirpative part of the RARC from the construction of the ICUD. The largest series of 100 robot-assisted ICUDs, by Azzouni and colleagues,[7] reported a median overall operative time and diversion time of 352 and 123 minutes, respectively. The median estimated blood loss was 300 mL. The diversion time showed a decreasing trend from the first 25 to the last 25 patients. Infection was the most common complication (51 cases). The highest Clavien grade for the infectious cases was 2. Most of the infections (34 cases) were reported in the early postoperative period (1–30 days). The gastrointestinal (GI) tract was the second most common organ system involved in the complications (36 cases). Despite being the second common cause of complications, no GI or anastomotic leak was reported in the series, which could have been related to the ICUD. A decline in high-grade complications was noted over the relevant period (first 25 to last 25 cases), in contrast with an increase in low-grade complications. To date, this remains the largest single-institution ICUD series. In contrast, the International Robotic Cystectomy Consortium (IRCC) reported 106 ICIC when comparing the ICUD with extracorporeal urinary diversion

(ECUD) in the IRCC dataset.[9] With 61 cases of ICNB, the 90-day complication rate, readmission rate, and mortality favored ICUD. There were fewer high-grade complications reported in the patients having ICUD, with significantly fewer GI and infectious complications. Type of diversion (ICUD vs ECUD) was not associated with 90-day complications and mortality on multivariable analysis.

Collins and colleagues[10] reported their outcomes of ICUD, with 43 cases of ICIC. The median overall operative time for ICIC was 292 minutes, with 1 case converted to open. The most common 30-day complication was ureteroileal leak (21%) categorized as a high-grade complication. This complication was specific to the diversion. GI complications were 14%, with most of them being conservatively managed. In the late follow-up period (30–90 days) diversion-related complications included 1 case each of ureteroileal anastomosis stricture and ureteroenteric fistula.

Other series of fewer cases of ICIC have been reported (**Table 1**, **Tables 3** and **4**). The operative times have shown a decreasing trend over the years, highlighting the improvements in operative standards for ICIC. However, this improvement is not specific to diversion time, so such an observation should be treated with caution.

Intracorporeal Neobladder

Tyritzis and colleagues[11] reported the outcomes of the largest series of patients having ICNB. The median operative time for these 70 patients was 420 minutes with a conversion rate of 5.7%. Urosepsis (9%) and urinary tract infections (UTIs) (7%) were the most common causes of early and late complications, respectively. Three patients (4%) developed ureteroileal leak, whereas GI complications were reported in 4 patients within 30 days of ICNB. One patient had the reservoir rupture during retrograde urethrography. The causes of diversion-related long term complications (>30 days) included reservoir stones (2), ureteroileal anastomosis stricture (2), bowel obstruction (1), and urethrovaginal fistula (1).

In a series of 25 cases (23 neobladder and 2 ileal conduit), Canda and colleagues[12] reported a mean operative time of 594 minutes with mean estimated blood loss of 429 mL. They reported 2 cases of ureteroileal leak as early complications, whereas 5 patients had GI- complications. Among late complications, 1 case each of urinary fistula and ileus was reported. The highest Clavien grade was 3b. In their series of 12 cases (3 neobladder and 9 ileal conduit), Pruthi and colleagues[13] reported that the mean operative time was 318 minutes, mean estimated blood loss was 221 mL, and mean length of stay was 4.5 days. One patient experienced UTI and 1 patient experienced migrated ureteral stent, within 30 days of surgery.

In a series of 15 cases (7 ileal conduit and 8 neobladder) Goh and colleagues[8] reported median operative time (450 minutes for the conduit and 450 minutes for the neobladder), median estimated blood loss (200 mL for the conduit and 225 mL for the neobladder), and median length of hospital stay (9 days for ileal conduit and 8 days for the neobladder). Infection was the most common complication, with 5 (33%) reported cases. Two cases were bacteremia, 1 sepsis, 1 emphysematous pyelitis, and 1 UTI. The highest Clavien grade was 4b. All of the infections were in the early postoperative period. Genitourinary (GU) complications were 26% (anastomotic urinary leak, urinary fistula, ureteral stricture, and azotemia). The highest Clavien grade was 3b. Half of them were reported early and half were reported late after surgery. Four GI complications were reported. Three of them were ileus and there was 1 case of *Clostridium difficile* colitis. The highest Clavien grade was 2. All of them were reported in the early postoperative period (**Tables 2–4**).

Table 1
Perioperative outcomes for ICIC

Series	Patients (n)	EBL (mL), Median (Range)	OOT (min), Median (Range)	Conversion	LOS (d), Median (Range)
Azzouni et al,[7] 2013	100	300	352	0	9
Jonsson et al,[5] 2011	9	350 (200–2200)	460 (325–561)	0	17 (6–72)
Rehman et al,[2] 2011	9	258[a] (200–500)	346.2[a] (210–480)	0	14[a] (10–27)
Bishop et al,[19] 2013	8	225	360	0	9
Goh et al,[8] 2012	7	200 (50–400)	450 (300–600)	0	9 (5–27)
Balaji et al,[21] 2004	3	250[a] (50–500)	691[a] (616–828)	0	7.3[a] (5–10)

Abbreviations: EBL, estimated blood loss; LOS, length of stay; OOT, overall operative time.
[a] Mean.
Data from Refs.[2,5,7,8,20,21]

Table 2
Perioperative outcomes for intracorporeal neobladder

Series	Patients (n)	EBL (mL), Median, (Range)	OOT (min), Median (Range)	Conversion	LOS (d), Median (Range)
Collins et al,[19] 2014	67	500 (100–2200)	415 (265–760)	4	9 (4–78)
Jonsson et al,[5] 2011	36	625 (200–2200)	480 (330–760)	2	9 (4–78)
Goh et al,[8] 2012	8	225 (100–700)	450 (420–780)	—	8 (5–27)
Sala et al,[22] 2006	1	100	720	—	5
Beecken et al,[4] 2003	1	200	510	—	—

Data from Refs.[4,5,8,19,22]

FUNCTIONAL OUTCOMES

Health-related QoL

Understanding the impact of treatment of bladder cancer and losing an organ is of utmost importance and ICUD is no exception. This understanding is achieved by using validated QoL questionnaires to identify the effects on relevant aspects of life.[14] However, limited data exist for the type of diversion and the method (intracorporeal vs extracorporeal). In addition, there remains a lack of comparison between open and robot-assisted approaches. Yuh and colleagues[15] reported QoL outcomes measured by using the Functional Assessment of Cancer Therapy-Bladder (FACT-BL) validated questionnaire. The study reported that QoL parameters returned to baseline by 6 months. Using the Bladder Cancer Index (BCI) questionnaire, Poch and colleagues[16] similarly reported return of urinary domain function to baseline within 1 month. About half of the patients had undergone ICUD (53%), and the BCI scores for ICUD returned to baseline sooner that the patients who had ECUD. In addition, the estimation of body image perception was better for patients who underwent ICUD using the validated Body Image Scale (BIS). Aboumohammed and colleagues recently reported QoL for patients having open and robot-assisted radical cystectomy.[17] The study reported no difference in QoL outcomes between open and robot-assisted approaches. In addition, in the comparison of the diversion type (ie, ECUD vs ICUD), both groups returned to their baseline scores by 6 months. The important aspect of this study was the 30-month follow-up duration, which allowed the assessment to be performed after an adequate perisurgical period to ensure a reliable understanding of QoL, as advocated in other studies for ORC.[18]

Continence and Sexual Outcomes

The success of RARC with ICNB also needs to assessed, based on functional outcomes in terms of continence rates and sexual outcomes. As, ICNB is being performed in selective centers across the world, limited data are available. Tyritzis and colleagues[11] reported functional outcomes of their 70 patients having ICNB. At 12-month follow-up, daytime and nighttime continence rates were 88% and 73% respectively. In addition, 81% of patients with nerve-sparing cystectomy were potent at 12 months, with 67% of women being sexually active after surgery. In their experience of 23 ICNB, Canda and colleagues[12] reported daytime and nighttime continence rates of 67% and 18% respectively. Most of these patients had nerve-sparing cystectomy (92%), despite low continence rates being noted. This may imply that nerve-sparing surgery has little effect on continence. Tyritzis and colleagues,[11] found no difference in continence rates for patients having

Table 3
Perioperative outcomes for ICIC and neobladder (data reported combined)

Series	Patients (n) (Neobladder + Ileal Conduit)	EBL (mL), Mean (Range)	OOT (min), Mean (Range)	LOS (d), Mean (Range)
Schumacher et al,[23] 2011	45 (36 + 9)	669 (200–2200)	476 (325–760)	14 (4–78)
Canda et al,[12] 2012	25 (23 + 2)	429 (100–1200)	594 (426–744)	10.5 (7–36)
Pruthi et al,[13] 2010	12 (3 + 9)	221 (50–400)	318 (258–438)	4.5

Data from Refs.[12,13,23]

Table 4
Diversion-related complications (organ system categories, Clavien grade, and early/late complications)

Series	Type of Diversion (n)	Total No. (%)	Complication as per Organ System: GU (n)	GI (n)	Infectious (n)	Clavien Grade (Highest)	Early and Late Complications (n)	
Azzouni et al,[7] 2013	Ileal conduit (100)	Infectious 51 (31) GI 36 (22) GU 18 (11)	Hydronephrosis (6) Epididymitis (1)	Ileus (16) Intestinal fistula (1) Liver dysfunction (1) GI bleeding (1)	UTI (21) Fungal infection (5)	GI (3) GU (3) Infectious (2)	GI (31) GU (14) Infectious (34)	GI (5) GU (4) Infectious (17)
Goh et al,[8] 2012	Ileal conduit (7) Neobladder (8)	Infectious 5 (33) GU 4 (26) GI 4 (27)	Anastomotic urinary leak (1) Urinary fistula (1) Ureteral stricture (1) Azotemia (1)	Ileus (3) *C difficile* colitis (1)	Bacteremia (2) Sepsis (1) Emphysematous pyelitis (1) UTI (1)	GU (3b) GI (2) Infectious (4b)	GU (2) GI (4) Infectious (5)	GU (2)
Schumacher et al,[23] 2011	Ileal conduit (9) Neobladder (36)	GU 11 GI 2 Infectious 1	Ureteric stricture (3) Urethrovaginal fistula (1) Enterocyle per vagina (1)	Small bowel insufficiency (1) Aortojejunal fistula (1)	Abscess (1)	GU (3b) GI (3b) Infectious (3a)	GU (4) GI (1) Infectious (1)	GU (7) GI (1)
Canda et al,[12] 2012	Ileal conduit (2) Neobladder (23)	GI 5 Infectious 4 GU 3	Anastomotic urinary leak (2) Urinary fistula (1)	Nausea and vomiting (3) Ileus (2)	UTI (4)	GU (3b) GI (3b) Infectious (2)	GU (1) GI (3) Infectious (3)	GU (2) GI (2) Infectious (1)
Collins et al,[19] 2014	Neobladder (67)	Infectious 19 GU 15 GI 4	Ureteroileal stricture (3) Hydronephrosis (3) High residual urine	Paralytic ileus (2) Obstructive ileus (2)	Urosepsis (6) Wound infection (1)	GU (3b) GI (3b) Infectious (4b)	GU (5) GI (3) Infectious (12)	GU (10) GI (1) Infectious (7)
Bishop et al,[20] 2013	Ileal conduit (8)	GI 4	—	Ileus (2) *C difficile* colitis (1) Ulcerative colitis (1)	—	GI (2)	—	—
Rehman et al,[2] 2011	Ileal conduit (9)	GI 1	—	Necrosis of ileal conduit (1)	—	GI (3b)	—	—
Pruthi et al,[13] 2010	Ileal conduit (9) Neobladder (3)	GU 1 Infectious 1	Migrated ureteral stent (1)	—	UTI (1)	—	GU (1) Infectious (1)	—
Balaji et al,[21] 2004	Ileal conduit (3)	GI 1	—	Ileus (1)	—	—	—	—

Data from Refs.[2,7,8,12,13,19–21,23]

nerve-sparing and non–nerve-sparing ICNB (88.2% vs 88.9%).

LEARNING CURVE

Rapid adoption of ICUD requires clear understanding of the learning curve associated with this technique. The way to succeed in effectively including ICUD in the armamentarium of a minimally invasive surgeon is by approaching it in 2 steps. First and foremost is to gain expertise at performing the extirpative part of the procedure and overcome the learning curve of RARC. Reduction in the cystectomy time and intraoperative complications, should be followed by adopting a mentored approach to perform ICUD. A nonmentored approach is likely to take additional time at establishing the skills for ICUD.

The largest series of ICIC, by Azzouni and colleagues,[7] reported a decreasing diversion time with subsequent cases. Although no cutoff number of cases for flattening the learning curve was determined, a decrease in diversion time from the first 25 to the last 25 cases was noted. This decrease means that subsequent cases improve understanding of the technique, not only for the surgeon but also for the operating room staff, which results in a smooth flow of the procedure and reduces diversion time.

Collins and colleagues[19] evaluated the learning curve for ICNB for 2 surgeons at a single center. The junior surgeon was mentored during his 20 cases. There was a decline in operative time, and conversion and complication rates from the first 10 to the last 10 cases. However, the study did not report and analyze the duration of diversion separately, and was unable to specify the numbers required to overcome the learning curve and achieve adequate outcomes. Despite the shortcomings, the study clearly showed that dedicated mentored training in a high-volume center can affect the outcomes of ICNB.

FUTURE DIRECTIONS

Encouraging results from data presented to date clearly highlight the direction in which progress needs to be made for performing ICUD. Future studies are needed to explore the learning curve for ICUD. Surgeons need to report diversion times separately, along with complications specific to urinary diversions. It is critical to identify the factors affecting the learning curve for ICUD, and the number of cases with acceptable outcomes. Functional outcomes and QoL assessment need to be performed in larger cohorts of patients for better understanding. Randomized studies could provide better answers to some of these concerns. Improving the techniques of robotic surgery remains an area for all robotic surgeons to work on and accelerate the incorporation of ICUD into RARC, making it a complete minimally invasive procedure.

SUMMARY

Current data report better outcomes for ICUD in terms of perioperative, complications and functional outcomes. Sequential case numbers and mentored training can help achieve the desired goals. Nerve-sparing cystectomy with ICNB can help patients retain better sexual functions. Despite initial difficulties, ICUD has come a long way since the early days of RARC, and is likely to become a permanent part of minimally invasive radical cystectomy.

REFERENCES

1. Menon M, Hemal AK, Tewari A, et al. Nerve-sparing robot-assisted radical cystoprostatectomy and urinary diversion. BJU Int 2003;92:232–6.
2. Rehman J, Sangalli MN, Guru K, et al. Total intracorporeal robot-assisted laparoscopic ileal conduit (Bricker) urinary diversion: technique and outcomes. Can J Urol 2011;18:5548–56.
3. Huang GJ, Stein JP. Open radical cystectomy with lymphadenectomy remains the treatment of choice for invasive bladder cancer. Curr Opin Urol 2007; 17:369–75.
4. Beecken WD, Wolfram M, Engl T, et al. Robotic-assisted laparoscopic radical cystectomy and intra-abdominal formation of an orthotopic ileal neobladder. Eur Urol 2003;44:337–9.
5. Jonsson MN, Adding LC, Hosseini A, et al. Robot-assisted radical cystectomy with intracorporeal urinary diversion in patients with transitional cell carcinoma of the bladder. Eur Urol 2011;60: 1066–73.
6. Poch MA, Raza J, Nyquist J, et al. Tips and tricks to robot-assisted radical cystectomy and intracorporeal diversion. Curr Opin Urol 2013;23:65–71.
7. Azzouni FS, Din R, Rehman S, et al. The first 100 consecutive, robot-assisted, intracorporeal ileal conduits: evolution of technique and 90-day outcomes. Eur Urol 2013;63:637–43.
8. Goh AC, Gill IS, Lee DJ, et al. Robotic intracorporeal orthotopic ileal neobladder: replicating open surgical principles. Eur Urol 2012;62:891–901.
9. Ahmed K, Khan SA, Hayn MH, et al. Analysis of intracorporeal compared with extracorporeal urinary diversion after robot-assisted radical cystectomy: results from the International Robotic Cystectomy Consortium. Eur Urol 2014;65(2):340–7.

10. Collins JW, Tyritzis S, Nyberg T, et al. Robot-assisted radical cystectomy: description of an evolved approach to radical cystectomy. Eur Urol 2013;64: 654–63.
11. Tyritzis SI, Hosseini A, Collins J, et al. Oncologic, functional, and complications outcomes of robot-assisted radical cystectomy with totally intracorporeal neobladder diversion. Eur Urol 2013;64:734–41.
12. Canda AE, Atmaca AF, Altinova S, et al. Robot-assisted nerve-sparing radical cystectomy with bilateral extended pelvic lymph node dissection (PLND) and intracorporeal urinary diversion for bladder cancer: initial experience in 27 cases. BJU Int 2012;110:434–44.
13. Pruthi RS, Nix J, McRackan D, et al. Robotic-assisted laparoscopic intracorporeal urinary diversion. Eur Urol 2010;57:1013–21.
14. Guru KA, Wilding GE, Piacente P, et al. Robot-assisted radical cystectomy versus open radical cystectomy: assessment of postoperative pain. Can J Urol 2007;14:3753–6.
15. Yuh B, Butt Z, Fazili A, et al. Short-term quality-of-life assessed after robot-assisted radical cystectomy: a prospective analysis. BJU Int 2009;103:800–4.
16. Poch MA, Stegemann AP, Rehman S, et al. Short-term patient reported health-related quality of life (HRQL) outcomes after robot-assisted radical cystectomy (RARC). BJU Int 2014;113:260–5.
17. Aboumohamed AA, Raza SJ, Al-Daghmin A, et al. Health-related quality of life outcomes after robot-assisted and open radical cystectomy using a validated bladder-specific instrument: a multi-institutional study. Urology 2014;83(6):1300–8.
18. Ng CK, Kauffman EC, Lee MM, et al. A comparison of postoperative complications in open versus robotic cystectomy. Eur Urol 2010;57:274–81.
19. Collins JW, Tyritzis S, Nyberg T, et al. Robot-assisted radical cystectomy (RARC) with intracorporeal neobladder - what is the effect of the learning curve on outcomes? BJU Int 2014;113:100–7.
20. Bishop CV, Vasdev N, Boustead G, et al. Robotic intracorporeal ileal conduit formation: initial experience from a single UK centre. Adv Urol 2013;2013: 642836.
21. Balaji KC, Yohannes P, McBride CL, et al. Feasibility of robot-assisted totally intracorporeal laparoscopic ileal conduit urinary diversion: initial results of a single institutional pilot study. Urology 2004;63:51–5.
22. Sala LG, Matsunaga GS, Corica FA, et al. Robot-assisted laparoscopic radical cystoprostatectomy and totally intracorporeal ileal neobladder. J Endourol 2006;20:233–5 [discussion: 236].
23. Schumacher MC, Jonsson MN, Hosseini A, et al. Surgery-related complications of robot-assisted radical cystectomy with intracorporeal urinary diversion. Urology 2011;77:871–6.

Emerging Technologies to Improve Techniques and Outcomes of Robotic Partial Nephrectomy

Striving Toward the Pentafecta

L. Spencer Krane, MD,
Ashok K. Hemal, MD, MCh, FAMS, FACS, FRCS(Glasg)*

KEYWORDS

• Robotics • Partial nephrectomy • Kidney • Pentafecta • Emerging technology

KEY POINTS

- Robotic partial nephrectomy is no longer an emerging field but has been widely accepted as a safe and appropriate management technique for small renal masses.
- Future directions for robotic partial nephrectomy include identifying patient-specific outcomes to measure improvement. The pentafecta assessing both early and late outcomes may provide this road map for comparison.
- The usage of technologic advances, patient selection, and pathway creation will provide further implementation of this technology and continue to improve surgical results.

Robotic partial nephrectomy (RPN) has been widely adopted for the management of renal masses amenable to extirpative surgery. Its role in providing the advantages of a minimally invasive procedure while still safely sparing nephrons has led to increased adoption.[1] As this technology has been adapted in many high-volume institutions, several techniques and technologies have been implemented to provide improved outcomes; the nomenclature to ensure obtaining these goals is also evolving. **Fig. 1** demonstrates a timeline of advances that have occurred throughout the development of RPN.

The *trifecta* is an established gambling term for describing prediction of the exact order of the first 3 horses finishing a race. This terminology has been adapted to describe outcomes of patients undergoing RPN. As described from the University of Southern California Group, the trifecta in RPN includes negative margins, no urologic complications, and a minimal decrease in renal function postoperatively. They found a trend toward an increased rate of trifecta with their most recent patients; however, the range of patients achieving this outcome was between 44% and 68%.[2] Early reports of trifecta outcomes demonstrate that using the robotic platform seems to improve the likelihood of obtaining these. Khalifeh and colleagues[3] note that RPN is much more likely to produce trifecta outcomes than a strict laparoscopic approach with an increase from 32% to 59% of patients.

Although the achievement of a trifecta may provide early indicators of surgical success, patients inevitably requires further follow-up to assess the success of these elements. Negative cancer

Disclosures: None.

Department of Urology, Wake Forest University School of Medicine, 1 Medical Center Boulevard, Winston-Salem, NC 27157, USA
* Corresponding author. Wake Forest Medical School & Baptist Medical, Medical Center Boulevard, Winston-Salem, NC 27157.
E-mail address: ahemal@wakehealth.edu

Urol Clin N Am 41 (2014) 511–519
http://dx.doi.org/10.1016/j.ucl.2014.07.006

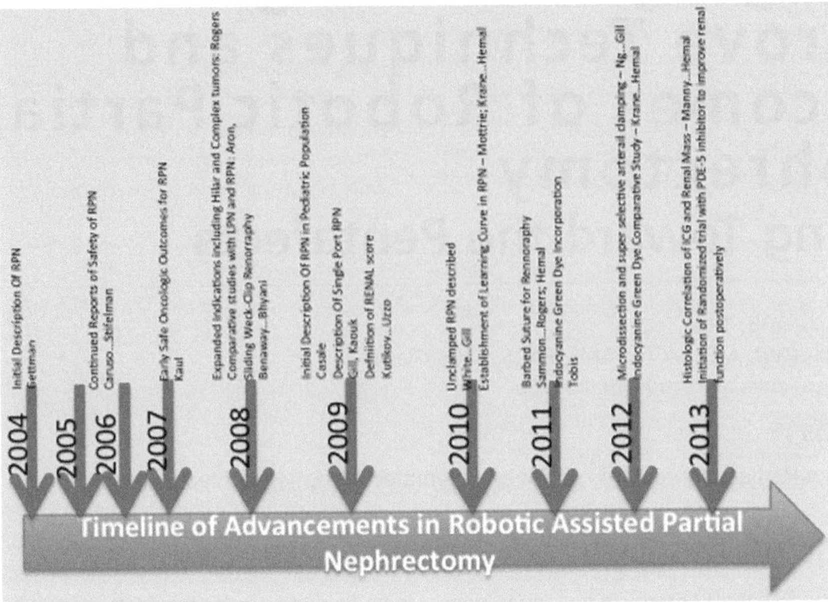

Fig. 1. Overall timeline for RPN. ICG, indocyanine green; LPN, laparoscopic partial nephrectomy; PDE-5, phosphodiesterase type 5.

margins do not necessarily correlate with long-term oncologic control. Although minimizing urologic complications is a goal, patients who experience any complication may not feel as if they have received a trifecta-worthy procedure. The authors, therefore, think the goal of performing RPN should be a pentafecta, which encompasses not only the trifecta but also includes long-term maintenance of preoperative renal function and freedom from cancer recurrence. In addition, avoidance of all complications is required not just pertaining to the urologic subset. In order to achieve a pentafecta outcome, there are several necessary components: a technically sound procedure, an appropriate patient selection, care pathway–guided perioperative management, and long-term continuity of care and follow-up. This review highlights these emerging techniques and their role in improving patient outcomes for RPN, particularly in establishing outcomes leading to a pentafecta.

PATIENT SELECTION AND IMMEDIATE PERIOPERATIVE MANAGEMENT FOR PREVENTION OF COMPLICATIONS

With only 80% of small renal masses identified on computerized tomography being malignant lesions, identifying the appropriate patients to undergo surgical procedures would minimize undue morbidity. Although it was initially reported that there was a poor concordance between renal mass biopsy and final pathology, recent reports have demonstrated improved diagnostic accuracy of the renal biopsy in establishing a pathologic diagnosis. An agreement between biopsy and final pathology was 92% in a recent publication by Halverson and colleagues,[4] and this was associated with 100% positive predictive values for a treatment algorithm based on the biopsy.

In optimizing outcomes, the perioperative patient management also plays a significant role in ensuring safe and reliable care. Several groups have established care pathways, creating standardization in perioperative management and smooth transitions for patients between the hospital and their return home. Abaza and Shah[5] described a pathway including the minimization of narcotics, cessation of drain usage, immediate postoperative ambulation, early induction of a clear-liquid diet, and urethral catheter removal on postoperative day 1 following RPN. Through the use of the pathway, 97% of patients could be discharged from the hospital on postoperative day 1, with only a 2.7% readmission rate. The implementation of the pathway and date of surgery, as noted in the series from Patel and colleagues,[6] was the only predictor of early discharge. In these patients, once again, a low readmission rate was documented.

Complication rates following RPN are in the 15% to 25% range based on the definition of complication used, whether this is a strict deviation from the clinical course or if this is only a complication requiring further management.[7,8] Pentafecta achievement requires a smooth perioperative course by minimizing deviation from the established clinical course and understanding the potential complications before their development.

MINIMIZING WARM ISCHEMIA TIME

The role of minimizing ischemic time during tumor excision has been an evolving process. Historically, a maximum of 30 minutes of warm ischemia time was the goal, although data supporting this time point are poorly substantiated.[9] Clinical evidence in a porcine model demonstrates safety up to 90 minutes with selective clamping[10]; in humans, outcomes with 55 minutes of ischemia seem to have minimal long-term functional loss.[11]

In the authors' experience, they noted 5 Qs responsible for the maintenance of renal function: (1) quality of residual tissue, (2) quantity of residual nephron mass, (3) quickness in resection, (4) quality noncompressing renal reconstruction, and (5) qualitative use in clamping techniques. These Qs are highlighted to ensure adequate long-term renal functional outcomes and are of particular concern in solitary kidneys or in patients with preexisting chronic kidney disease. Smith et al.[12] reported zero ischemia or unclamped procedures in open partial nephrectomy. Gill and colleagues[13] pioneered these techniques in minimally invasive surgery, although this initially required a complicated coordinated effort with the anesthesiologists involving pulmonary artery monitoring and transesophageal echocardiography with which they were able to create hypotension that corresponded to resection of the deepest part of the tumor. In this early cohort of patients, they found no change in serum creatinine or estimated glomerular filtration rate (eGFR) at the time of discharge. Subsequent descriptions of zero ischemia did not include the invasive monitoring or temporal hypotension. Rizkala and colleagues[14] have used a preplaced suture that is used during an unclamped procedure when bleeding is encountered. Novak and colleagues[15] have noted that, in 22 patients without hilar clamping, there was only one transfusion and most patients were stable for discharge on postoperative day 1. Krane and colleagues[16] performed an unclamped RPN and compared outcomes with clamped procedures and did not note any increase in perioperative morbidity.

Techniques for surgical excision with selective versus global ischemia have also been described. Using the high 10 × magnification of the daVinci surgical system, there is an ability to perform tumor-specific devascularization without global ischemia to the kidney. In a recent multi-institutional analysis, Desai et al note that in patients undergoing selective devascularization, the percentage decrease in the estimated decrease in glomerular filtration rate was 17% for the global ischemia group versus 11% in the selective devascularization. They did find a increase in transfusion rate (24% vs 6%) and operative duration (71 minutes) for the super selective clamping, and also noted similar renal parenchymal preservation between the two groups.[17]

An initial multi-institutional analysis of selective ischemia also found that this could improve early renal functional outcomes.[18] Hsi and colleagues[19] also reported that, in the immediate postoperative period, the renal functional was better preserved in the selective ischemia group; however, at a median of 6.6 months of follow-up, there was no statistical difference between global and selective ischemia.

Whether or not short-duration ischemia truly impacts renal function postoperatively has been the subject of intense debate. Recent publications have highlighted that the most important determinant of long-term renal function is volume preservation. The authors' group assessed unclamped partial nephrectomies in a nonrandomized fashion. They did not find a statistically significant difference in the long-term follow-up for unclamped versus clamped (either with artery and vein or simply the artery) procedures.[16] No randomized trials have been created to assess the long-term renal functional data or oncologic outcomes in order to assess the overall superiority or inferiority of an unclamped or selective devascularization procedure compared with the clamping technique.

To improve perioperative renal function, other adjuncts have been used. Rogers and colleagues[20] have described intraoperative cold ischemia. Using a gel-port, they were successful in placing ice slush directly on the kidney during hilar clamping and tumor excision. An added benefit of this technique is the ability to remove the tumor very quickly through this port, allowing for immediate pathologic analysis with margin assessment. Olweny and colleagues[21] have adopted the use of hyperspectral light imaging to assess renal oxygenation during RPN. They found that baseline renal hemoglobin oxygenation was inversely associated with preoperative eGFR and eGFR at the most recent follow-up, opening the door for more exploratory studies with this technology. The authors' group is currently investigating pharmacologic treatment to minimize the deleterious effects of warm ischemia. They are in the midst of assessing the role of immediate preoperative oral sildenafil in a randomized placebo-controlled trial with a primary end point of the difference between groups in terms of the 3-month change in eGFR. The role of statins in the prevention of early and long-term renal functional outcomes has also been described.[22]

INDOCYANINE GREEN DYE AND NEAR-INFRARED FLUORESCENCE FOR IDENTIFICATION OF RENAL VASCULATURE, MINIMIZING ISCHEMIA, AND DECREASING MARGIN RATE

Indocyanine green (ICG) dye is a well-described adjunct to surgical procedures, having been used in hepatic and ophthalmologic surgeries extensively. The incorporation of a near-infrared fluorescent camera on the daVinci Si robotic platform has allowed this technology to be introduced into minimally invasive urologic oncology. ICG is a water-soluble dye, which is highly protein bound following intravascular injection. When bound to protein, it is almost completely restricted to the intravascular space. Additionally, ICG is hepatically cleared; it poses no threat to renal functional outcomes and it is not restricted in patients with renal insufficiency.

The intravascular distribution of the ICG makes it an ideal molecule for selective arterial clamping. Following injection of the dye, within seconds, the kidney is hyperfluorescent with intravascular ICG. Therefore, injection following selective or superselective clamping of the tertiary or quaternary arteries demonstrates perfusion to the remainder of the kidney but not the areas supplied by the clamped artery. This practice ensures only regional rather than global ischemia. Borofsky and colleagues[18] performed a multi-institutional retrospective analysis of this procedure and described the feasibility of this. In addition, they noted that in match-paired analysis comparing ICG with selective clamping to patients with global ischemia, there were significantly improved short-term renal functional outcomes with a decrease of −1.8% of GFR with ICG versus −14.9% without ICG and selective clamping. Harke and colleagues[23] have performed a similar matched-pair analysis with 22 patients undergoing selective arterial clamping and, once again, found a short-term decrease in eGFR to be statistically significantly less following ICG injection and selective clamping.

Bilitranslocase is a transporter molecule located on the proximal tubule, and it has been reported to be downregulated in small renal masses. Following injection of the ICG, these masses appear hypofluorescent when compared with the normal renal parenchyma. An image of a clear cell renal carcinoma before and after ICG administration is seen in **Fig. 2**. The reliability of this downregulation and the ability for ICG to routinely identify malignancy has been called into question. In their retrospective analysis of 100 consecutive cases with ICG administration, Manny and colleagues[24] found that, in hypofluorescent masses, the sensitivity was only 84% and the specificity was just 57%. For clear cell renal carcinoma, there was 96% concordance noted with hypofluorescence; this was also seen from another institution.[25]

ICG has proven to be a useful surgical adjunct to the RPN, but the true utility in terms of patient outcomes is still debated. In 94 patients, Krane and colleagues[26] performed the largest comparative study of ICG in a nonrandomized retrospective analysis. There was a statistically significant improvement in warm ischemia time from 17 to 15 minutes, but the clinical utility of this is debatable as the margin rate and complications were similar in both cohorts. ICG is clearly an emerging technology in RPN, but how this technology will fit into improving specific patient outcomes has not been fully identified.[27]

SINGLE PORT AND LAPROENDOSCOPIC SINGLE SITE SURGERY (LESS) RPN

The utility of the robotic format for adapting single-site surgery has been adopted by multiple groups. Single-site laproendoscopic surgery has been advocated because of the improved cosmesis and potential for earlier return to normal daily activities. In this technique, however, there is an

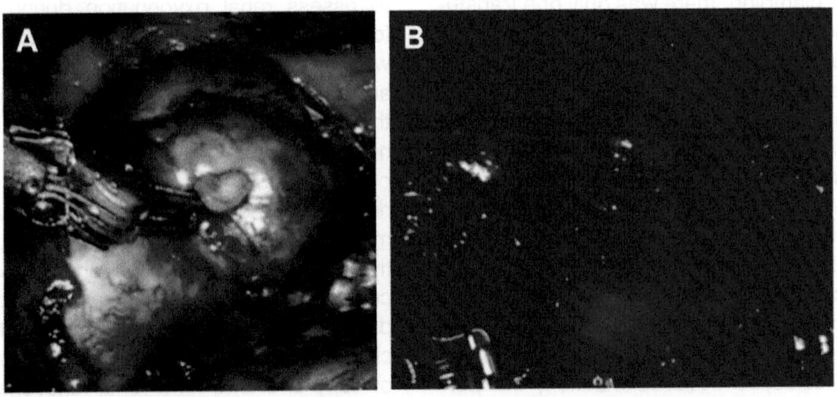

Fig. 2. A clear cell renal carcinoma seen on white light (*A*) remains hypofluorescent following injection of ICG (*B*).

increased risk for collision of the robotic arms; often retraction is compromised because of the lack of a fourth arm. Pneumoperitoneal leakage is also reported. The initial studies for applying LESS to RPN were successfully demonstrated by the Cleveland Clinic team.[28]

Thereafter, adoption of this into a robotic platform has been reported by several centers. Tiu and colleagues[29] described robotic single-site surgery in 67 consecutive patients. In their analysis, which compared 20 patients with renal masses greater than 4 cm to 47 with smaller masses, they found no difference in the risk of perioperative complications or positive surgical margin. However, in a retrospective study, they did find that in these larger mass tumors, the single-site RPN does not alter changes in postoperative renal function between the two tumor size groups; but they did have a slight increase in warm ischemia time for the larger masses. The only group to describe intermediate-term outcomes for Robotic-LESS surgery was Tiu and colleagues.[29] They noted that at a minimum of a 2-year follow-up, there was no statistically significant change in eGFR and also that there was only one positive surgical margin in their cohort of 39 patients.

In a multi-institutional retrospective analysis of patients undergoing conventional RPN versus single-incision RPN, Komninos and colleagues[30] found that the likelihood of obtaining a trifecta outcome was significantly less likely in the single-site RPN, with only 25.6% of single site versus 42.7% of conventional robotic nephrectomy patients obtaining this result. In this study, the authors report that, in patients who had a single-site incision, there was a statistically significant increase in operative time (25 minutes), 6 more minutes of warm ischemia time, and a 7% larger decrease in long-term eGFR when compared with conventional RPN.

As with other advances and emerging techniques for RPN, the utility of this approach in affecting patient outcomes has not been fully described. Additionally, none of these studies have been conducted with the newest version of the daVinci Xi. As the robotic technologies continue to evolve, the safety and efficacy of single-site RPN will need to be constantly updated to ensure surgeons continue to hold themselves to the high standards previously established.

INTRAOPERATIVE ULTRASOUND AND TILE-PRO

Intraoperative ultrasound is a critical adjunct to provide information concerning renal tumor anatomy, depth of penetration into the parenchyma, vascular anatomy, and the relationship of the pelvicaliceal system on the robotic console using the Tile-Pro integrated software. Ultrasound guidance is helpful in identifying the tumor margin which is then scored at the capsule around the tumor prior to resection. The ultrasound also allows the surgeon assess quality of tissue surrounding the renal mass, viewing the real time images within the surgical console.[31] The development of the ProArt drop-in robotic ultrasound probe has provided new technology for the surgeon to use during RPN. The wristed instruments associated with the robotic platform have rendered the drop-in robotic probe more useful in providing surgeon autonomy.[32,33] This autonomy prevents instrument clashes between the surgeon and bedside assistant.

Further evaluations of the role of intraoperative ultrasound for RPN have demonstrated many potential uses. In the first description of using contrast-enhanced ultrasound, Rao and collaborators[34] used this technology to assess the feasibility of selective arterial clamping. Using SonoVue, they were able to assess the success of selective arterial clamping, document the lack of perfusion in the renal mass at the time of excision, and avoid global ischemia during tumor excision.

RECONSTRUCTION OF RENAL DEFECT

Initial reports of renorraphy were described using a sliding Weck clip (Teleflex, Research Triangle Park, NC) technique, which allowed for bolstering of the defect with the use of rolled Surgicel (Ethicon, Somerville, NJ) bolsters.[35] The LapraTy (Ethicon) absorbable clip helped in the performance of renorraphy.[36] The initial use of the Surgicel bolster technique in the closure of parenchymal defects has evolved and is no longer used. Kaouk and colleagues,[37] in the series of 252 RPNs, reported minimal bolster usage and continue to have no change in outcomes.

By no longer using plastic nonabsorbable clips, the authors have been able to prevent clip migration following the dissolution of the absorbable suture. Clip migration has been associated with the development of nephrolithiasis[38] and bowel migration in several reports.[39] In addition, nonabsorbable clips could produce imaging characteristics that could produce difficult radiologic interpretations.[40]

Cohen and colleagues[41] have evaluated the use of fibrin sealants in perioperative outcomes. In this study, they did not find any adverse or advantageous effects of sealants and, therefore, recommended against their routine use. Surgicel placement could produce imaging abnormalities, including the appearance of a gas-containing infection in the authors' experience. In addition, it can induce granuloma formation or other toxicities.[42]

Sundaram and colleagues have registered a clinical trial assessing the need for renorraphy. They are performing a randomized trial comparing the usage of just a base-layer running stitch with a formal renorraphy with a barbed suture. Their primary outcome is the percentage of renal volume loss observed at 4 months following the procedure; however, renal functional changes and perioperative safety will also be assessed.

As mentioned earlier, in order to achieve the 5 Qs responsible for the maintenance of renal function, the authors' current technique of reconstruction of renal defects involves a 3-layer closure. Following cold tumor excision, the base of the parenchymal defect and any entry into the pelvicaliceal system is closed using a running 3-0 poliglecaprone 25 suture on an small half circle needle. This practice serves the purpose of oversewing any open vessels, or running a suture at the base takes care of all bleeders at the base that were feeding the excised tumor; this is the most important suture in this repair. It also allows for approximating the pelvicaliceal system, which prevents urinary leakage and urinoma.

If there are large feeding vessels and major caliceal infundibulum, it can also be tackled with laproclip (Covidien, Dublin), which is an absorbable clip. When there is a large tumor base, it is advisable to sew vessels separately from pelvicaliceal system. The renal parenchymal defect is then brought together using additionally poliglecaprone suture or barbed suture (V-Loc, Covidien). Then the renal parenchyma is approximated with a 0 poliglecaprone suture on a CT-1 needle. The sliding Laproclips are used to support the parenchymal closure on opposing ends. The authors have not found it important to cinch the repair very tightly to compress the parenchyma.

The final layer is a reapproximation of the perirenal and Gerota fascia covering the repaired kidney defect. The preferred suture for this is a barbed suture. In some case when complete mobilization of the kidney is undertaken, especially in thin patients, the authors think pexing kidney to ensure anatomic replacement of the kidney. The authors use hemostatic agents and surgical bolsters only sparingly. Ureteral catheterization is avoided in almost all cases.

EXPANDING THE INDICATIONS FOR RPN

Although initially described as a useful adjunct in the management of small renal masses, experienced robotic surgeons continue to expand its role for difficult cases. The utility of RPN in pT1b or larger tumors is well described. Several small series from single institutions have documented the safety in performing these procedures. The oncologic results have been promising in a short-term follow-up. Gupta and colleagues[43] reported a case series of 19 patients and noted no recurrences in 22 months. In a large multi-institutional series from 4 centers of excellence encompassing 83 patients with renal masses larger than 4 cm, there was only one local recurrence noted in a patient with a pT3a tumor who had a negative margin.[44] A pT1b clear cell renal cell carcinoma that underwent an RPN at the authors' institution is seen in **Fig. 3**A.

With the classification of renal masses using the RENAL nephrometry score, the standardization of the complexity of renal masses has been attempted. By using this system, investigators have noted that even highly complex tumors (RENAL score of 10 or greater) or hilar tumors can be safely removed using robotic assistance. Eyraud and colleagues[45] compared RPN for 70 hilar tumors with 294 patients with polar or nonhilar tumors. Although the operative time, warm ischemia time, and estimated blood loss were statistically higher in the hilar group, multivariate analysis did not demonstrate that the hilar location was associated with an increased risk of complication or change in renal function.[45] Hilar tumors amenable to RPN are noted in **Fig. 3**B, C. For hilar tumors, Abreu and colleagues[46] reported that an unclamped procedure can be performed safely.

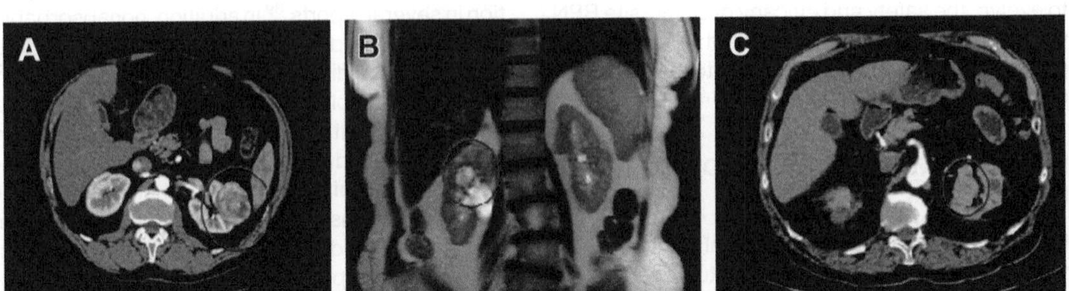

Fig. 3. Large (*A*) and hilar (*B, C*) tumors (*red circle*) amenable to RPN at the authors' institution.

Abaza and Angell[47] also described the utility of RPN in patients with tumor thrombus. In 4 patients with either intraparenchymal renal vein tributary or main rein vein thrombus, the safe performance of RPN has been described. The intermediate-term oncologic results of this procedure did demonstrate that there were 2 of 4 patients who developed metastatic disease during their follow-up. Increasing the utility of RPN in all patient subtypes has also been a goal; investigators have published results on elderly patients, obese patients,[48] and children.[49]

RPN has been used in removing multiple tumors from a single kidney. In a cohort of patients, most of whom had a hereditary renal cancer syndrome, Boris and colleagues[50] found that they could safely perform multiple tumor excisions and were even successful in performing one-third of these without any renal vascular clamping. Abreu and colleagues[51] compared the outcomes of a matched comparison of 33 single versus multiple renal tumor resections for patients undergoing minimally invasive partial nephrectomy.[51] They found that, although there was a small increase in the duration of both the surgical procedure and postoperative hospital stay, the overall complication rate and postoperative eGFR were similar.

AUGMENTED REALITY IN RPN

Using augmented reality, one can overcome the loss of haptic feedback in robotic surgery by using preoperative imaging to superimpose onto the surgical field of view. This technique provides the surgeon the ability to incorporate visual information from the operative field with images previously obtained. Most of the early studies on this have been feasibility assessments; however, several in vivo studies produce exciting possibilities.[52,53]

Teber and colleagues[54] were able to fuse images from a mobile C-arm initially in a porcine model and subsequently a laparoscopic model to aid in port placement. In 10 patients, they found excellent concordance between images and patient anatomy and performed margin-negative partial nephrectomy in all cases. Cheung and colleagues[55] found that when comparing conventional visualization and a fusion system using ultrasound, a faster planning time for resection was achieved using the fusion visualization system in a simulated partial nephrectomy.

NEW ROBOTIC SYSTEM

The new daVinci Xi platform has been released. The Xi robot has boom-mounted, laser-guided arms for precise port placement, which could potentially reduce the difficulties found with arm collision. Other advantages may be seen in patients with extreme body habitus, including obesity. Combined with new-energy-source integration and continuously changing instruments, the technologic platforms are routinely improving.

SUMMARY

The technique of RPN continues to evolve, but the goals remain the same. The achievement of pentafecta outcomes is difficult to obtain; however, surgeons should continue to strive for this standard of excellence. The future continues to be bright for patients and surgeons alike in continuing to perform RPN.

REFERENCES

1. Kim SP, Shah ND, Weight CJ, et al. Contemporary trends in nephrectomy for renal cell carcinoma in the United States: results from a population based cohort. J Urol 2011;186(5):1779–85. http://dx.doi.org/10.1016/j.juro.2011.07.041.
2. Hung AJ, Cai J, Simmons MN, et al. "Trifecta" in partial nephrectomy. J Urol 2013;189(1):36–42. http://dx.doi.org/10.1016/j.juro.2012.09.042.
3. Khalifeh A, Autorino R, Hillyer SP, et al. Comparative outcomes and assessment of trifecta in 500 robotic and laparoscopic partial nephrectomy cases: a single surgeon experience. J Urol 2013;189(4):1236–42. http://dx.doi.org/10.1016/j.juro.2012.10.021.
4. Halverson SJ, Kunju LP, Bhalla R, et al. Accuracy of determining small renal mass management with risk stratified biopsies: confirmation by final pathology. J Urol 2013;189(2):441–6. http://dx.doi.org/10.1016/j.juro.2012.09.032.
5. Abaza R, Shah K. A single overnight stay is possible for most patients undergoing robotic partial nephrectomy. Urology 2013;81(2):301–6. http://dx.doi.org/10.1016/j.urology.2012.08.067.
6. Patel A, Golan S, Razmaria A, et al. Early discharge after laparoscopic or robotic partial nephrectomy: care pathway evaluation. BJU Int 2014;113(4):592–7. http://dx.doi.org/10.1111/bju.12278.
7. Spana G, Haber GP, Dulabon LM, et al. Complications after robotic partial nephrectomy at centers of excellence: multi-institutional analysis of 450 cases. J Urol 2011;186(2):417–21. http://dx.doi.org/10.1016/j.juro.2011.03.127.
8. Krane LS, Manny TB, Mufarrij PW, et al. Does experience in creating a robot-assisted partial nephrectomy (RAPN) programme in an academic centre impact outcomes or complication rate? BJU Int 2013;112(2):207–15. http://dx.doi.org/10.1111/bju.12160.
9. Patel AR, Eggener SE. Warm ischemia less than 30 minutes is not necessarily safe during partial nephrectomy: every minute matters. Urol Oncol

2011;29(6):826–8. http://dx.doi.org/10.1016/j.urolonc.2011.02.015.

10. Benway BM, Baca G, Bhayani SB, et al. Selective versus nonselective arterial clamping during laparoscopic partial nephrectomy: impact upon renal function in the setting of a solitary kidney in a porcine model. J Endourol 2009;23(7):1127–33. http://dx.doi.org/10.1089/end.2008.0605.
11. Parekh DJ, Weinberg JM, Ercole B, et al. Tolerance of the human kidney to isolated controlled ischemia. J Am Soc Nephrol 2013;24(3):506–17. http://dx.doi.org/10.1681/ASN.2012080786.
12. Smith GL, Kenney PA, Lee Y, et al. Non-clamped partial nephrectomy: techniques and surgical outcomes. BJU Int 2011;107(7):1054–8. http://dx.doi.org/10.1111/j.1464-410X.2010.09798.x.
13. Gill IS, Eisenberg MS, Aron M, et al. "Zero ischemia" partial nephrectomy: novel laparoscopic and robotic technique. Eur Urol 2011;59(1):128–34. http://dx.doi.org/10.1016/j.eururo.2010.10.002.
14. Rizkala ER, Khalifeh A, Autorino R, et al. Zero ischemia robotic partial nephrectomy: sequential preplaced suture renorrhaphy technique. Urology 2013; 82(1):100–4. http://dx.doi.org/10.1016/j.urology.2013.03.042.
15. Novak R, Mulligan D, Abaza R. Robotic partial nephrectomy without renal ischemia. Urology 2012; 79(6):1296–301. http://dx.doi.org/10.1016/j.urology.2012.01.065.
16. Krane LS, Mufarrij PW, Manny TB, et al. Comparison of clamping technique in robotic partial nephrectomy: does unclamped partial nephrectomy improve perioperative outcomes and renal function? Can J Urol 2013; 20(1):6662–7. Available at: http://www.ncbi.nlm.nih.gov/pubmed/23433142. Accessed July 7, 2014.
17. Desai MM, de Castro Abreu AL, Leslie S, et al. Robotic partial nephrectomy with superselective versus main artery clamping: a retrospective comparison. Eur Urol 2014. http://dx.doi.org/10.1016/j.eururo.2014.01.017. pii:S0302-2838(14)00068-2.
18. Borofsky MS, Gill IS, Hemal AK, et al. Near-infrared fluorescence imaging to facilitate super-selective arterial clamping during zero-ischaemia robotic partial nephrectomy. BJU Int 2013;111(4):604–10. http://dx.doi.org/10.1111/j.1464-410X.2012.11490.x.
19. Hsi RS, Macleod LC, Gore JL, et al. Comparison of selective parenchymal clamping to hilar clamping during robotic-assisted laparoscopic partial nephrectomy. Urology 2014;83(2):339–44. http://dx.doi.org/10.1016/j.urology.2013.09.033.
20. Rogers CG, Ghani KR, Kumar RK, et al. Robotic partial nephrectomy with cold ischemia and on-clamp tumor extraction: recapitulating the open approach. Eur Urol 2013;63(3):573–8. http://dx.doi.org/10.1016/j.eururo.2012.11.029.
21. Olweny EO, Faddegon S, Best SL, et al. Renal oxygenation during robot-assisted laparoscopic partial nephrectomy: characterization using laparoscopic digital light processing hyperspectral imaging. J Endourol 2013;27(3):265–9. http://dx.doi.org/10.1089/end.2012.0207.
22. Krane LS, Sandberg JM, Rague JT, et al. Do statin medications impact renal functional or oncologic outcomes for robotic partial nephrectomy? J Endourol 2014. http://dx.doi.org/10.1089/end.2014.0276. [Epub ahead of print].
23. Harke N, Schoen G, Schiefelbein F, et al. Selective clamping under the usage of near-infrared fluorescence imaging with indocyanine green in robot-assisted partial nephrectomy: a single-surgeon matched-pair study. World J Urol 2013. http://dx.doi.org/10.1007/s00345-013-1202-4. [Epub ahead of print].
24. Manny TB, Krane LS, Hemal AK. Indocyanine green cannot predict malignancy in partial nephrectomy: histopathologic correlation with fluorescence pattern in 100 patients. J Endourol 2013;27(7): 918–21. http://dx.doi.org/10.1089/end.2012.0756.
25. Angell JE, Khemees TA, Abaza R. Optimization of near infrared fluorescence tumor localization during robotic partial nephrectomy. J Urol 2013;190(5):1668–73. http://dx.doi.org/10.1016/j.juro.2013.04.072.
26. Krane LS, Manny TB, Hemal AK. Is near infrared fluorescence imaging using indocyanine green dye useful in robotic partial nephrectomy: a prospective comparative study of 94 patients. Urology 2012;80(1):110–6. http://dx.doi.org/10.1016/j.urology.2012.01.076.
27. Krane LS, Hemal AK. Surgery: is indocyanine green dye useful in robotic surgery? Nat Rev Urol 2014; 11(1):12–4. http://dx.doi.org/10.1038/nrurol.2013.303.
28. Stein RJ, White WM, Goel RK, et al. Robotic laparoendoscopic single-site surgery using GelPort as the access platform. Eur Urol 2010;57(1):132–6. http://dx.doi.org/10.1016/j.eururo.2009.03.054.
29. Tiu A, Shin TY, Kim KH, et al. Robotic laparoendoscopic single-site transumbilical partial nephrectomy: functional and oncologic outcomes at 2 years. Urology 2013;82(3):595–9. http://dx.doi.org/10.1016/j.urology.2013.05.010.
30. Komninos C, Shin TY, Tuliao P, et al. R-LESS partial nephrectomy trifecta outcome is inferior to multiport robotic partial nephrectomy: comparative analysis. Eur Urol 2013. http://dx.doi.org/10.1016/j.eururo.2013.10.058. pii:S0302-2838(13)01196-2.
31. Rogers CG, Laungani R, Bhandari A, et al. Maximizing console surgeon independence during robot-assisted renal surgery by using the fourth arm and tilepro. J Endourol 2009;23(1):115–21. http://dx.doi.org/10.1089/end.2008.0416.
32. Kaczmarek BF, Sukumar S, Petros F, et al. Robotic ultrasound probe for tumor identification in robotic partial nephrectomy: initial series and outcomes. Int J Urol 2013;20(2):172–6. http://dx.doi.org/10.1111/j.1442-2042.2012.03127.x.

33. Kaczmarek BF, Sukumar S, Kumar RK, et al. Comparison of robotic and laparoscopic ultrasound probes for robotic partial nephrectomy. J Endourol 2013;27(9):1137–40. http://dx.doi.org/10.1089/end.2012.0528.
34. Rao AR, Gray R, Mayer E, et al. Occlusion angiography using intraoperative contrast-enhanced ultrasound scan (CEUS): a novel technique demonstrating segmental renal blood supply to assist zero-ischaemia robot-assisted partial nephrectomy. Eur Urol 2013;63(5):913–9. http://dx.doi.org/10.1016/j.eururo.2012.10.034.
35. Benway BM, Wang AJ, Cabello JM, et al. Robotic partial nephrectomy with sliding-clip renorrhaphy: technique and outcomes. Eur Urol 2009;55(3):592–9. http://dx.doi.org/10.1016/j.eururo.2008.12.028.
36. Shalhav AL, Orvieto MA, Chien GW, et al. Minimizing knot tying during reconstructive laparoscopic urology. Urology 2006;68(3):508–13. http://dx.doi.org/10.1016/j.urology.2006.03.071.
37. Kaouk JH, Hillyer SP, Autorino R, et al. 252 robotic partial nephrectomies: evolving renorrhaphy technique and surgical outcomes at a single institution. Urology 2011;78(6):1338–44. http://dx.doi.org/10.1016/j.urology.2011.08.007.
38. Lee Z, Reilly CE, Moore BW, et al. Stone formation from nonabsorbable clip migration into the collecting system after robot-assisted partial nephrectomy. Case Rep Urol 2014;2014:397427. http://dx.doi.org/10.1155/2014/397427.
39. Wu SD, Rios RR, Meeks JJ, et al. Rectal Hem-o-Lok clip migration after robot-assisted laparoscopic radical prostatectomy. Can J Urol 2009;16(6):4939–40. Available at: http://www.ncbi.nlm.nih.gov/pubmed/20003674. Accessed July 7, 2014.
40. Lucioni A, Valentin C, Gong EM, et al. Computed tomography appearance of the Lapra-Ty and Weck hem-o-lok clips in patients who recently underwent laparoscopic urologic surgery. J Comput Assist Tomogr 2006;30(5):784–6. http://dx.doi.org/10.1097/01.rct.0000228153.81151.ea.
41. Cohen J, Jayram G, Mullins JK, et al. Do fibrin sealants impact negative outcomes after robot-assisted partial nephrectomy? J Endourol 2013;27(10):1236–9. http://dx.doi.org/10.1089/end.2013.0136.
42. Agarwal MM, Mandal AK, Agarwal S, et al. Surgicel granuloma: unusual cause of "recurrent" mass lesion after laparoscopic nephron-sparing surgery for renal cell carcinoma. Urology 2010;76(2):334–5. http://dx.doi.org/10.1016/j.urology.2009.06.070.
43. Gupta GN, Boris R, Chung P, et al. Robot-assisted laparoscopic partial nephrectomy for tumors greater than 4 cm and high nephrometry score: feasibility, renal functional, and oncological outcomes with minimum 1 year follow-up. Urol Oncol 2013;31(1):51–6. http://dx.doi.org/10.1016/j.urolonc.2010.10.008.
44. Petros F, Sukumar S, Haber GP, et al. Multi-institutional analysis of robot-assisted partial nephrectomy for renal tumors >4 cm versus ≤4 cm in 445 consecutive patients. J Endourol 2012;26(6):642–6. http://dx.doi.org/10.1089/end.2011.0340.
45. Eyraud R, Long JA, Snow-Lisy D, et al. Robot-assisted partial nephrectomy for hilar tumors: perioperative outcomes. Urology 2013;81(6):1246–51. http://dx.doi.org/10.1016/j.urology.2012.10.072.
46. Abreu AL, Gill IS, Desai MM. Zero-ischaemia robotic partial nephrectomy (RPN) for hilar tumours. BJU Int 2011;108(6 Pt 2):948–54. http://dx.doi.org/10.1111/j.1464-410X.2011.10552.x.
47. Abaza R, Angell J. Robotic partial nephrectomy for renal cell carcinomas with venous tumor thrombus. Urology 2013;81(6):1362–7. http://dx.doi.org/10.1016/j.urology.2013.01.052.
48. Naeem N, Petros F, Sukumar S, et al. Robot-assisted partial nephrectomy in obese patients. J Endourol 2011;25(1):101–5. http://dx.doi.org/10.1089/end.2010.0272.
49. Lee RS, Sethi AS, Passerotti CC, et al. Robot assisted laparoscopic partial nephrectomy: a viable and safe option in children. J Urol 2009;181(2):823–8. http://dx.doi.org/10.1016/j.juro.2008.10.073 [discussion: 828–9].
50. Boris R, Proano M, Linehan WM, et al. Initial experience with robot assisted partial nephrectomy for multiple renal masses. J Urol 2009;182(4):1280–6. http://dx.doi.org/10.1016/j.juro.2009.06.036.
51. Abreu AL, Berger AK, Aron M, et al. Minimally invasive partial nephrectomy for single versus multiple renal tumors. J Urol 2013;189(2):462–7. http://dx.doi.org/10.1016/j.juro.2012.09.039.
52. Hughes-Hallett A, Mayer EK, Marcus HJ, et al. Augmented reality partial nephrectomy: examining the current status and future perspectives. Urology 2014;83(2):266–73. http://dx.doi.org/10.1016/j.urology.2013.08.049.
53. Herrell SD, Galloway RL, Su LM. Image-guided robotic surgery: update on research and potential applications in urologic surgery. Curr Opin Urol 2012;22(1):47–54. http://dx.doi.org/10.1097/MOU.0b013e32834d4ce5.
54. Teber D, Guven S, Simpfendörfer T, et al. Augmented reality: a new tool to improve surgical accuracy during laparoscopic partial nephrectomy? Preliminary in vitro and in vivo results. Eur Urol 2009;56(2):332–8. http://dx.doi.org/10.1016/j.eururo.2009.05.017.
55. Cheung CL, Wedlake C, Moore J, et al. Fused video and ultrasound images for minimally invasive partial nephrectomy: a phantom study. Med Image Comput Comput Assist Interv 2010;13(Pt 3):408–15. Available at: http://www.ncbi.nlm.nih.gov/pubmed/20879426. Accessed July 7, 2014.

Robot-Assisted Surgery for the Treatment of Upper Urinary Tract Urothelial Carcinoma

Susan Marshall, MD*, Michael Stifelman, MD

KEYWORDS

• Robot-assisted surgery • Upper urinary tract • Urothelial carcinoma • Nephroureterectomy

KEY POINTS

- Robotic nephroureterectomy with excision of the bladder cuff using a 2-docking approach is safe and feasible in treating upper urinary (UUTUC) tract urothelial carcinoma.
- The robotic approach for UUTUC may offer increased visualization of vascular anatomy for an accurate lymphadenectomy.
- Robotic distal ureterectomy and reimplantation using the 4-arm technique is safe and feasible and adheres to all principles of oncology and reconstruction.

INTRODUCTION

Upper urinary tract urothelial carcinoma (UUTUC) is an uncommon malignancy composing only 5% to 10% of all urothelial cancers.[1] However, it is often invasive on first presentation (60%), requiring radical surgery for treatment.[1,2] The gold standard for the treatment of UUTUC is an open radical nephroureterectomy (NU) with en bloc excision of the bladder cuff including the ureteral orifice. In 1991, Clayman and colleagues[3] first described the laparoscopic radical NU, which was introduced as a minimally invasive alternative to open surgery. Despite its learning curve, laparoscopic NU offered less morbidity and improved cosmesis, with comparable oncologic outcomes.[4–6] As minimally invasive surgery evolves and improves, robotic surgery is increasingly adopted into urologic oncology. Robotic surgery alleviated the technical challenges of laparoscopic instrument manipulation and offered the feasibility of performing a variety of complex urologic surgeries.[7]

Robot-assisted laparoscopic NU (RNU) is still a new procedure. Upper tract transitional cell carcinoma (TCC) is a rare disease, so reported studies have few patient numbers and only short-term follow-up. No randomized studies have compared RNU with its open or laparoscopic counterparts. Although intermediate- and long-term data are scarce, RNU does seem to offer comparable advantages to open and laparoscopic approaches. RNU can maintain sound oncologic principles with the feasibility to perform en bloc excision of the kidney and ureter with bladder cuff to avoid tumor spillage and an accurate retroperitoneal or pelvic extended lymph node dissection.[6] Better visualization of the vascular anatomy and recapitulation of open surgery suturing techniques also make reconstruction feasible, potentially improving functional outcomes and decreasing morbidity.[8]

Here the authors review the robotic surgical management of upper urinary tract urothelial

Department of Urology, NYU Langone Medical Center, 150 East 32nd Street, 2nd Floor, New York, NY 10016, USA
* Corresponding author.
E-mail address: Susan.Marshall@nyumc.org

Urol Clin N Am 41 (2014) 521–537
http://dx.doi.org/10.1016/j.ucl.2014.07.007

carcinoma, with a review of the steps and tips on making this robotic approach more widely adoptable.

PREOPERATIVE PREPARATION

Preoperative Workup

UUTUC can present as hematuria, flank pain, or without any symptoms. Computed tomography (CT) urography is now well established as a diagnostic tool to evaluate UUTUC, with the presence of a filling defect suggesting a urothelial mass. In addition, CT allows for a staging evaluation of local extension and nodal involvement as well as distant metastases.[9] Magnetic resonance imaging (MRI) urography is an alternative diagnostic imaging tool to assess for urothelial tumors. In those cases when renal function is compromised, MRI may offer a useful alternative to intravenous contrast for CT. Moreover, recent advances in multiparametric MRI have made this modality advantageous in differentiating renal pelvis urothelial carcinoma from central/hilar renal cell carcinoma.[10] A combination of size and qualitative metrics on MRI urogram has demonstrated its capability in predicting higher-grade urothelial cancers in the bladder.[11]

Retrograde pyelography can confirm the radiologic findings. Ureteroscopy with ureteral biopsy should be performed at the same setting. Selective cytology and barbotage from each ureter and renal pelvis may be performed if a discrete mass to biopsy is lacking or to confirm the diagnosis.[12,13] In those cases of sessile tumors not evident on radiologic studies, or in case of carcinoma in situ without a discrete mass, brush biopsy and cytology can yield the diagnosis. Selective ureteral cytology has a 43% to 78% sensitivity, whereas the false-negative rate ranges from 25% to 50%, based on the tumor grade.[12,13] UUTUC biopsy is strongly concordant with pathologic grade (80%–90%).[12,13]

In the authors' institution, they follow the following algorithm in the preoperative workup of an upper tract urothelial cancer:

1. Obtain CT urogram or MRI urogram
2. Obtain urine cytology and urine fluorescence in situ hybridization to confirm suspicion of TCC
3. Perform ureteroscopy with ureteral biopsy to differentiate low-grade from high-grade TCC
4. If the lesion is above the iliac vessels and high grade, medical oncology is consulted for neoadjuvant chemotherapy (NC) before surgery.
    a. Neoadjuvant cisplatin-based combination chemotherapy has shown a 15% to 25% improvement in survival benefit for bladder cancer of clinical stage T2-T4aN0, according to 2 prospective trials and a meta-analysis.[14–16] Although there is no level 1 evidence in upper tract TCC, similar beneficial effects are assumed for upper tract TCC. The advantages of NC for UUTUC are potentially the following: the ability to treat micrometastatic, nonclinically evident disease, tumor downstaging and shrinking before NU, and the ability to give more effective doses of chemotherapy before renal loss and before surgical deconditioning.[14,17] The downsides of NC are potentially the following: increased surgical complexity with fibrosis/disrupted surgical planes, increased postoperative morbidity, and overtreatment (treating those who did not need chemotherapy).[18] However, 2 studies have shown no difference in operative outcomes (estimated blood loss, operative time, complications, hospital stay) between those who received or did not receive NC before radical NU.[16,19]
5. If the lesion is above the iliac vessels, low grade, and without indications for endoscopic treatment (Strong indications for endoscopic treatment include solitary kidney, renal insufficiency, and weak preoperative performance status.), radical NU is performed. Endoscopic or conservative treatment can be considered in low-grade, small-sized, unifocal lesions and when there is no evidence of infiltrative disease in compliant patients who accept close follow-up.[14]
6. If the lesion (high grade or low grade) is below the iliac vessels, in the authors' institution, a distal ureterectomy (DU) with bladder cuff and ureteral reimplant are performed.
    a. Several studies of T1-2N0 and some select cases of T3-4N0 have reported no difference in cancer control outcomes between DU versus radical NU.[20–22]
    b. High-grade patients are referred to medical oncology postoperatively for adjuvant chemotherapy, as they have preserved renal function from nephron-sparing surgery.

Preoperative Planning

- Remove stent if possible 3 to 7 days before procedure
- Full bowel prep
- Sterilize urine
- Consent for both a DU and an NU and all possibilities of reconstruction

A ureteral stent, if present, is removed 3 to 7 days before surgery. In the authors' experience, they have found that removing the stent before surgery decreases the periureteral inflammation and edema that is caused by the stent. Tissue edema and inflammation disrupts normal tissue planes and, hence, can make dissection more challenging.

All patients receive a mechanical bowel preparation, usually with polyethylene 3350 and electrolyte oral solution oral solution or oral magnesium citrate. Preoperative intravenous antibiotics are given as per the current American Urologic Association's guidelines.

NU

Radical RNU should maintain sound oncologic principles to achieve comparative outcomes with open and laparoscopic NU. These principles include en bloc excision of the kidney and ureter with bladder cuff to avoid tumor spillage and perihilar with retroperitoneal or pelvic extended lymph node dissection, based on the location and stage of the tumor.[6] The ureterovesical junction and intravesical ureter are excised with a margin of bladder cuff and closed in a 2-layered sutured repair adhering to open principles.

The initial RNU procedures were performed using 2 different modalities, with a robotic nephrectomy and ureteral dissection, followed by an open or laparoscopic approach to remove the distal ureter and bladder cuff.[23] Several groups have incorporated techniques to eliminate using the open or laparoscopic approach to the bladder cuff portion, such as the hybrid port technique[23] and/or a combination of 5 to 6 ports.[24,25]

Eandi and colleagues[26] then described their technique of repositioning patients and redocking the robot for the pelvic portion of the case. Because the kidney is located in the upper abdomen, whereas the distal ureter and bladder are located deep in the pelvis, careful planning of port placement is crucial. Strategic planning may even allow for not having to reposition or redock the robot at all.[23,27,28] Redraping and/or redocking the robot can add up to 50 minutes of additional operative time.[29]

Hemal and colleagues[30] and Lee and colleagues[31] have reported their single-robot-docking techniques of performing RNU with bladder cuff excision in a single position, without redocking or repositioning. In the authors' experience, they have found that their 2-robot-docking technique is effective, time efficient, and feasible.[32] With a skilled robotics team, redocking the robot can be done in less than 10 minutes.

The authors' technique of positioning patients in a modified flank with a low lithotomy position enables them to perform the procedure without repositioning patients on the bed. It saves operative time and preserves the operative field. They do place an additional port inferior to the umbilicus on the contralateral side, and redock the robot, for better access to the distal ureter.

Here, the authors outline their technique of performing a radical RNU and bladder cuff excision using the 2-robot-docking approach.

PART 1: NEPHRECTOMY

Positioning

The authors have found it most optimal to position patients in the following manner. Patients are placed in a low lithotomy, lateral decubitus position. Two gel rolls are placed behind patients to support and angle the torso to a 45° angle. The legs are placed in stirrups, with each leg pointing toward the contralateral shoulder. The sole of the feet should be bearing the weight of the leg (**Fig. 1**A). Patients are secured to the bed using 3-in cloth tape across their chest. The contralateral lower arm is placed on an arm board. The ipsilateral arm can be placed in either of 2 ways. It can be placed on a thoracic arm board over the body onto the contralateral side. The second, and the authors' current position of choice, is keeping the ipsilateral arm straight on the ipsilateral side of their torso. A rolled-up foam pad is tucked in the patients' waist to support the arm, which is cradled in 2 foam pads (see **Fig. 1**B). The arm is then secured to the side of patients with 3-in cloth tape from the bed to their chest and from the bed to the patients' hip.

Once the position is confirmed, the kidney position is checked by airplaning the table toward the

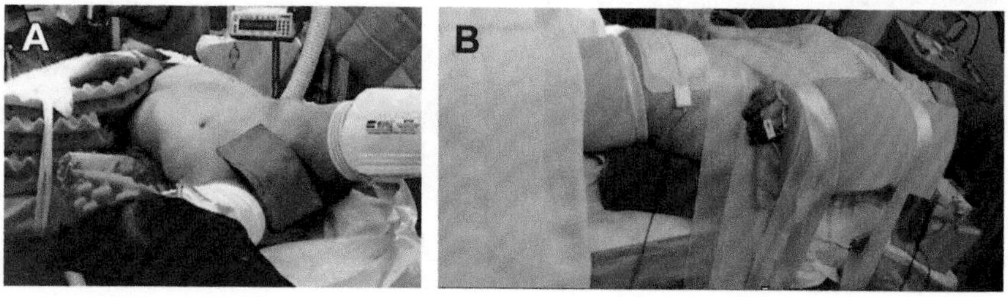

Fig. 1. (*A*) Arm positioned over the contralateral side. (*B*) The authors' current arm positioning at the side.

surgeon (patients' contralateral side) to confirm there is no slippage of the patients and that all pressure points are padded. To check the position for the ureteral/bladder cuff portion of the case, the table is airplaned away from the surgeon to a supine position and placed in Trendelenburg position to confirm there is no slippage and that all pressure points are padded.

The benefits of this low lithotomy, lateral decubitus position are several. First, the assistant surgeon has direct access to the bladder, if a simultaneous cystoscopy or bladder filling is needed. Second, this position allows for the robot to be redocked for the bladder portion of the surgery without having to reposition the patients on the bed. Patients can also be airplaned freely in either direction and can also be placed in Trendelenburg position. In this way, the authors think that this position facilitates access to both the upper abdomen and the pelvis in a time-efficient and safe manner.

Port Placement

The robot is brought in perpendicular to the patients (**Fig. 2**). This docking position is facilitated by the placement of the authors' triangle of ports as high up (cephalad) as possible. In doing so, they avoid having to dock the robot obliquely over the shoulder, which would be required if the triangle of ports was lower on the abdomen to allow room for the fourth arm. The authors' technique for a robotic partial nephrectomy has been previously published, and their positioning and port placement for a radical nephrectomy is the same.[7] They place the camera port 12 cm above the umbilicus, in the epigastric region. The left arm is right below the costal margin, and the right arm is 6 to 8 cm apart from the camera. They place the fourth arm port most lateral (see **Fig. 2**). The key points of their port placement are the same for a NU. They place the triangle of the left arm, right arm, and camera port as high up (cephalad) as possible, to allow the fourth arm to placed in the lower lateral quadrant (**Fig. 3**). The only modification for an NU is that the fourth arm is placed more cephalad and lateral to help with the bladder portion of the case.

In preparation for the ureterectomy/bladder portion of the case, an additional robotic port is placed at the level of or just below the umbilicus in the contralateral lower quadrant (**Fig. 4**). For right-sided tumors, an additional 5-mm port can be placed laterally at the anterior axillary line for a self-retaining liver retractor. For this maneuver, the authors' use a triangle liver retractor to elevate the liver and attach it to a self-retaining retractor arm on the side rails of the bed.

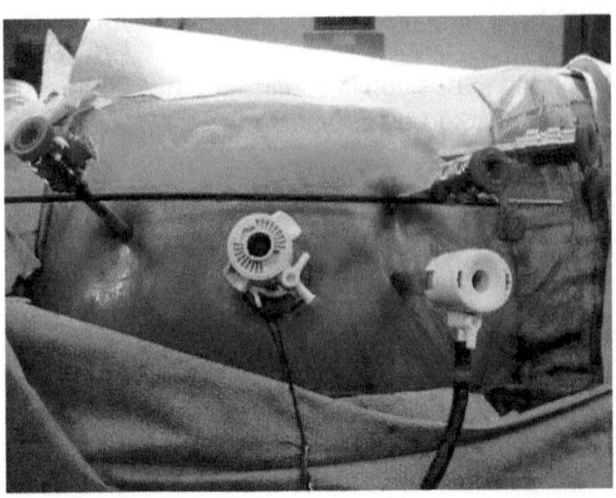

Fig. 2. Triangle of ports.

Exposure and Entry into the Retroperitoneal Space

First, an incision is made lateral to the colon in its attachments to Gerota fascia, to reflect the colon medially and to access the retroperitoneum. If the appropriate plane is found, it should be an avascular plane (**Fig. 5**). The mobilization will first go caudad and then cephalad. The borders of the colon mobilization are the iliac and gonadal vessels inferiorly, the adrenal gland superiorly, and the aorta medially (**Fig. 6**). It is important not to incise too laterally along the abdominal sidewall to prevent incising the lateral attachments of the kidney itself. If this were to happen, the kidney can fall medially, obstructing the view of the hilum.

Left side

The next step is mobilization of the spleen. The lateral attachments of the spleen are sharply divided. Then, with the back of the left robotic arm instrument, the spleen is tented up cephalad, with the right arm (or suction) pushing the kidney down caudad (**Fig. 7**). In doing so, the spleen should be rotated medially and cephalad. On coming medially with the dissection, the tail of the pancreas should peel off revealing a plane of dissection. However, care must be taken to be

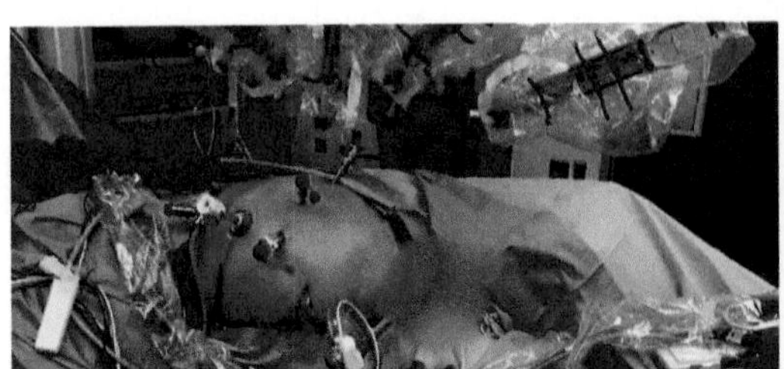

Fig. 3. Port and robot placement for left-sided case.

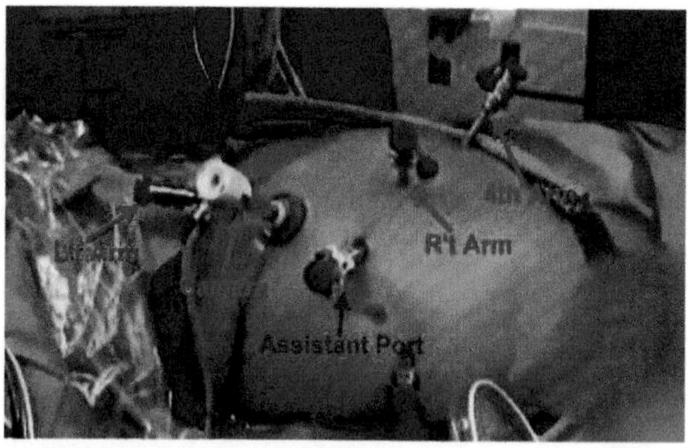

Fig. 4. Trocars labeled for left-sided case.

aware of the splenic vein and artery coursing through the fat, as one's dissection comes across the top of the kidney.

Right side

For a right-sided case, through the additional 5-mm lateral port, the liver retractor is introduced and positioned to lift the liver cephalad, taking care not to put too much tension under the liver, which will cause bleeding. Once the exposure is created, the peritoneum is reflected off the Gerota fascia in the same manner as described earlier. The mobilization will first go caudad and then cephalad. The incision on the peritoneum should go transversely across and below the underside of the liver. The liver retractor can then be readjusted to produce greater retraction as the liver is mobilized and freed to be lifted up. The superior border of the colon mobilization is the location of the adrenal gland. On coming medially with the dissection, care must be taken to avoid injury to the duodenum, which must also be lifted off the underlying plane. The authors mobilize adequately enough to be able to see the inferior vena cava medially.

Hilar Dissection

The second step is the hilar dissection. Attention is turned to the lower pole of the kidney. The best location to find the gonadal vein is at the lower pole of the kidney, which would then lead to the renal hilum. Sharp dissection is carried out right on top of the gonadal vein and moved caudally toward the iliacs and cephalad to the renal vein. The fourth arm is used to lift up on the kidney laterally. In left-sided cases, the gonadal vein is ligated with bipolar electrocautery right at its entry to the left renal vein to allow for easier mobilization and retraction (**Fig. 8**). Next, the ureter is found coursing parallel to the gonadal vein, more laterally anatomically, and superior on the screen. Adequate tissue is left around the ureter to avoid injuring it inadvertently and to avoid compromising its blood supply. In addition, careful attention is paid to keeping the periureteric tissue with the ureter in order to allow an adequate margin in the event of ureteral invasion by malignancy.

Next, the gonadal vein is isolated away from the ureter laterally. The psoas is found, and the fat is cleaned and lifted up off the psoas muscle belly. The fourth arm is then brought in underneath the fat of the lower pole and the ureter and lifted up. A Weck clip is placed on the ureter to prevent spillage.

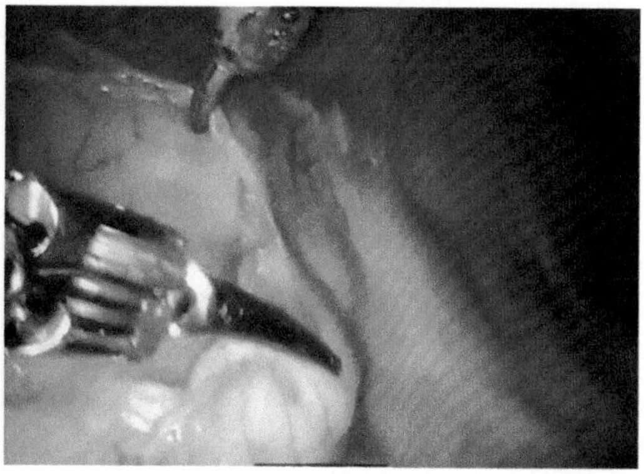

Fig. 5. Colon and peritoneum reflected off of Gerota fascia on an avascular plane.

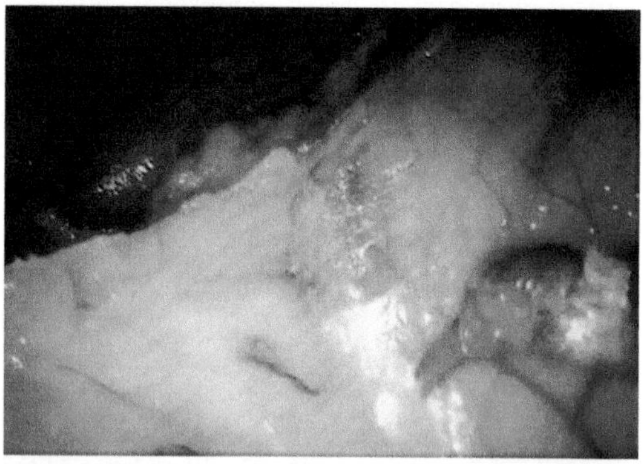

Fig. 6. Peritoneum with colon and pancreas (*left*) is reflected medially, approaching the upper pole of left kidney (*right*).

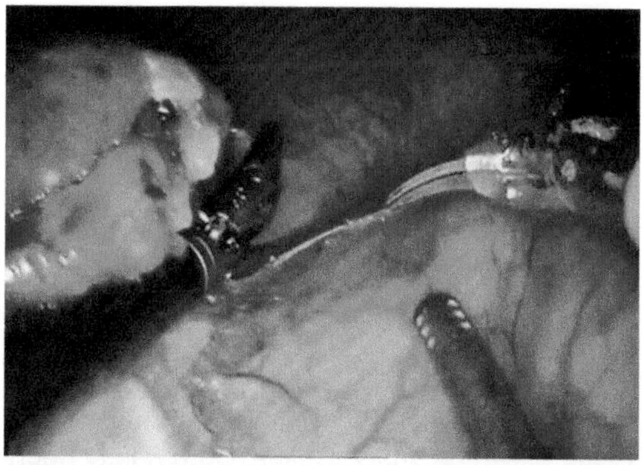

Fig. 7. Left arm instrument pushes up the spleen cephalad and medially to help with dissection off Gerota fascia (*right*).

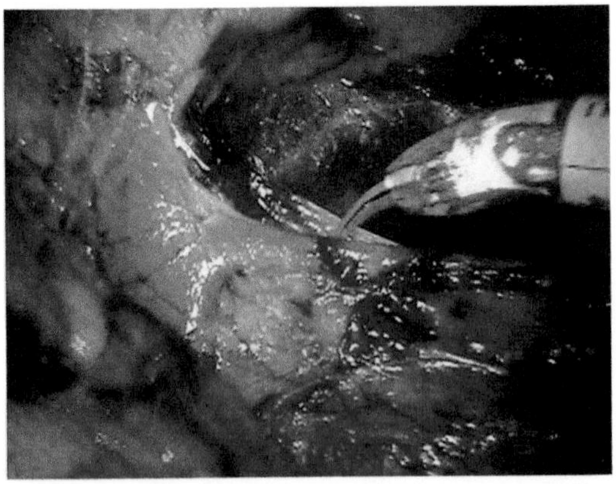

Fig. 8. Left gonadal vein at its entry into renal vein. The left gonadal vein is ligated.

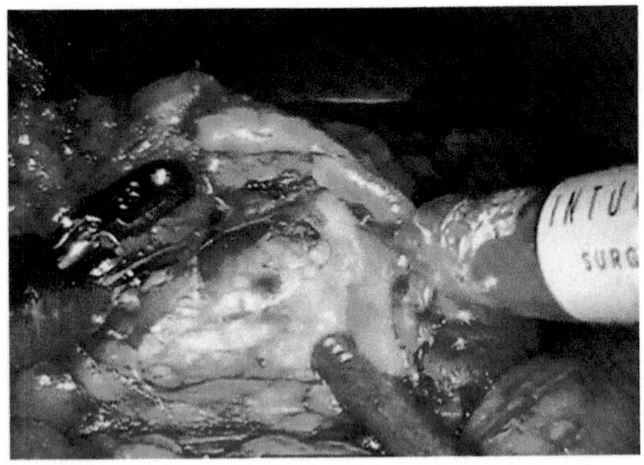

Fig. 10. Lymph node dissection down the anterior and lateral surface of the aorta.

At this time, the renal vein, which has already been isolated, is visible in the field. The renal artery is identified using a drop-in Doppler probe.

Retroperitoneal Lymph Node Dissection

Hilar dissection is carried out more medially at this time to perform the lymph node dissection anterior to the aorta (**Fig. 9**). Lymph node dissection is then carried out in a caudad direction until the bifurcation of the aorta is reached (**Figs. 10** and **11**). All lymph tissue anterior to and adjacent to the aorta is cleared off the aorta, recapitulating the split-and-roll technique of open surgery. The authors think that bipolar electrocautery is sufficient to close off the small lymphatics during dissection. The lymphatics are cleared off the aorta down to the level of the aortic bifurcation.

Attention is then turned back to the cephalad corner of the lymphadenectomy (LND) where it began near the hilum (**Fig. 12**). The renal artery ostium can be encountered as dissection is carried superiorly up the aorta. Although there is no standard template for lymph node dissection for upper tract TCC, the authors follow this algorithm at their institution: For a left-sided case, they remove preaortic and para-aortic nodes and interaortocaval if necessary. For a right-sided case, the precaval and paracaval nodes are removed. The authors keep the lymph node tissue en bloc with the kidney when possible for later removal with the specimen. Once the lymph node dissection is completed to this point, the hilar vessels are divided separately, using a vascular stapler on each (**Fig. 13**). Hemostasis should now be confirmed at the region of the hilum and aorta before proceeding.

Once the hilum is divided, the remainder of the lateral attachments of the kidney as well as the upper pole is sharply released, using bipolar electrocautery. The fourth arm can be very useful at this step by maneuvering it to stretch the kidney medially, cephalad, or caudad to facilitate the division of its remaining attachments. Care is taken to keep an adequate amount of perinephric tissue on the kidney for more accurate staging purposes.

At this time, any remaining mobilization of the ureter is done, if needed. The ureter should be

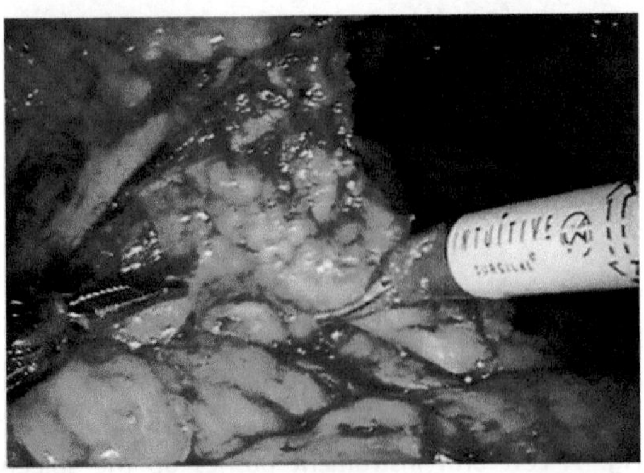

Fig. 9. Hilar adenopathy below renal vein, with renal artery posterior to it.

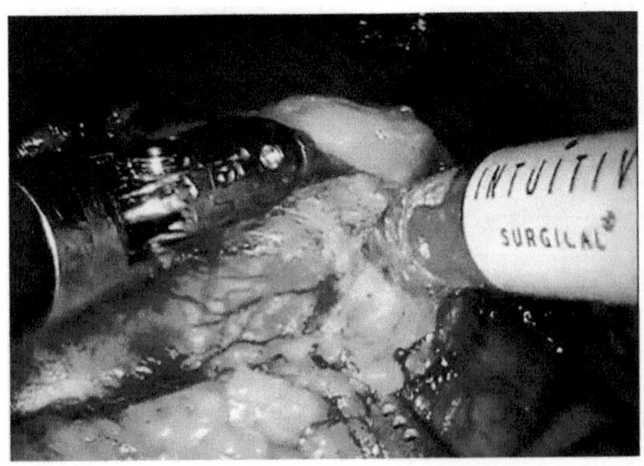

Fig. 11. Lymph node dissection reaches the aortic bifurcation.

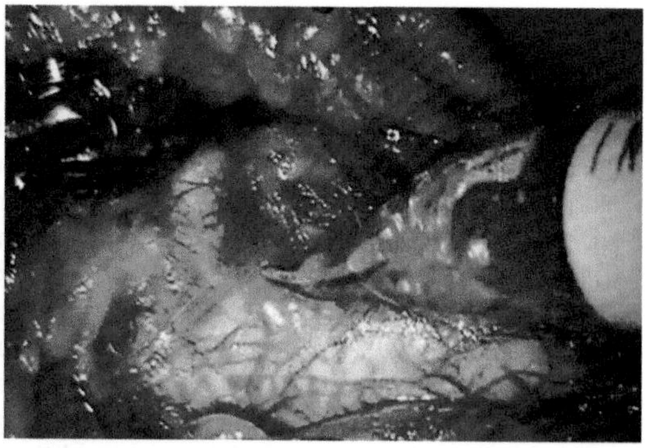

Fig. 12. After lymph node dissection, the aorta and renal artery is exposed, facilitating ligation of the artery.

isolated down to the level of the iliac vessels as a landmark. The gonadal vein is divided where it crosses the ureter.

Redocking the Robot

The robot is now undocked, and the bed is then airplaned toward the side of the lesion to make the patients parallel to the floor (supine); the bed is placed in the Trendelenburg position. The robot is then redocked, to come in obliquely over the ipsilateral hip/knee, called *side docking*. The robot comes in at a 45° angle to the patients, over their ipsilateral hip (**Fig. 14**). No repositioning of patients on the bed is done.

The port configuration will lend itself to a prostatectomy port configuration (except more cephalad) without having to place additional ports. The fourth arm on the robot will now be swung over and placed on the contralateral side of the robot because of the new redocked position from below. The previously right arm trocar will now function as the left arm trocar, and the previous assistant trocar will now function as the right arm (**Fig. 15**).

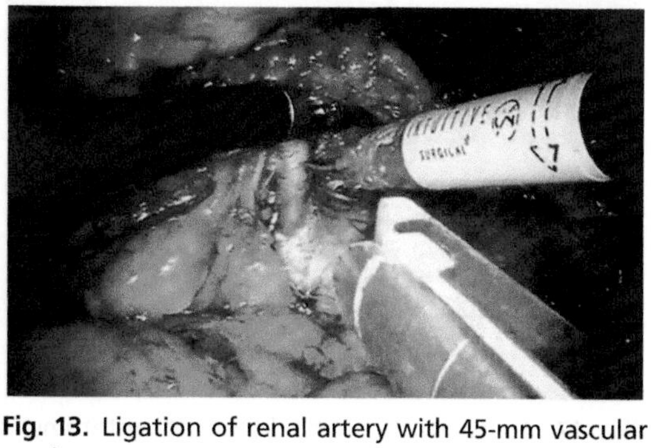

Fig. 13. Ligation of renal artery with 45-mm vascular stapler.

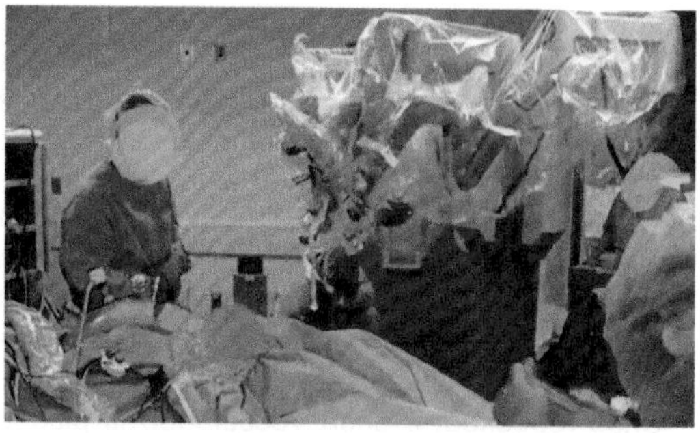

Fig. 14. Side docking: obliquely over the ipsilateral hip, at 45° to patient.

PART 2: BLADDER CUFF EXCISION

The authors think that RNU should adhere to strict oncologic principles in the management of the distal ureter and bladder cuff as open NU. The best approach to excising the distal ureter and bladder cuff still lacks consensus. The goal is to excise the kidney, ureter, and bladder cuff en bloc to prevent tumor spillage. Although an open approach is still the gold standard, minimally invasive approaches that mimic the open approach have reported comparable outcomes.[33] Xylinas and colleagues[34] compared 3 different methods of bladder cuff excision on oncologic outcomes (extravesical, intravesical, endoscopic). Among 2681 patients, 67.5% underwent the transvesical approach; 29.3% underwent the extravesical approach; and 3.2% had the endoscopic approach. There was no difference in terms of survival among the 3 distal ureteral management approaches, but patients with the endoscopic approach were at significantly higher risk of intravesical recurrence.

In the authors' experience, a transurethral incision of the bladder cuff is not performed. Instead, once the ureter is dissected down to the level of the bladder, the bladder cuff is sharply excised

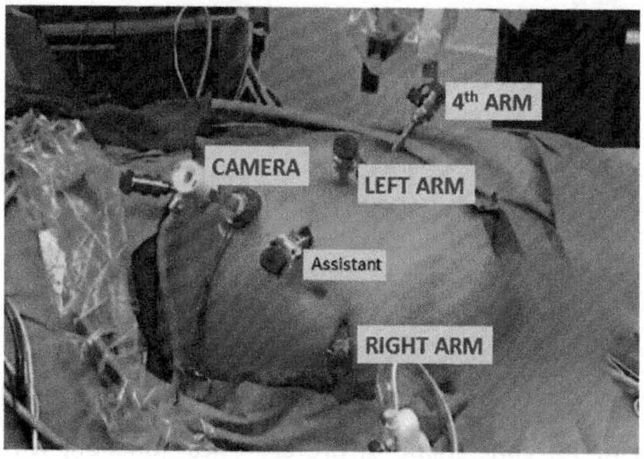

Fig. 15. Ports reassigned for bladder cuff excision.

with an adequate margin around the ureter. The authors advocate this technique because it is feasible, effective, time efficient, and maintains oncologic principles. The authors find that a sharp incision around the bladder cuff extravesically negates the need for a prior transurethral incision. It eliminates time spent on the endoscopic portion of the procedure. It also minimizes spillage, as it eliminates the ongoing diffusion of fluid from a prenephrectomy transurethral incision.

Once redocked, a short vessel loop is placed around the ureter with a Weck clip to help with retraction. The vas deferens is ligated as it crosses anterior to the ureter. The fourth arm is used to push the sigmoid colon medially, while a grasping forceps instrument is placed in the left robotic arm. Dissection and isolation of the ureter is carried down as distally as possible.

Once a cone shape of detrusor muscle is seen as the ureter is tented up, the ureterovesical junction at the bladder has been reached (**Fig. 16**). The authors make a 2-cm incision in the bladder cone at the 12-o'clock position just above the ureteral hiatus. An apical stitch is placed at the top of this incision as a handle to prevent the cystotomy from retracting. The authors use a 2-0 polyglactin 910 barbed stitch and tack it to the peritoneum on the anterior abdominal wall with a Weck clip, which provides exposure; the needle is left on the suture to save for later use. With the bladder open and exposure obtained, the ureteral orifice can be excised safely without the risk of inadvertently damaging the contralateral ureter or leaving the ureter behind.

The bladder is closed with the preplaced barbed suture in a running fashion. The cystotomy is then closed with a 2-0 polyglactin 910 suture in 2 layers. The bladder is filled through a urethral Foley catheter to test the closure for any leak. A Foley catheter is kept in for 1 week. The specimen bag can be introduced through the 12-mm assistant port, and it can be removed via a lower midline incision or a Pfannenstiel incision.

After the ureter and bladder cuff have been excised, the authors have found that an apical stitch is necessary to prevent the cystotomy from sinking below and underneath the bladder (**Fig. 17**). To maintain exposure, a 2-0 polyglactin 910 stitch is placed at the apex, at the 12-o'clock position, and tacked into the peritoneum on the anterior abdominal wall with a Weck clip (**Fig. 18**). The needle is left on the suture to save for later use. In the authors' experience, this sliding Weck technique has been useful, easy, and time efficient. The cystotomy is then closed with 2-0 polyglactin 910 suture in 2 layers (**Fig. 19**). The bladder can be filled through a urethral catheter to test the closure for any leak. A Foley catheter is kept in for 1 week. The specimen bag can be introduced through the 12-mm assistant port, and it can be removed through a Pfannenstiel incision (**Fig. 20**).

Take home points

1. Place the ports high up, to use the fourth arm.
2. Dissect the nodes en bloc with kidney.
3. Approach the distal ureter like a prostate, but use a side dock.

DU AND URETERAL REIMPLANT

In select patients, a DU and reimplant may be a treatment option. According to the National Comprehensive Cancer Network's guidelines, segmental ureterectomy (SU) should be reserved for low-grade mid to distal ureteral UUTUC. The European Association of Urology strongly recommends it for patients with a solitary kidney or bilateral low-stage cancers.[35] The major benefit of a DU is the preservation of renal function to maximize eligibility for future adjuvant cisplatin-based

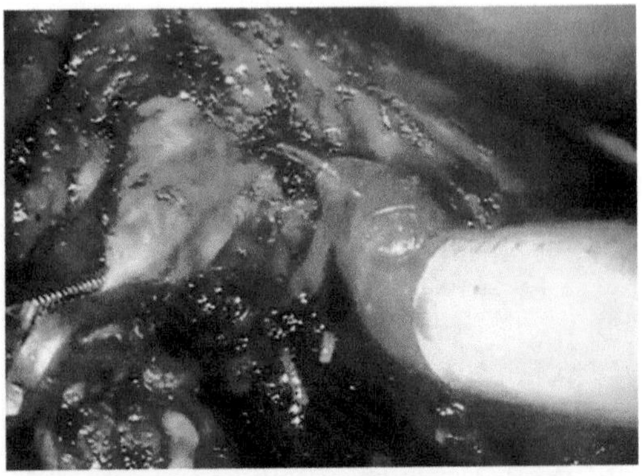

Fig. 16. Cone shape of ureterovesical junction, with ureter (*left*) grasped by Prograsp instrument.

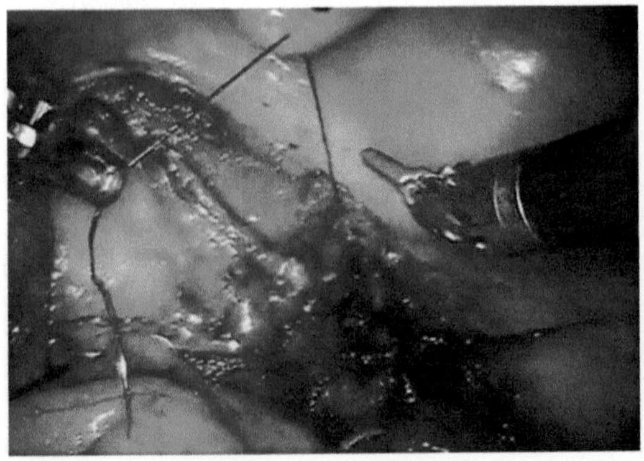

Fig. 17. Apical stitch on bladder cuff cystotomy is tacked to anterior abdominal wall, for traction.

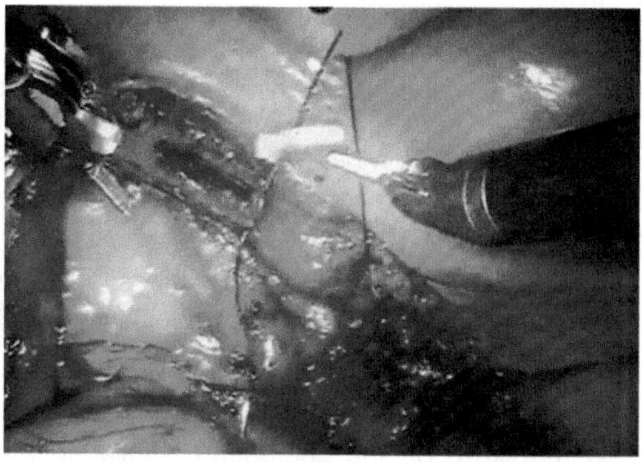

Fig. 18. Sliding Weck technique.

chemotherapy. DU also minimizes the morbidity associated with decreased renal function.

Several studies have reported no difference in oncologic outcomes between DU and radical NU. A large Surveillance, Epidemiology, and End Results Program (SEER) study of 2044 patients demonstrated that DU provides equally favorable outcomes as radical NU in locally advanced upper tract TCC.[20] The 5-year cancer-specific, mortality-free rates for SU versus radical NU with or without bladder cuff were 86.6% versus 82.2% versus 80.5%, respectively, without any significant differences.[20] Colin and colleagues,[22] in their multi-institutional cohort study of ureteral cancer, suggested that tumor location and surgery type were not independent prognostic factors for recurrence-free survival or cancer-specific mortality.

These results have been corroborated more recently by Hung and colleagues,[36] who compared oncologic outcomes between patients who underwent SU (n = 35) or radical NU (n = 77) for pure ureteral TCC. Advanced or non–organ confined (>T2) disease was present in 20% and 31% of the NU and SU groups, respectively. There was a 4-year follow-up period. No significant difference was found between SU and NU in terms of bladder

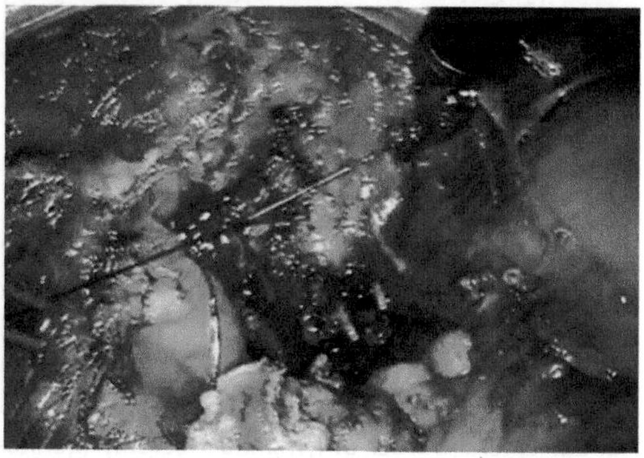

Fig. 19. Bladder closed in 2 layers.

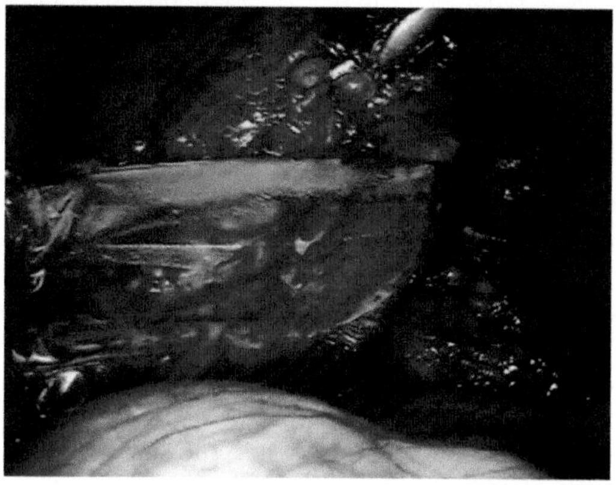

Fig. 20. Endoscopic specimen retrieval bag.

recurrences, local recurrences, distant metastasis, and cancer-specific survival rates. These data suggests that SU is not inferior to radical NU in oncologic outcomes and may also be of benefit to patients with high-grade or non–organ confined upper tract TCC.[36]

Robotic Approach

The robotic approach to DU and reimplant may have several advantages to open or laparoscopic approaches, including improved cosmesis, better visualization of vascular anatomy to perform an extended pelvic lymphadenectomy, and the ability to maintain all principles of oncology and reconstruction.

The first robotic distal ureteral reimplant with a psoas hitch was reported in 2007 by De Naeyer and colleagues[37] in a patient with distal ureteral stricture caused by endometriosis. Following this, other reports, by Mufarrij and colleagues[38] and Patil and colleagues,[39] reported the feasibility and safety of robotic reconstructive ureteral surgery. Glinianski and colleagues[40] then reported the use of robotic reimplantation for upper tract TCC in 9 patients. Although the data thus far are limited, published reports have demonstrated robotic ureterectomy and reimplantation to be technically safe and oncologically feasible. Here the authors describe their steps in performing this operation.

Port Placement and Docking

The robot is docked from the foot of the bed in a similar fashion to a robotic radical prostatectomy, except all ports are moved more cephalad to access the distal ureter and bladder (**Fig. 21**). Ports are placed in an inverted V shape using the following 5 to 6 trocars:

- 1 Hassan for camera
- 3 Robotic

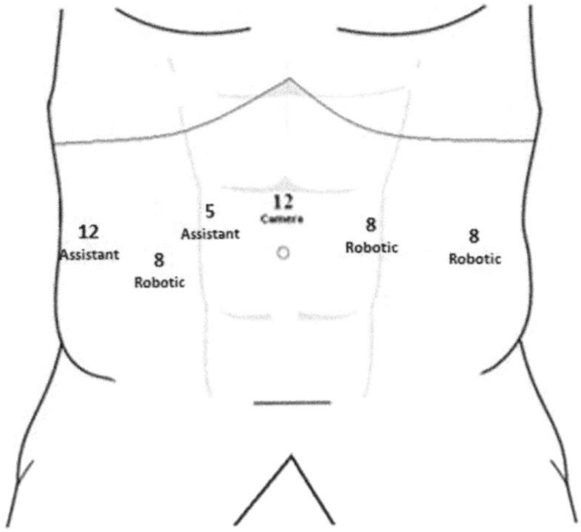

Fig. 21. Port placement for distal ureterectomy.

- 2 Accessory
  - 5 mm
  - 12 mm

A similar workup as described earlier is used to evaluate and confirm ureteral TCC. It is imperative that the entire ipsilateral renal unit is evaluated to confirm there is no proximal disease. This evaluation is best done preoperatively; but if it is unable to be done secondary to the obstructing mass, it may be performed intraoperatively with an ureteroscope placed through a trocar once the proximal ureteral margin is confirmed negative for TCC.

Ureteral dissection is performed, starting proximal to the expected area of tumor, to allow for enough mobilization of the ureter. Adequate periureteral tissue is left on the ureter to avoid inadvertent injury to the ureter and to maintain a sufficient margin around the ureter. Care is taken as to avoid disruption of the ureteral blood supply, which will be laterally sourced, in the distal ureter. Dissection of the bladder is also performed to allow for adequate mobilization of the bladder on its pedicle so that it can be brought up to the ureter tension free. A Weck clip is placed proximal to the distal ureteral lesion to prevent tumor spillage and also distal to prevent potential tumor spillage from above or below. In between these 2 clips, a segment of ureter is sent for frozen pathologic section to confirm that there is no cancer present. The distal ureter is then freed all the way to the bladder, and the affected ureter along with bladder cuff is excised as described previously.[8] The bladder is closed with a 2-0 polyglactin 910 barbed suture as described later.

Next, an extended pelvic lymph node dissection can be performed as described later. The authors use the same template as for bladder cancer, with the following borders: laterally to the genitofemoral nerve, superiorly to the aortic bifurcation, medially to the obturator nerve and iliac vessels, and inferiorly to the lymph node of Cloquet (**Figs. 22–25**).[41,42] The authors perform this on all their patients undergoing a DU. In addition, the authors confirm frozen sections are negative before preparing for the reimplant.

With the aforementioned procedure complete, the reimplant is begun. The clip on the ureter is removed, and the ureter is spatulated using robotic Potts scissors on the posterior side of the ureter for approximately 1.5 cm. The bladder is next mobilized off the peritoneum similar to the way the bladder is mobilized for a robotic radical prostatectomy. The goal is to allow the bladder to be hitched to either the sidewall or psoas muscle to allow for a tension-free anastomosis. If further bladder mobilization is required, the contralateral median umbilical ligament and bladder pedicle can be sacrificed.

For very distal ureterectomies, the authors typically hitch the bladder to the sidewall. For ureterectomies closer to the iliac vessels, the authors perform a classic psoas hitch. A robotic psoas hitch is feasible and effective, as reported in the recent literature.[43–46] When performing a psoas hitch, it is important to, when possible, identify the psoas tendon and use that for the hitch (**Fig. 26**). In addition, attention should be given to place sutures away from the genitofemoral and ilioinguinal nerves. Sutures should be placed in the psoas vertically to further decrease the risk of nerve entrapment, as the nerves course vertically and obliquely down. The authors use a 2-0 polyglactin 910 suture to perform the hitch and leave the bladder filled with 300 mL saline to confirm the sutures are not placed too deeply in (ie, through the mucosa) the bladder.

With the psoas hitch performed, the authors confirm there is adequate length for the ureter to

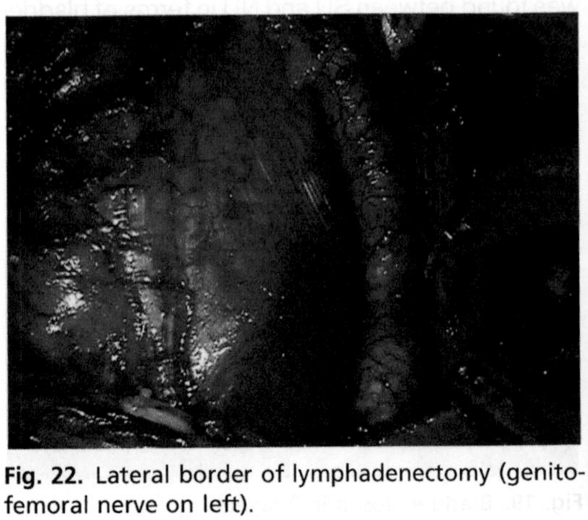

Fig. 22. Lateral border of lymphadenectomy (genitofemoral nerve on left).

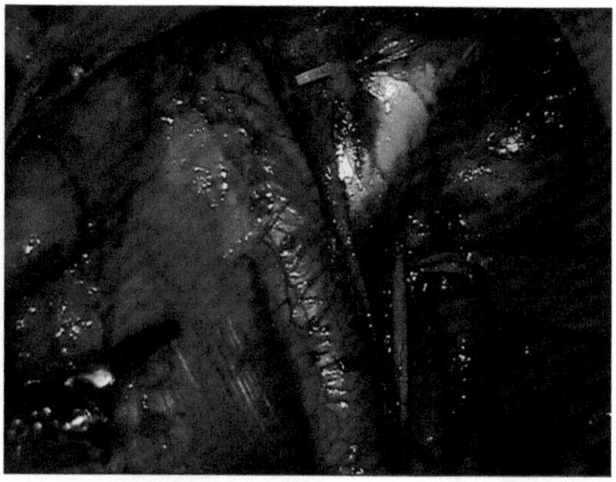

Fig. 23. Distal border.

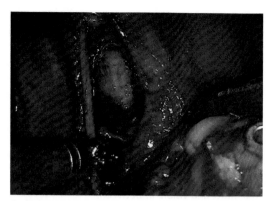

Fig. 25. Posterior border of dissection, showing hypogastric vessels

meet the dome of the bladder without any tension. Once confirmed, the bladder muscle is incised down to the level of, but not through, the mucosa for approximately 1.5 cm (**Fig. 27**), at which time the mucosa is opened and the bladder drained. A 4-0 polyglactin 910 suture is placed through each apex. The authors use a dyed suture on the lateral wall and an undyed suture on the medial wall to prevent inadvertent crossover. They run both sides and tie each suture to itself. At this point, a stent is placed over a wire up the ureter via the anastomosis, and the distal end of the ureteral stent is pushed into the bladder across the anastomosis. The superior edge of the anastomosis can be closed with either interrupted or a running suture. The serosa is now reapproximated over the anastomosis. The anastomosis is tested by refilling the bladder (**Figs. 28–30**). The authors prefer a refluxing anastomosis for all their patients because it allows for more accessible in-office surveillance with a flexible cystoscope passed into the refluxing ureter.

If a tension-free anastomosis cannot be completed because of inadequate length or reach, a Boari flap is required.

Boari Flap

The feasibility of a robotic Boari flap has been reported in the recent literature.[44,45,47,48] In the authors' experience, to create a Boari flap, a triangular flap is incised off the anterior surface of an adequately filled bladder (**Fig. 31**). It is crucial to keep the base of the flap wide and large (which would become the base of the tube). The flap is incised using minimal cautery to preserve the healthiness and vascularity of the tissue. An apical suture is placed at the vertex of the posteriorly spatulated ureter. It is also possible to tack the flap to the psoas with a suture to decrease tension. The anastomosis is performed in an onlay fashion. Interrupted stitches are used to close each side of the flap to the posteriorly spatulated ureter on-laid on to it. A stent is placed up with a wire inside of

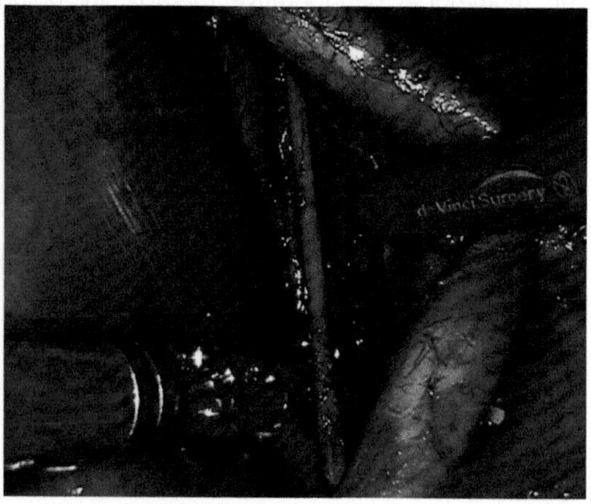

Fig. 24. Obturator nerve.

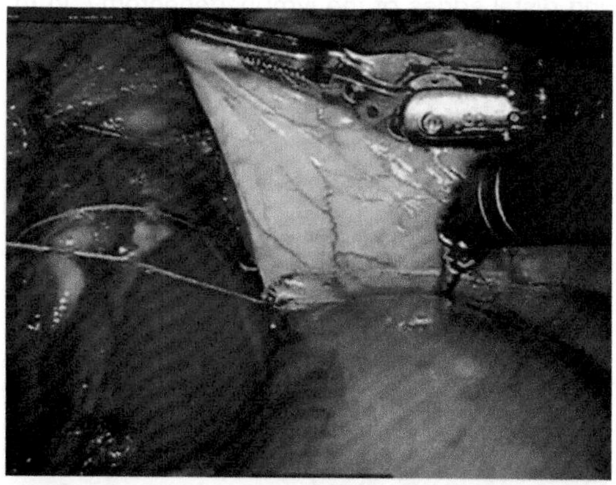

Fig. 26. Psoas hitch. Fourth arm pulls bladder laterally to assist.

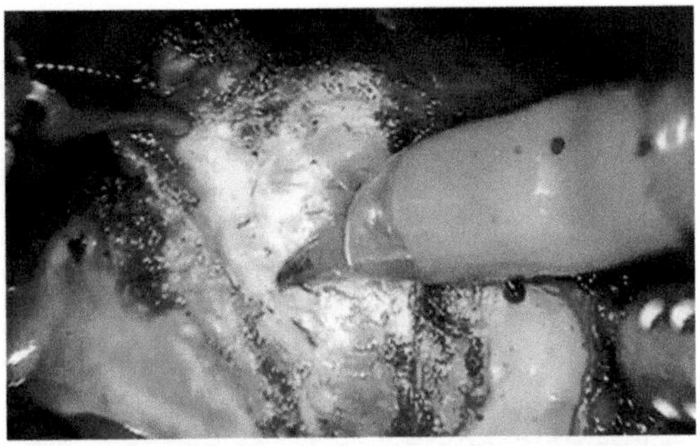

Fig. 27. Creation of detrusor flaps, with bladder mucosa intact and visible in between.

the stent. Then the running suture is used to close the proximal (cephalad) aspect of the Boari flap to tubularize it and complete the anastomosis. A V lock is used to close the caudal aspect in a running fashion. The tubular bladder is then reinforced with a second imbricating layer. The bladder is then retroperitonealize by closing the peritoneum over the bladder, which can be done easily with Weck clips (**Figs. 32–36**).

The benefit of a Boari flap is that it can gain additional length up to the midureter, more than a psoas hitch, to achieve a tension-free anastomosis. The downsides include greater operative time needed, more suturing, more complexity and reconstruction, and the risk of vascular compromise of the flap.[45,47]

LYMPHADENECTOMY

Pelvic Lymph Node Dissection with DU

An extended pelvic LND is performed using the same robotic and oncologic principles as described earlier for a retroperitoneal lymphadenectomy. The common iliac, external iliac, and internal iliac vessels are skeletonized of lymphatic tissue. Weck clips are used to clip the proximal and distal edges of the lymphadenectomy. In the authors' institution, lymph nodes are sent in separate packets labeled appropriately to distinguish each regional nodal group for a more accurate nodal count and accurate staging.[41] Lymph node (LN) yield can vary based on pathologic evaluation. The method by which LNs are submitted for pathologic review can affect the number of reported LNs (en bloc vs separate packets), with higher nodal counts seen with separate packets.[49]

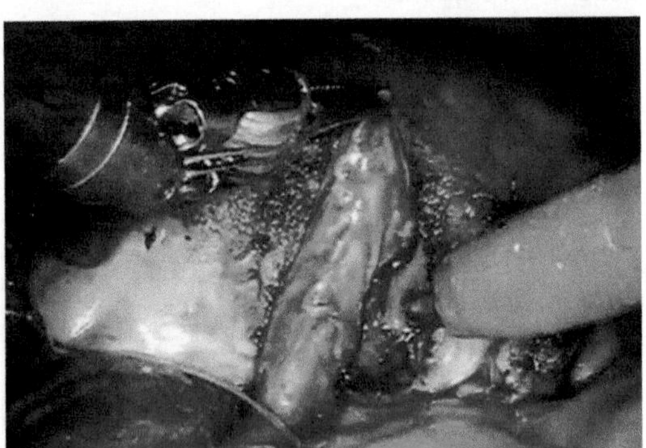

Fig. 28. The spatulated ureter will lie on the mucosa.

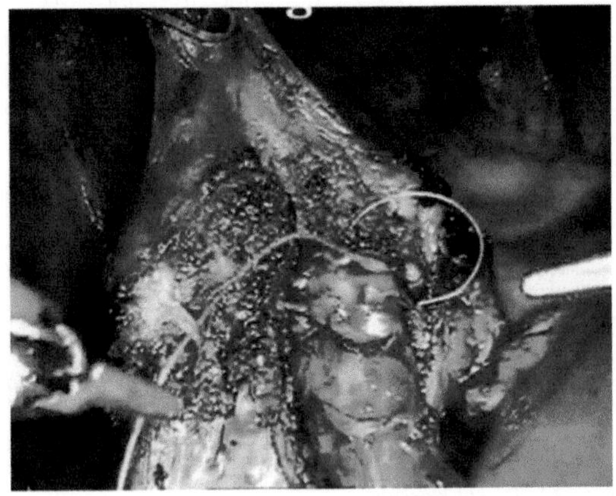

Fig. 29. Ureteral anastomosis to bladder.

LND for Upper Tract TCC

LND at the time of radical cystectomy for bladder cancer is the standard of care, both for its diagnostic and therapeutic benefit.[41] However, for upper tract TCC, an LND at the time of NU is still performed based on surgeon discretion because of a lack of level I data showing a clear survival benefit in upper tract TCC.[50] In a study of 151 patients with stage T2-3 UUTUC undergoing NU without LND, the median 2- and 5-year metastasis-free survival were 69.0% and 54.1%.[51] Although the evidence does not exist yet, multimodal perioperative therapy, including

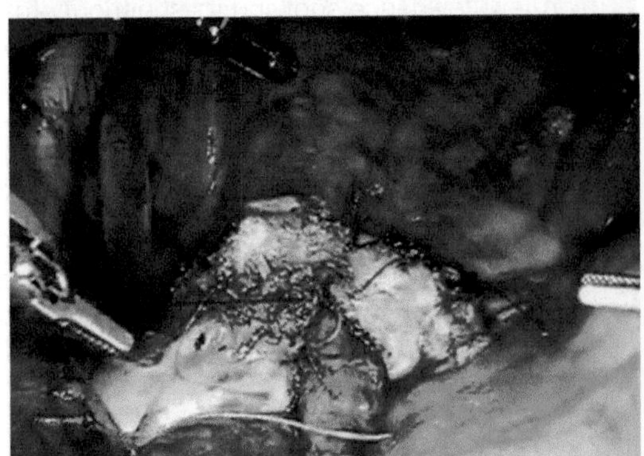

Fig. 30. Detrusor flaps closed over ureter.

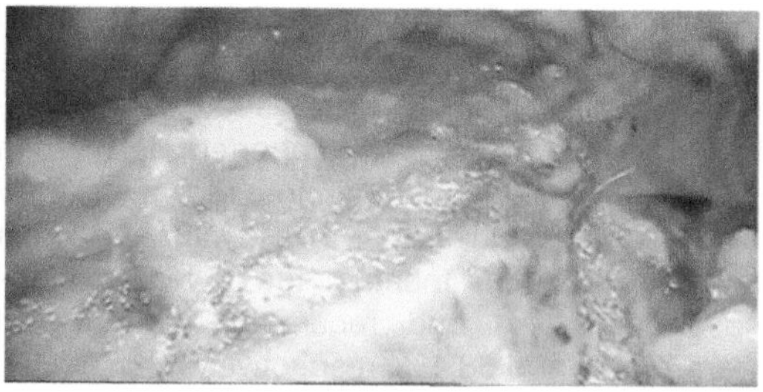

Fig. 31. Keep base of Boari flap wide.

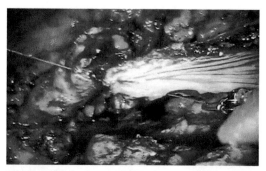

Fig. 33. Bladder flap (*right*) brought to apex of spatulated ureter (*left*) with a stitch.

NC, for UUTUC may be critical because kidney loss after NU will preclude some patients from receiving adjuvant chemotherapy after surgery. More data are needed to determine if LND performed at the time of NU would be a crucial component of maximal multimodal therapy. LND can both complement the benefits of NC and also measure its therapeutic benefits.

The challenge of LND for upper tract TCC as compared with bladder cancer is the variation in lymphatic drainage of the ureter. Because of the multiple potential locations of tumor in the urothelial tract, targeted LND depends largely on the location of the primary tumor, as in patients undergoing only DU.[52]

Hemal and colleagues[30] and Lee and colleagues[31] both reported their experience with retroperitoneal LND, with 2 to 35 lymph nodes removed, similar in extent and node count to open series.[24,53,54] For right-sided cancers, precaval and retrocaval nodes were removed. In left-sided cancers, para-aortic and retroaortic nodes were removed. Interaortocaval nodes were removed only if indicated. In both studies, the LND extended superiorly from adrenal or superior renal hilum distally to the aortic bifurcation or common iliac bifurcation.

In Roscigno and colleagues's[53] study of LND for upper tract TCC, the number of lymph nodes removed seemed to be associated with cancer-specific mortality. Longer survival was observed in patients in whom at least 8 LNs had been removed. In contrast, Kondo and colleagues[55] found that the number of LN removed showed minimal influence on survival, whereas the template extent of LND was significant.

In Kondo's more recent multi-institutional prospective study of 77 patients with UUTUC of pT2 or greater, patients with renal pelvis TCC who received an LND resulted in significantly higher cancer-specific survival (89.8% vs 51.7%) and overall survival (86.1% vs 48.0%) than the no LND group.[56] Disease-free survival was also higher in the LND group (77.8%). In contrast, those with ureteral TCC showed no difference in cancer-specific survival between the LND and no LND groups.[56]

OUTCOMES

RNU has been shown to be feasible and safe in multiple studies, but data on intermediate- to long-term oncologic outcomes are still lacking. Minimally invasive surgery has benefits in functional outcomes. RNU has demonstrated less blood loss compared with open and laparoscopic surgeries, likely because of better visualization of the vascular anatomy and shorter operative time.

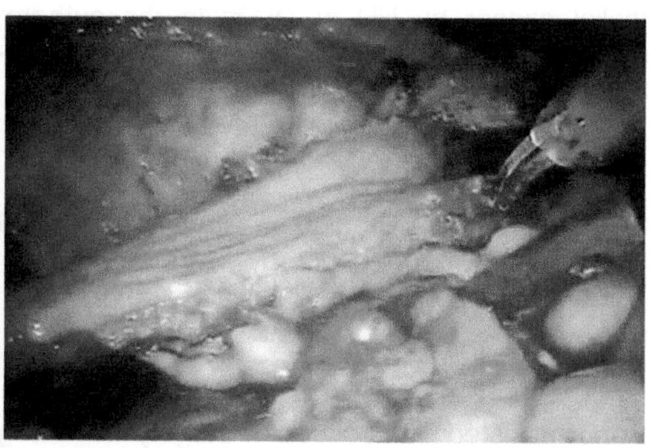

Fig. 32. Bladder flap freed.

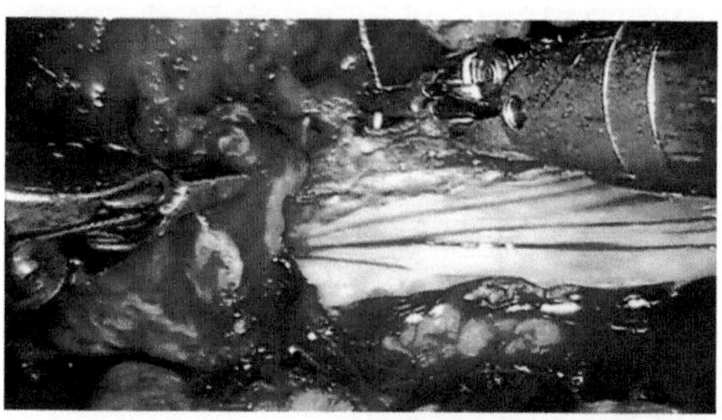

Fig. 34. Bladder-ureteral anastomosis performed in an onlay fashion with the posteriorly spatulated ureter (*left*) on the bladder flap (*right*).

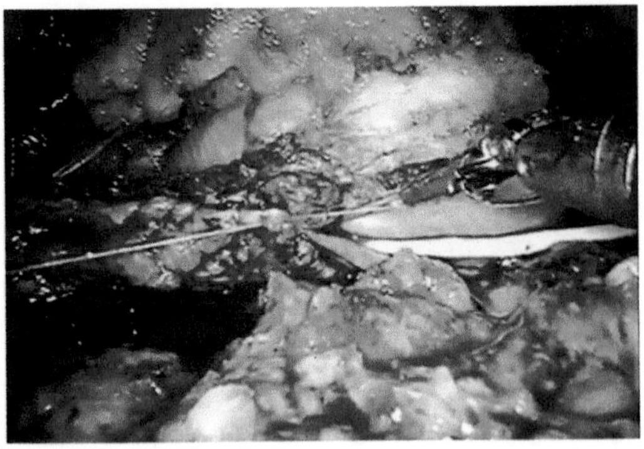

Fig. 35. Closing Boari flap with ureteral double-J stent in place.

Blood loss during RNU has been shown to range from 75 to 270 mL, which was less compared with open NU (299.6–750.0 mL) and also to laparoscopic NU (144–580 mL).[33] The mean hospital stay has also been shown to be comparable, if not improved, for recent RNU compared with its open and laparoscopic counterparts. The mean hospital stay ranged from 2.7 to 8.4 days for RNU compared with 2.3 to 21.1 days for LNU and open NU combined.[33] In a more recent, contemporary series by Khemees and colleagues[57] of 29 patients, 27 patients were discharged on postoperative day 1.

RNU reports have also demonstrated comparable operative times. The mean operative time in studies ranged from 161 to 326 minutes. Repositioning patients added approximately 50 to 100 minutes to the operative time, with studies requiring repositioning having a mean operative time of 300 minutes.[23,28,29] A meta-analysis comparing operative times of LNU and open RNU ranged from 156 to 426 minutes.[28,50] RNU operative times were comparable, ranging from 161 to 326 minutes.[33]

Intermediate- to long-term data are still lacking in oncologic outcomes for RNU, both because of the rarity of the disease and the short-term follow-up in this relatively new surgical technique. Earlier published series demonstrating the feasibility of the procedure reported less than 18 months in follow-up time. In a recent study by Lim and colleagues[25] of RNU with a median follow-up of 45.5 months, the 5-year cancer-specific survival and recurrence-free survival were 75.8% and 68.1%, respectively. These rates for RNU are promising, and comparable with published open and laparoscopic series. The 5-year tumor-free survival rates after open NU range from 51.2% to 76.0%; after laparoscopic NU, they range from 71.6% to 79.0%.[58–61] These results suggest that RNU may have comparable intermediate-term oncologic outcomes to its open and laparoscopic counterparts.

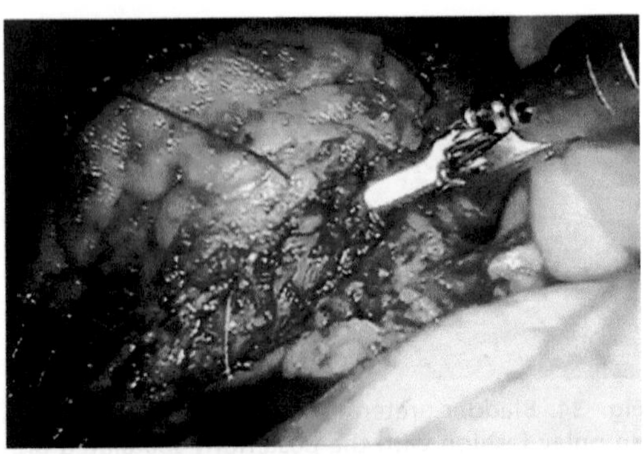

Fig. 36. Boari flap closed in 2 layers.

DU Versus NU

In the large SEER study of 2044 patients, Jeldres and colleagues[20] reported no decline in cancer control outcome among those who received SU versus those who underwent a NU with or without bladder cuff excision. This finding was also true in select patients with T3 tumors. At 5 years, cancer-specific mortality-free rates for SU versus NU with or without bladder cuff removal were 86.6% versus 82.2% versus 80.5%, respectively. The median follow-up time was 30 months.[21] In a French multicenter study by Colin and colleagues,[22] 52 patients were treated with SU and 416 with radical NU. There was no statistical difference between the radical NU and SU groups for the 5-year probability of cancer-specific survival, recurrence-free survival, and metastasis-free survival. Several other studies have shown similar findings, with no difference in cancer control outcome between SU and NU for T1-T2 organ-confined cancer.[20,62,63]

DU Follow-up Algorithm

Aggressive surveillance for bladder cancer is critical after the surgical treatment of upper tract urothelial cancer by NU or DU.[64] In the authors' center, they have developed the following surveillance protocol after a DU:

- Ureteroscopy every 6 months × 2 years, followed by every 1 year
- Upper tract imaging alternating every 6 months with ureteroscopy
- Cystoscopy and cytology every 3 months

SUMMARY

Robot-assisted laparoscopic surgery is being increasingly used in urologic oncologic surgery.

RNU is still a relatively new technique as reported in the literature. As upper tract TCC is a rare disease, reported studies have few patients; there are no randomized studies comparing RNU with open or laparoscopic NU. Although intermediate- and long-term outcome data are scarce, RNU does seem to offer some advantages in addition to decreased morbidity. While maintaining sound oncologic principles, RNU can offer the surgeon the feasibility to perform an en bloc excision of the kidney and ureter with bladder cuff and a DU. Better visualization of the vascular anatomy may make a complex operation more amenable to accurate retroperitoneal and pelvic lymph node dissections. Randomized, prospective studies will be needed to determine the long-term outcomes of RNU.

REFERENCES

1. Sun M, Abdo A, Abdollah F, et al. Management of upper urinary tract urothelial carcinoma. Expert Rev Anticancer Ther 2010;10(12):1955–65.
2. Roupret M, Babjuk M, Comperat E, et al. European guidelines on upper tract urothelial carcinomas: 2013 update. Eur Urol 2013;63(6):1059–71.
3. Clayman RV, Kavoussi LR, Figenshau RS, et al. Laparoscopic nephroureterectomy: initial clinical case report. J Laparoendosc Surg 1991;1(6):343–9.
4. Simone G, Papalia R, Guaglianone S, et al. Laparoscopic versus open nephroureterectomy: perioperative and oncologic outcomes from a randomised prospective study. Eur Urol 2009;56(3):520–6.
5. Ni S, Tao W, Chen Q, et al. Laparoscopic versus open nephroureterectomy for the treatment of upper urinary tract urothelial carcinoma: a systematic review and cumulative analysis of comparative studies. Eur Urol 2012;61(6):1142–53.
6. Margulis V, Shariat SF, Matin SF, et al. Outcomes of radical nephroureterectomy: a series from the Upper Tract Urothelial Carcinoma Collaboration. Cancer 2009;115(6):1224–33.
7. Phillips CK, Taneja SS, Stifelman MD. Robot-assisted laparoscopic partial nephrectomy: the NYU technique. J Endourol 2005;19(4):441–5 [discussion: 445].
8. Phillips EA, Wang DS. Current status of robot-assisted laparoscopic ureteral reimplantation and reconstruction. Curr Urol Rep 2012;13(3):190–4.
9. Browne RF, Meehan CP, Colville J, et al. Transitional cell carcinoma of the upper urinary tract: spectrum of imaging findings. Radiographics 2005;25(6): 1609–27.
10. Wehrli NE, Kim MJ, Matza BW, et al. Utility of MRI features in differentiation of central renal cell carcinoma and renal pelvic urothelial carcinoma. AJR Am J Roentgenol 2013;201(6):1260–7.
11. Rosenkrantz AB, Haghighi M, Horn J, et al. Utility of quantitative MRI metrics for assessment of stage and grade of urothelial carcinoma of the bladder: preliminary results. AJR Am J Roentgenol 2013; 201(6):1254–9.
12. Assimos DG, Hall MC, Martin JH. Ureteroscopic management of patients with upper tract transitional cell carcinoma. Urol Clin North Am 2000; 27(4):751–60.
13. Skolarikos A, Griffiths TR, Powell PH, et al. Cytologic analysis of ureteral washings is informative in patients with grade 2 upper tract TCC considering endoscopic treatment. Urology 2003;61(6): 1146–50.
14. Cordier J, Sonpavde G, Stief CG, et al. Oncologic outcomes obtained after neoadjuvant and adjuvant chemotherapy for the treatment of urothelial carcinomas of the upper urinary tract: a review. World J Urol 2013;31(1):77–82.
15. Griffiths G, Hall R, Sylvester R, et al. International phase III trial assessing neoadjuvant cisplatin, methotrexate, and vinblastine chemotherapy for muscle-invasive bladder cancer: long-term results of the BA06 30894 trial. J Clin Oncol 2011;29(16): 2171–7.
16. Grossman HB, Natale RB, Tangen CM, et al. Neoadjuvant chemotherapy plus cystectomy compared with cystectomy alone for locally advanced bladder cancer. N Engl J Med 2003; 349(9):859–66.
17. Kaag MG, O'Malley RL, O'Malley P, et al. Changes in renal function following nephroureterectomy may affect the use of perioperative chemotherapy. Eur Urol 2010;58(4):581–7.
18. Hellenthal NJ, Shariat SF, Margulis V, et al. Adjuvant chemotherapy for high risk upper tract urothelial carcinoma: results from the Upper Tract Urothelial Carcinoma Collaboration. J Urol 2009;182(3):900–6.
19. Rajput MZ, Kamat AM, Clavell-Hernandez J, et al. Perioperative outcomes of laparoscopic radical nephroureterectomy and regional lymphadenectomy in patients with upper urinary tract urothelial carcinoma after neoadjuvant chemotherapy. Urology 2011;78(1):61–7.
20. Jeldres C, Lughezzani G, Sun M, et al. Segmental ureterectomy can safely be performed in patients with transitional cell carcinoma of the ureter. J Urol 2010;183(4):1324–9.
21. Lughezzani G, Jeldres C, Isbarn H, et al. Nephroureterectomy and segmental ureterectomy in the treatment of invasive upper tract urothelial carcinoma: a population-based study of 2299 patients. Eur J Cancer 2009;45(18):3291–7.
22. Colin P, Ouzzane A, Pignot G, et al. Comparison of oncological outcomes after segmental ureterectomy or radical nephroureterectomy in urothelial carcinomas of the upper urinary tract: results

from a large French multicentre study. BJU Int 2012;110(8):1134–41.
23. Rose K, Khan S, Godbole H, et al. Robotic assisted retroperitoneoscopic nephroureterectomy – first experience and the hybrid port technique. Int J Clin Pract 2006;60(1):12–4.
24. Roscigno M, Brausi M, Heidenreich A, et al. Lymphadenectomy at the time of nephroureterectomy for upper tract urothelial cancer. Eur Urol 2011; 60(4):776–83.
25. Lim SK, Shin TY, Kim KH, et al. Intermediate-term outcomes of robot-assisted laparoscopic nephroureterectomy in upper urinary tract urothelial carcinoma. Clin Genitourin Cancer 2013;11(4):515–21.
26. Eandi JA, Nelson RA, Wilson TG, et al. Oncologic outcomes for complete robot-assisted laparoscopic management of upper-tract transitional cell carcinoma. J Endourol 2010;24(6):969–75.
27. Nanigian DK, Smith W, Ellison LM. Robot-assisted laparoscopic nephroureterectomy. J Endourol 2006;20(7):463–5 [discussion: 465–6].
28. Hu JC, Silletti JP, Williams SB. Initial experience with robot-assisted minimally-invasive nephroureterectomy. J Endourol 2008;22(4):699–704.
29. Park SY, Jeong W, Ham WS, et al. Initial experience of robotic nephroureterectomy: a hybrid-port technique. BJU Int 2009;104(11):1718–21.
30. Hemal AK, Stansel I, Babbar P, et al. Robotic-assisted nephroureterectomy and bladder cuff excision without intraoperative repositioning. Urology 2011; 78(2):357–64.
31. Lee Z, Cadillo-Chavez R, Lee DI, et al. The technique of single stage pure robotic nephroureterectomy. J Endourol 2013;27(2):189–95.
32. Pugh J, Parekattil S, Willis D, et al. Perioperative outcomes of robot-assisted nephroureterectomy for upper urinary tract urothelial carcinoma: a multi-institutional series. BJU Int 2013;112(4): E295–300.
33. Rai BP, Shelley M, Coles B, et al. Surgical management for upper urinary tract transitional cell carcinoma (UUT-TCC): a systematic review. BJU Int 2012;110(10):1426–35.
34. Xylinas E, Rink M, Cha EK, et al. Impact of distal ureter management on oncologic outcomes following radical nephroureterectomy for upper tract urothelial carcinoma. Eur Urol 2014;65(1): 210–7.
35. Oosterlinck W, Solsona E, van der Meijden AP, et al. EAU guidelines on diagnosis and treatment of upper urinary tract transitional cell carcinoma. Eur Urol 2004;46(2):147–54.
36. Hung SY, Yang WC, Luo HL, et al. Segmental ureterectomy does not compromise the oncologic outcome compared with nephroureterectomy for pure ureter cancer. Int Urol Nephrol 2014;46(5): 921–6.
37. De Naeyer G, Van Migem P, Schatteman P, et al. Case report: pure robot-assisted psoas hitch ureteral reimplantation for distal-ureteral stenosis. J Endourol 2007;21(6):618–20.
38. Mufarrij PW, Shah OD, Berger AD, et al. Robotic reconstruction of the upper urinary tract. J Urol 2007;178(5):2002–5.
39. Patil NN, Mottrie A, Sundaram B, et al. Robotic-assisted laparoscopic ureteral reimplantation with psoas hitch: a multi-institutional, multinational evaluation. Urology 2008;72(1):47–50 [discussion: 50].
40. Glinianski M, Guru KA, Zimmerman G, et al. Robot-assisted ureterectomy and ureteral reconstruction for urothelial carcinoma. J Endourol 2009;23(1): 97–100.
41. Marshall SJ, Hayn MH, Stegemann AP, et al. Impact of surgeon and volume on extended lymphadenectomy at the time of robot-assisted radical cystectomy: results from the International Robotic Cystectomy Consortium (IRCC). BJU Int 2013; 111(7):1075–80.
42. Youssef RF, Raj GV. Lymphadenectomy in management of invasive bladder cancer. Int J Surg Oncol 2011;2011:758189.
43. Kozinn SI, Canes D, Sorcini A, et al. Robotic versus open distal ureteral reconstruction and reimplantation for benign stricture disease. J Endourol 2012; 26(2):147–51.
44. Musch M, Hohenhorst L, Pailliart A, et al. Robot-assisted reconstructive surgery of the distal ureter: single institution experience in 16 patients. BJU Int 2013;111(5):773–83.
45. Allaparthi S, Ramanathan R, Balaji KC. Robotic distal ureterectomy with Boari flap reconstruction for distal ureteral urothelial cancers: a single institutional pilot experience. J Laparoendosc Adv Surg Tech A 2010;20(2):165–71.
46. Uberoi J, Harnisch B, Sethi AS, et al. Robot-assisted laparoscopic distal ureterectomy and ureteral reimplantation with psoas hitch. J Endourol 2007; 21(4):368–73 [discussion: 372–3].
47. Schimpf MO, Wagner JR. Robot-assisted laparoscopic Boari flap ureteral reimplantation. J Endourol 2008;22(12):2691–4.
48. Yang C, Jones L, Rivera ME, et al. Robotic-assisted ureteral reimplantation with Boari flap and psoas hitch: a single-institution experience. J Laparoendosc Adv Surg Tech A 2011;21(9): 829–33.
49. Stein JP, Penson DF, Cai J, et al. Radical cystectomy with extended lymphadenectomy: evaluating separate package versus en bloc submission for node positive bladder cancer. J Urol 2007;177(3): 876–81 [discussion: 881–2].
50. Ouzzane A, Colin P, Ghoneim TP, et al. The impact of lymph node status and features on oncological outcomes in urothelial carcinoma of the upper

urinary tract (UTUC) treated by nephroureterectomy. World J Urol 2013;31(1):189–97.
51. Colin P, Ghoneim TP, Nison L, et al. Risk stratification of metastatic recurrence in invasive upper urinary tract carcinoma after radical nephroureterectomy without lymphadenectomy. World J Urol 2014; 32(2):507–12.
52. Green DA, Rink M, Xylinas E, et al. Urothelial carcinoma of the bladder and the upper tract: disparate twins. J Urol 2013;189(4):1214–21.
53. Roscigno M, Shariat SF, Margulis V, et al. The extent of lymphadenectomy seems to be associated with better survival in patients with nonmetastatic upper-tract urothelial carcinoma: how many lymph nodes should be removed? Eur Urol 2009; 56(3):512–8.
54. Mason RJ, Kassouf W, Bell DG, et al. The contemporary role of lymph node dissection during nephroureterectomy in the management of upper urinary tract urothelial carcinoma: the Canadian experience. Urology 2012;79(4):840–5.
55. Kondo T, Hashimoto Y, Kobayashi H, et al. Template-based lymphadenectomy in urothelial carcinoma of the upper urinary tract: impact on patient survival. Int J Urol 2010;17(10):848–54.
56. Kondo T, Hara I, Takagi T, et al. Template-based lymphadenectomy in urothelial carcinoma of the renal pelvis: a prospective study. Int J Urol 2014; 21(5):453–9.
57. Khemees TA, Nasser SM, Abaza R. Clinical pathway after robotic nephroureterectomy: omission of pelvic drain with next-day catheter removal and discharge. Urology 2014;83(4):818–23.
58. Roupret M, Hupertan V, Sanderson KM, et al. Oncologic control after open or laparoscopic nephroureterectomy for upper urinary tract transitional cell carcinoma: a single center experience. Urology 2007;69(4):656–61.
59. Capitanio U, Shariat SF, Isbarn H, et al. Comparison of oncologic outcomes for open and laparoscopic nephroureterectomy: a multi-institutional analysis of 1249 cases. Eur Urol 2009;56(1):1–9.
60. Manabe D, Saika T, Ebara S, et al. Comparative study of oncologic outcome of laparoscopic nephroureterectomy and standard nephroureterectomy for upper urinary tract transitional cell carcinoma. Urology 2007;69(3):457–61.
61. Waldert M, Remzi M, Klingler HC, et al. The oncological results of laparoscopic nephroureterectomy for upper urinary tract transitional cell cancer are equal to those of open nephroureterectomy. BJU Int 2009;103(1):66–70.
62. Simonato A, Varca V, Gregori A, et al. Elective segmental ureterectomy for transitional cell carcinoma of the ureter: long-term follow-up in a series of 73 patients. BJU Int 2012;110(11 Pt B):E744–9.
63. Simhan J, Smaldone MC, Egleston BL, et al. Nephron-sparing management vs radical nephroureterectomy for low- or moderate-grade, low-stage upper tract urothelial carcinoma. BJU Int 2014;114(2):216–20.
64. Raman JD, Sosa RE, Vaughan ED Jr, et al. Pathologic features of bladder tumors after nephroureterectomy or segmental ureterectomy for upper urinary tract transitional cell carcinoma. Urology 2007;69(2):251–4.

Robot-Assisted Adrenalectomy (Total, Partial, & Metastasectomy)

Mark W. Ball, MD[a,*], Mohamad E. Allaf, MD[b]

KEYWORDS

• Adrenalectomy • Robotic surgery • Partial adrenalectomy • Metastasectomy

KEY POINTS

- Robotic adrenalectomy has been shown to be feasible and safe for resection multiple types of adrenal tumors.
- Compared with traditional laparoscopic adrenalectomy, robotic adrenalectomy is associated with lower blood loss and length of stay but at an increased cost per surgery.
- The role of partial adrenalectomy is currently limited to patients with familial syndromes but may be facilitated by a robotic approach.
- Resection of metastases to the adrenal gland seems safe and feasible using a robotic approach.
- Large prospective studies comparing laparoscopic and robotic adrenalectomy are still needed to define the benefit of robotics.

INTRODUCTION

Minimally invasive adrenalectomy became the gold standard treatment of benign adrenal neoplasms after the initial report of laparoscopic adrenalectomy was described by Gagner and colleagues[1] in 1992. Multiple series have demonstrated decreased pain, lower blood loss, faster convalescence, less ileus, and shorter hospital stays compared with open surgery.[2–10] More recently, robotic surgery has been increasingly used as an alternative to laparoscopic surgery. Multiple feasibility studies have demonstrated the safety and feasibility of robotic adrenalectomy.[11–17] The perceived advantages of robotic over traditional laparoscopy include stereoscopic vision, improved magnification, and greater range of motion.[18] As experience with robotic adrenalectomy has increased, robotic adrenalectomy has been used for progressively more difficult operations, including resection of large tumors,[16] pheochromocytomas,[19] and adrenocortical carcinomas (ACC).[20] Additionally, recent studies also support the role of a robotic-assisted approach during partial adrenalectomy[21] and adrenal metastasectomy.[22]

In this article, the authors review the evolution of robotic adrenal surgery, discuss the evaluation of adrenal lesions, indications for robotic adrenalectomy, and describe the surgical technique. Indications for robotic partial adrenalectomy and metastasectomy are also reviewed along with early outcomes for these procedures.

EVALUATION

Radiographic Evaluation

Adrenal tumors are frequently diagnosed, with incidental adrenal tumors found in 3.4% to 7.0%

Conflicts of Interest: None.

[a] Urological Surgery, Department of Urology, The James Buchanan Brady Urological Institute, The Johns Hopkins University School of Medicine, 600 North Wolfe Street, Marburg 134, Baltimore, MD 21287, USA; [b] Department of Urology, The James Buchanan Brady Urological Institute, The Johns Hopkins University School of Medicine, 600 North Wolfe Street, Marburg 134, Baltimore, MD 21287, USA

* Corresponding author.

E-mail address: mark.ball@jhmi.edu

Urol Clin N Am 41 (2014) 539–547
http://dx.doi.org/10.1016/j.ucl.2014.07.008
0094-0143/14/$ – see front matter

of patients on imaging studies.[23] Although adrenal masses were historically diagnosed based on sequelae from hormone-secreting tumors, most masses are now found based on imaging alone. Meaningful clinical information may be gleaned from the imaging evaluation. Besides size, which can drive surgical management, enhancement characteristics can help differentiate adenomas from other lesions. Hamrahian and colleagues,[24] from the Cleveland Clinic, evaluated 290 patients and found that adrenal adenomas had significantly lower mean Hounsfield unit (HU) attenuation (16.2) than ACC (36.9), adrenal metastases (39.2), or pheochromocytoma (38.6). The high intracytoplasmic fat content of adenomas causes this difference in attenuation. Furthermore, a cutoff of 10 HU was associated with a 100% specificity to differentiate adenomas from nonadenomas, though the sensitivity was only 40%. Therefore, although lesions with 10 HU or less are almost universally adenomas, lesions with greater than 10 HU attenuation may require further evaluation, as 30% of adrenal adenomas are fat poor.[25] In these cases, the pattern of intravenous contrast washout can be helpful. Adenomas have faster washout of enhancement than other lesions like metastases or pheochromocytomas, which retain contract for longer periods. A washout of 40% to 60% at 10 min is typical of adenomas, with specificity approaching 100%.[26]

Although computed tomography (CT) studies can identify most adrenal adenomas, magnetic resonance imaging (MRI) can also be a useful adjunct. In opposed-phase MRI, lesions with intracellular lipid may be identified by loss of signal intensity on out-of-phase images.[27]

ENDOCRINE EVALUATION

A full hormonal evaluation is necessary in all patients with adrenal lesions to determine if the mass is functionally active. This evaluation is particularly important in preoperative planning, as blood pressure control, electrolyte status, and volume resuscitation should be tailored in patients with functionally active lesions. The American Association of Clinical Endocrinologists (AACE) and the American Association of Endocrine Surgeons (AAES) recently released a comprehensive review of the management of adrenal incidentalomas, including hormonal workup.[28] The guidelines recommend all patients with an adrenal incidentaloma to undergo clinical, biochemical, and radiographic evaluation for signs and symptoms of hypercortisolism, aldosteronism, pheochromocytoma, or a malignant tumor. The recommend screening results are described later and summarized in **Table 1**.

Hypercortisolism

Hypercortisolism, or Cushing syndrome, is characterized by excess circulating glucocorticoid. The signs and symptoms of hypercortisolism include hypertension, truncal obesity, moon facies, hirsutism, mood disturbance, osteopenia, diabetes mellitus, and easy bruising.[29] Although there are multiple causes of Cushing syndrome, including exogenous steroid use and corticotropin-secreting pituitary tumors, the cause germane to this review is a cortisol-secreting adrenal tumor. The simplest screening test recommended by the AACE/AAES is the 1-mg overnight dexamethasone suppression test.[28] In patients with clinical suspicion because of

Table 1
Endocrine workup of an incidentally discovered adrenal mass

Lesion/Syndrome to Rule Out	Screening Test	Confirmatory Tests
Hypercortisolism	Overnight 1 mg dexamethasone suppression Urine-Free Cortisol	Late-night salivary cortisol, 24-h urine-free cortisol
Primary aldosteronism	Morning plasma aldosterone and renin to calculate an aldosterone-to-renin ratio	Aldosterone suppression test with salt loading Adrenal vein sampling used to distinguish an adrenal mass from bilateral adrenal hyperplasia when unclear radiographically and in patients >40 y
Pheochromocytoma	Plasma fractionated metanephrines/normetanephrines or 24-h total urinary metanephrines	Routine confirmation unnecessary with an abnormal screening test Iodine-123 metaiodobenzylguanidine used to rule out extra-adrenal pheochromocytoma

hypertension, obesity, diabetes, or osteoporosis, 3 tests including the late-night salivary cortisol and urine-free cortisol in addition to the dexamethasone suppression test may be administered to confirm the diagnosis.

Primary Aldosteronism

Primary aldosteronism, or Conn syndrome, is characterized by elevated serum aldosterone levels. Hyperaldosteronism results in increased total-body sodium, which causes hypertension and sometimes mild hypernatremia, as well as decreased potassium, which can cause muscle weakness and paresthesias.[29] Standard laboratory evaluation may reveal hypernatremia and hypokalemia, although these may be masked by drugs including potassium-sparing diuretics. Screening for hyperaldosteronism should be performed in patients with adrenal lesions and hypertension, and screening can be omitted in patients without hypertension.[28] Before screening, hypokalemia should be corrected; mineralocorticoid receptor antagonists should be stopped at least 6 weeks before screening. Screening is performed by obtaining an aldosterone-to-renin ratio (ARR). An ARR greater than 20 suggests hyperaldosteronism, which can be confirmed by demonstrating a lack of aldosterone suppression with salt loading on a 24-hour urine study. A high-resolution CT scan can distinguish aldosteronomas from adrenal hyperplasia in many people; but aldosteronomas may be very small and not always readily apparent. In these cases, and in most patients older than 40 years, adrenal vein sampling is recommended to lateralize the lesion.[28]

Pheochromocytoma

Pheochromocytoma is a catecholamine-producing tumor of the adrenal medulla. Symptoms include hypertension, headache, diaphoresis, and tremor.[29] Screening for pheochromocytoma should include the measurement of plasma fractionated metanephrines and normetanephrines or 24-hour total urinary metanephrines. Additionally, genetic counseling should be offered, as up to 25% of patients with pheochromocytoma has associated familial syndrome, including von Hippel-Lindau, multiple endocrine neoplasia type 2, neurofibromatosis type I, or succinate dehydrogenase mutations.

SURGICAL INDICATIONS

In general, indications for adrenalectomy include hormonally active adrenal tumors, enlarging lesions, masses with concerning radiographic characteristics, and large lesions greater than 4 to 6 cm, as the risk of ACC increases over this threshold.[28] Hormonally inactive tumors less than 3 cm are almost uniformly benign adrenal adenomas that do not require intervention, unless signs of hormonal activity develop or they increase in size. Indications for robotic adrenalectomy in particular mirror those of laparoscopic adrenalectomy and include most adrenal tumors, except those concerning for ACC, which should still be approached with open surgery. For larger tumors found to be locally invasive or otherwise concerning for ACC during minimally invasive adrenalectomy, most investigators recommend an open conversion.[30,31]

SURGICAL TECHNIQUE

Positioning, Approach, and Port Placement

Patients are placed in the modified left or right flank position with the side of the lesion facing up. All pressures points are carefully padded with a combination of pillows and foam, and patients are secured to the surgical table with tape. The patients' arms are placed in a mildly flexed position either over a double arm board or tucked next to the body.

Multiple surgical approaches have been described to access the adrenal gland, but the 2 most common approaches are the lateral transabdominal adrenalectomy (LTA) and the posterior retroperitoneoscopic adrenalectomy (PRA).

LTA is the most common transperitoneal approach. This approach allows greater working space than the retroperitoneal approach, which can be beneficial for larger tumors and obese patients.[32] Patients are placed in the flank position with the side of the tumor facing up, allowing gravity to retract the abdominal contents medially.

LTA port placement is illustrated in **Fig. 1**. After initiating pneumoperitoneum with a Veress needle, a 12-mm camera port is placed superolateral to the umbilicus. Next, two 8-mm robotic ports are placed under vision, 1 below the costal margin at the later border of the rectus and the other cephalad to the anterosuperior iliac spine. All robotic ports should have at least 8 cm of distance between them to prevent clashing. A 12-mm assistant port is place between the camera port and lower robotic port. For right-sided cases, a 5-mm port can be placed below the xiphoid process to place a liver retractor. Finally, the robot is docked coming over the patients' ipsilateral shoulder.

PRA is the most common retroperitoneal approach.[33] This approach allows avoidance of entering the peritoneal cavity, which may be beneficial in patients with prior abdominal surgery. However, there is often less working room and

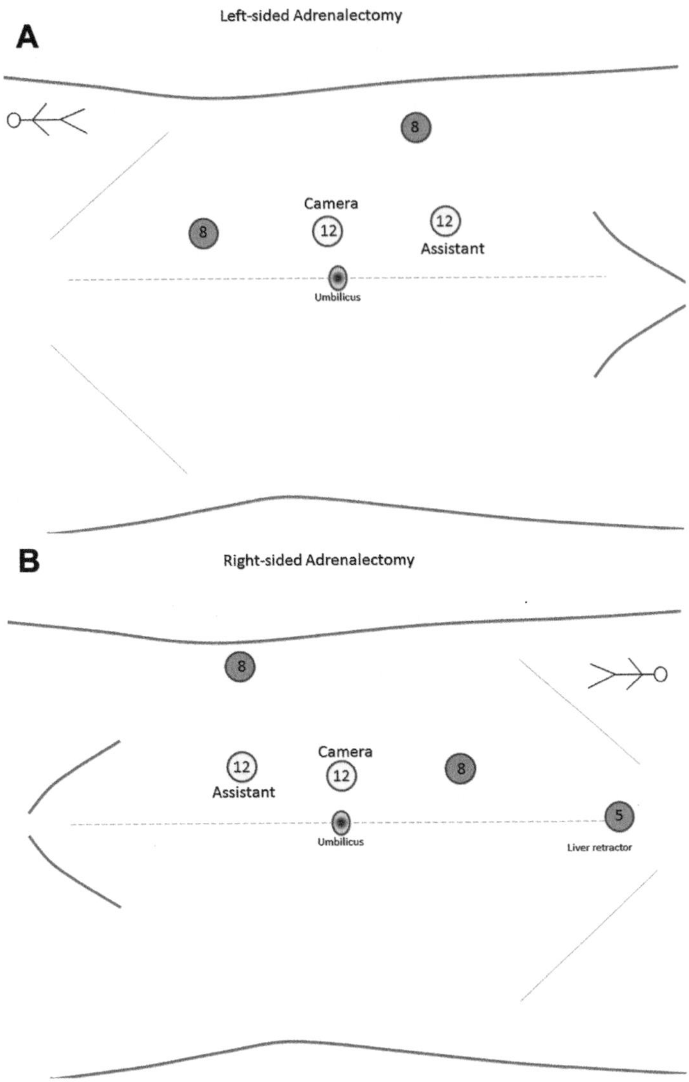

Fig. 1. Port placement for (*A*) left-sided and (*B*) right-sided robotic adrenalectomy.

anatomic landmarks may be unfamiliar compared with the transperitoneal view. Access to the retroperitoneum is gained inferolateral to the tip of the 12th rib by perforation the dorsal lumbar fascia and with finger dissection of the retroperitoneal space.[11] Next, two 8-mm incisions for the robotic working arms are made medial and lateral to the camera port with finger guidance to ensure they are positioned in the retroperitoneum. A balloon can be used to dissect and inflate the retroperitoneal space; the ports are placed; and the robotic is docked.

In a systematic review and meta-analysis comparing LTA and PRA during laparoscopic adrenalectomy, there was no difference in operative time, blood loss, time to ambulation, oral intake, or complication rate between techniques, with equivocal findings for hospital length of stay (LOS) and convalescence time.[34] A more recent meta-analysis found no difference in any perioperative outcome, including operative time, blood loss, hospital stay, time to oral intake, overall and major morbidity, and mortality.[35]

SURGICAL STEPS

For left-sided tumors, the splenorenal and splenocolic ligaments are divided and the spleen, colon, and pancreas are medialized to visualize the adrenal gland. Next, the renal hilum is identified and the left renal vein is dissected to identify the left adrenal vein (**Fig. 2**).

For right-sided adrenal tumors, the triangular ligament of the liver is released and the liver is retracted superiorly to exposure the adrenal gland. Minimal to no reflection of the colon is needed

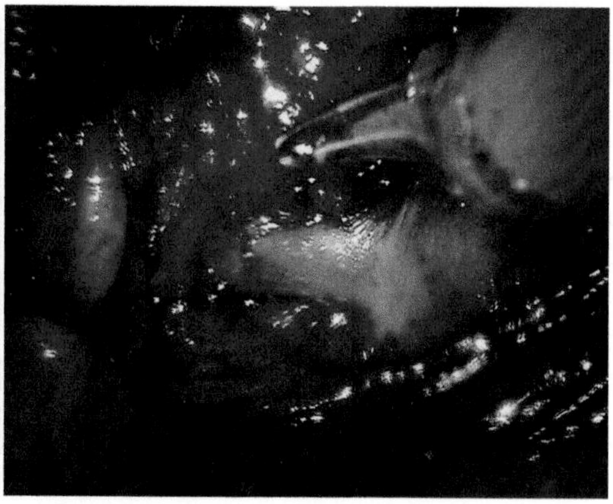

Fig. 2. Identification of the left adrenal vein draining into the left renal vein.

on the right side. Next the duodenum is Kocherized to expose the inferior vena cava and the right adrenal vein is identified.

Once the adrenal vein is identified, it is clipped and ligated (**Fig. 3**). Next the adrenal gland is dissected circumferentially, first by dissecting the gland off of the upper pole of the kidney and working medially. The arterial blood supply can be controlled with clips or a bipolar tissue-sealing device. Gerota's fat on the upper pole of the kidney can be taken with the adrenal gland to avoid direct manipulation of the gland itself. Once the adrenal is completely dissected, it is placed in an entrapment sac and removed by extending one of the port sites. Routine placement of a drain is not required. The robotic is undocked, and the abdomen is closed in the standard fashion.

OUTCOMES

Several studies have evaluated the safety and feasibility of robotic adrenalectomy, which are summarized in **Table 2**.[36–42] The first study from Winter and colleagues[39] in 2006 reported outcomes of 30 robotic adrenalectomies using an LTA approach. In this initial series, they reported an operating room (OR) time of 185 minutes, no conversions, a 7% complication rate, and a median LOS of 2 days. Subsequent studies demonstrated shorter OR times, with otherwise similar outcomes as shown in **Table 2**.

There have been multiple series comparing outcomes of robotic and laparoscopic adrenalectomy. The initial series, reported by Morino and colleagues,[43] compared outcomes of 10 robotic and 10 laparoscopic cases. In this early series, the investigators found that the laparoscopic approach had a shorter OR time (115 vs 169 minutes), more conversions (4 vs 0), and longer LOS (5.7 vs 5.4 days). Brunaud and colleagues[44] evaluated a larger cohort of 50 robotic and 59 laparoscopic adrenalectomies. Although the OR time was again longer in the robotic cohort (189 vs 159 minutes), the estimated blood loss (EBL) was less (49 vs 71 mL) and the LOS was shorter in the robotic cohort (6.3 vs 6.9 days), whereas conversions were similar (4 vs 4). Agcaoglu and colleagues[16] compared outcomes in patients with large adrenal tumors. The investigators evaluated 24 patients in the robotic cohort and 38 in the laparoscopic group with a mean tumor size of more than 6 cm. The investigators found favorable outcomes in the robotic arm in all domains evaluated: shorter OR time (159.4 vs 187.2 minutes), lower EBL (836.6 vs 166.6 mL), less conversions (1 vs 4), and shorter LOS (1.4 vs 1.9 days). The same group also evaluated robotic versus laparoscopic PRA.[42] Again, a robotic approach was associated with a shorter OR time (163.2 vs 165.7 minutes), less EBL (25.3 vs 35.6 mL), and similar LOS (1 vs 1 day).

Comparative robotic and laparoscopic series have also been reported for specific patient cohorts. Aksoy and coauthors[45] compared outcomes in obese patients.[45] Evaluating 42 robotic patients and 57 laparoscopic, the investigators found similar OR times (186.1 vs 187.3), less EBL (50.3 vs 76.6 mL), and shorter LOS (1.2 vs 1.7 days). Aliyev and colleagues[19] reported outcomes in patients undergoing 25 robotic and 40 laparoscopic adrenalectomies for pheochromocytoma. The investigators found that patients undergoing robotic surgery had shorter OR time (149 vs 178 minutes), less EBL (36 vs 43 mL), fewer conversions (1 vs 3), and shorter LOS (1.2 vs 1.7 days).

Because of the disparate outcomes from the single-institution comparative series discussed earlier, Brandao and colleagues[46] performed a systematic review and meta-analysis of robotic versus

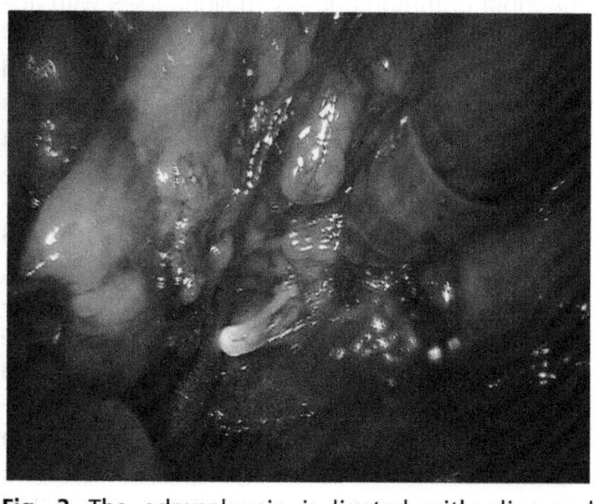

Fig. 3. The adrenal vein is ligated with clips and divided.

Table 2
Robotic adrenalectomy feasibility series

Series	n	OR Time (min)	Mean Tumor Size (cm)	LOS (d)	Conversions (%)	Complications (%)
Winter et al,[39] 2006	30	185	2.4	2.0	0	7
Brunaud et al,[36] 2008	100	99	2.9	6.4	5	10
Giulianotti et al,[37] 2011	42	118	5.5	4.0	0	4.8
Raman et al,[41] 2012	40	117	7.0	3.2	4	10
Nordenström et al,[40] 2011	100	113	5.3	NR	7	13
Agcaoglu et al,[42] 2012	31	163.2	3.1	1.0	0	0
Karabulut et al,[38] 2012	50	166	3.9	1.1	1	1

Abbreviations: NR, not reported; OR, operating room.
Data from Refs.[36–42]

laparoscopic adrenalectomy. This meta-analysis of 9 studies included 600 patients (277 in the robotic group and 323 in the laparoscopic). They found no difference in conversion rates, OR time, or postoperative complications. However, LOS and EBL were less in the robotic group. **Table 3** summarizes the outcomes of the robotic and laparoscopic comparative series.

Partial Adrenalectomy

Although the standard of care for most adrenal lesions is total adrenalectomy, there are a few situations in which partial adrenalectomy is an option. The indications include patients with heredity cancer syndromes (von Hippel-Lindau, multiple endocrine neoplasia type 2, neurofibromatosis type I, or succinate dehydrogenase mutations)[21] and in a solitary adrenal glands.[22] The technique for robotic partial adrenalectomy was initially described by Kumar and colleagues[22] from New York University as well as Boris and colleagues[21] from the National Cancer Institute. Port placement and adrenal exposure are similar to total adrenalectomy. The adrenal vein is clipped and divided for right-sided tumors but can be spared for some left-sided disease depending on the tumor locations. Intraoperative ultrasound is used to identify the tumor. In the case of pheochromocytoma, lesions appear as well-demarcated, homogenous, hypoechoic lesions. The tumor pseudocapsule is identified, and the tumor is enucleated with blunt dissection. Care is taken to preserve the adrenal by limiting superomedial dissection. Hemostasis is obtained with clips or cautery.

Asher and colleagues[47] reported outcomes for robotic partial adrenalectomy for pheochromocytoma in 15 patients. In that series, 4 patients had solitary adrenal glands. The mean OR time was 163 minutes, and the mean EBL was 161 mL. The median tumor size was 2.7 cm. One patient required elective conversion to an open procedure. At a median follow-up of 17.3 months, there were no local or metastatic recurrences.

There have been no comparative series of robotic and laparoscopic partial adrenalectomy or prospective studies. More investigation is needed to fully define the role of partial adrenalectomy and the robotic approach.

Metastasectomy

Metastases are the second most common tumor of the adrenal gland after benign adenomas.[25] The most common primary malignancies with adrenal metastases are lung, kidney, breast, and colon.[48] Although most adrenal metastases occur in the setting of diffuse metastatic disease, patients with isolated adrenal metastases may have a benefit from surgical resection.[49] The largest survival benefit is generally seen in patients with solitary lesions, a long disease-free interval, and smaller tumor size.[50]

The role of minimally invasive adrenal metastasectomy has been established in multiple laparoscopic series.[51–53] In a study by Strong and colleagues[54] comparing 63 open and 31 laparoscopic adrenal metastasectomies, the median survival was similar between groups at 30 months, whereas a laparoscopic approach was associated with less OR time, LOS, EBL, and complications.

Table 3
Comparative robotic and laparoscopic adrenalectomy series

Series	n (Robotic vs Lap)	OR Time, min (Robotic vs Lap)	LOS, d (Robotic vs Lap)	EBL	Conversions, n (Robotic vs Lap)	Complications, n (Robotic vs Lap)
Morino et al,[43] 2004	10 vs 10	169 vs 114	5.7 vs 5.4	NR	4 vs 0	0 vs 0
Brunaud et al,[44] 2008	50 vs 59	189 vs 159	6.3 vs 6.9	49 vs 71	4 vs 4	5 vs 9
Agcaoglu et al,[16] 2012	24 vs 38	159 vs 187	1.4 vs 1.9	84 vs 167	1 vs 4	0 vs 0
Agcaoglu et al,[42] 2012	31 vs 31	163 vs 166	1 vs 1	25 vs 36	NR	0 vs 0
Karabulut et al,[38] 2012	50 vs 50	166 vs 164	1.1 vs 1.5	41 vs 41	1 vs 2	1 vs 5
Pineda-Solis et al,[15] 2013	30 vs 30	190 vs 160	1.3 vs 1.9	30 vs 55	0 vs 5	0 vs 0
Aksoy et al,[45] 2013	42 vs 57	186 vs 187	1.3 vs 1.6	50 vs 77	0 vs 3	1 vs 2
You et al,[55] 2013	15 vs 8	207 vs 183	5.8 vs 6.7	NR	0 vs 0	2 vs 2
Aliyev et al,[19] 2013	25 vs 40	149 vs 178	1.2 vs 1.7	36 vs 43	1 vs 3	1 vs 2

Abbreviation: NR, not reported.
Data from Refs.[15,16,19,38,42–45,55]

The role of robotic metastasectomy is still being defined. Kumar and colleagues[22] described the first robotic-assisted metastasectomy in a patient with an isolated adrenal metastasis from a renal primary. However, to date, no case series or comparative studies have evaluated robotic adrenal metastasectomy.

SUMMARY

Robotic adrenalectomy is a safe procedure with comparable perioperative outcomes to laparoscopic surgery. Robotic surgery is potentially advantageous in terms of shorter hospital LOS and less EBL, though these benefits may come at the cost of increased surgical expense. A robotic approach may offer technical advantageous for large tumors, pheochromocytomas or for partial adrenalectomy, though these observations from retrospective series should be confirmed. Ultimately, a well-conducted, prospective randomized controlled trial is needed to define the role of robotics in adrenal surgery. Until then, the widespread adoption of robotic technology may lead to decreased case cost. For the time being, laparoscopic adrenalectomy is the standard of care; but robotic adrenalectomy remains an option at centers adept at robotic surgery.

REFERENCES

1. Gagner M, Lacroix A, Bolte E. Laparoscopic adrenalectomy in Cushing's syndrome and pheochromocytoma. N Engl J Med 1992;327:1033.
2. Shen WT, Lim RC, Siperstein AE, et al. Laparoscopic vs open adrenalectomy for the treatment of primary hyperaldosteronism. Arch Surg 1999; 134:628.
3. Hallfeldt KK, Mussack T, Trupka A, et al. Laparoscopic lateral adrenalectomy versus open posterior adrenalectomy for the treatment of benign adrenal tumors. Surg Endosc 2003;17:264.
4. Kim HH, Kim GH, Sung GT. Laparoscopic adrenalectomy for pheochromocytoma: comparison with conventional open adrenalectomy. J Endourol 2004;18:251.
5. Ramachandran MS, Reid JA, Dolan SJ, et al. Laparoscopic adrenalectomy versus open adrenalectomy: results from a retrospective comparative study. Ulster Med J 2006;75:126.
6. Humphrey R, Gray D, Pautler S, et al. Laparoscopic compared with open adrenalectomy for resection of pheochromocytoma: a review of 47 cases. Can J Surg 2008;51:276.
7. Kirshtein B, Yelle JD, Moloo H, et al. Laparoscopic adrenalectomy for adrenal malignancy: a preliminary report comparing the short-term outcomes with open adrenalectomy. J Laparoendosc Adv Surg Tech A 2008;18:42.
8. Lubikowski J, Uminski M, Andrysiak-Mamos E, et al. From open to laparoscopic adrenalectomy: thirty years' experience of one medical centre. Endokrynol Pol 2010;61:94.
9. Mir MC, Klink JC, Guillotreau J, et al. Comparative outcomes of laparoscopic and open adrenalectomy for adrenocortical carcinoma: single, high-volume center experience. Ann Surg Oncol 2013; 20:1456.
10. Wang HS, Li CC, Chou YH, et al. Comparison of laparoscopic adrenalectomy with open surgery for adrenal tumors. Kaohsiung J Med Sci 2009; 25:438.
11. Ludwig AT, Wagner KR, Lowry PS, et al. Robot-assisted posterior retroperitoneoscopic adrenalectomy. J Endourol 2010;24:1307.
12. Park JH, Kim SY, Lee CR, et al. Robot-assisted posterior retroperitoneoscopic adrenalectomy using single-port access: technical feasibility and preliminary results. Ann Surg Oncol 2013;20:2741.
13. Park JH, Walz MK, Kang SW, et al. Robot-assisted posterior retroperitoneoscopic adrenalectomy: single port access. J Korean Surg Soc 2011; 81(Suppl 1):S21.
14. D'Annibale A, Lucandri G, Monsellato I, et al. Robotic adrenalectomy: technical aspects, early results and learning curve. Int J Med Robot 2012;8:483.
15. Pineda-Solis K, Medina-Franco H, Heslin MJ. Robotic versus laparoscopic adrenalectomy: a comparative study in a high-volume center. Surg Endosc 2013;27:599.
16. Agcaoglu O, Aliyev S, Karabulut K, et al. Robotic versus laparoscopic resection of large adrenal tumors. Ann Surg Oncol 2012;19:2288.
17. Dickson PV, Alex GC, Grubbs EG, et al. Robotic-assisted retroperitoneoscopic adrenalectomy: making a good procedure even better. Am Surg 2013;79:84.
18. Hyams ES, Stifelman MD. The role of robotics for adrenal pathology. Curr Opin Urol 2009;19:89.
19. Aliyev S, Karabulut K, Agcaoglu O, et al. Robotic versus laparoscopic adrenalectomy for pheochromocytoma. Ann Surg Oncol 2013;20:4190.
20. Zafar SS, Abaza R. Robot-assisted laparoscopic adrenalectomy for adrenocortical carcinoma: initial report and review of the literature. J Endourol 2008; 22:985.
21. Boris RS, Gupta G, Linehan WM, et al. Robot-assisted laparoscopic partial adrenalectomy: initial experience. Urology 2011;77:775.
22. Kumar A, Hyams ES, Stifelman MD. Robot-assisted partial adrenalectomy for isolated adrenal metastasis. J Endourol 2009;23:651.
23. Nieman LK. Approach to the patient with an adrenal incidentaloma. J Clin Endocrinol Metab 2010; 95:4106.

24. Hamrahian AH, Ioachimescu AG, Remer EM, et al. Clinical utility of noncontrast computed tomography attenuation value (Hounsfield units) to differentiate adrenal adenomas/hyperplasias from nonadenomas: Cleveland Clinic experience. J Clin Endocrinol Metab 2005;90:871.
25. Uberoi J, Munver R. Surgical management of metastases to the adrenal gland: open, laparoscopic, and ablative approaches. Curr Urol Rep 2009;10:67.
26. Heinz-Peer G, Memarsadeghi M, Niederle B. Imaging of adrenal masses. Curr Opin Urol 2007; 17:32.
27. Israel GM, Korobkin M, Wang C, et al. Comparison of unenhanced CT and chemical shift MRI in evaluating lipid-rich adrenal adenomas. Am J Roentgenol 2004;183:215.
28. Zeiger MA, Thompson GB, Duh QY, et al. American Association of Clinical Endocrinologists and American Association of Endocrine Surgeons medical guidelines for the management of adrenal incidentalomas. Endocr Pract 2009;15:1.
29. Young WF Jr. The incidentally discovered adrenal mass. N Engl J Med 2007;356:601.
30. Henry JF, Sebag F, Iacobone M, et al. Results of laparoscopic adrenalectomy for large and potentially malignant tumors. World J Surg 2002;26:1043.
31. Shen WT, Sturgeon C, Duh QY. From incidentaloma to adrenocortical carcinoma: the surgical management of adrenal tumors. J Surg Oncol 2005;89:186.
32. Bickenbach KA, Strong VE. Laparoscopic transabdominal lateral adrenalectomy. J Surg Oncol 2012; 106:611.
33. Callender GG, Kennamer DL, Grubbs EG, et al. Posterior retroperitoneoscopic adrenalectomy. Adv Surg 2009;43:147.
34. Constantinides VA, Christakis I, Touska P, et al. Systematic review and meta-analysis of retroperitoneoscopic versus laparoscopic adrenalectomy. Br J Surg 2012;99:1639.
35. Nigri G, Rosman AS, Petrucciani N, et al. Meta-analysis of trials comparing laparoscopic transperitoneal and retroperitoneal adrenalectomy. Surgery 2013;153:111.
36. Brunaud L, Ayav A, Zarnegar R, et al. Prospective evaluation of 100 robotic-assisted unilateral adrenalectomies. Surgery 2008;144:995.
37. Giulianotti P, Buchs N, Addeo P, et al. Robot-assisted adrenalectomy: a technical option for the surgeon? Int J Med Robot 2011;7:27.
38. Karabulut K, Agcaoglu O, Aliyev S, et al. Comparison of intraoperative time use and perioperative outcomes for robotic versus laparoscopic adrenalectomy. Surgery 2012;151:537.
39. Winter J, Talamini M, Stanfield C, et al. Thirty robotic adrenalectomies: a single institution's experience. Surg Endosc 2006;20:119.
40. Nordenström E, Westerdahl J, Hallgrimsson P, et al. A prospective study of 100 robotically assisted laparoscopic adrenalectomies. J Robot Surg 2011;5:127.
41. Raman SR, Shakov E, Carnevale N, et al. Robotic adrenalectomy by an open surgeon: are outcomes different? J Robot Surg 2012;6:207.
42. Agcaoglu O, Aliyev S, Karabulut K, et al. Robotic vs laparoscopic posterior retroperitoneal adrenalectomy. Arch Surg 2012;147:272.
43. Morino M, Beninca G, Giraudo G, et al. Robot-assisted vs laparoscopic adrenalectomy: a prospective randomized controlled trial. Surg Endosc 2004; 18:1742.
44. Brunaud L, Bresler L, Ayav A, et al. Robotic-assisted adrenalectomy: what advantages compared to lateral transperitoneal laparoscopic adrenalectomy? Am J Surg 2008;195:433.
45. Aksoy E, Taskin HE, Aliyev S, et al. Robotic versus laparoscopic adrenalectomy in obese patients. Surg Endosc 2013;27:1233.
46. Brandao LF, Autorino R, Laydner H, et al. Robotic versus laparoscopic adrenalectomy: a systematic review and meta-analysis. Eur Urol 2014;65: 1154–61.
47. Asher KP, Gupta GN, Boris RS, et al. Robot-assisted laparoscopic partial adrenalectomy for pheochromocytoma: the National Cancer Institute technique. Eur Urol 2011;60:118.
48. Castillo OA, Vitagliano G, Kerkebe M, et al. Laparoscopic adrenalectomy for suspected metastasis of adrenal glands: our experience. Urology 2007;69:637.
49. Kim SH, Brennan MF, Russo P, et al. The role of surgery in the treatment of clinically isolated adrenal metastasis. Cancer 1998;82:389.
50. Gittens PR Jr, Solish AF, Trabulsi EJ. Surgical management of metastatic disease to the adrenal gland. Semin Oncol 2008;35:172–6.
51. Marangos IP, Kazaryan AM, Rosseland AR, et al. Should we use laparoscopic adrenalectomy for metastases? Scandinavian multicenter study. J Surg Oncol 2009;100:43.
52. Cobb WS, Kercher KW, Sing RF, et al. Laparoscopic adrenalectomy for malignancy. Am J Surg 2005;189:405.
53. Abel EJ, Karam JA, Carrasco A, et al. Laparoscopic adrenalectomy for metachronous metastases after ipsilateral nephrectomy for renal-cell carcinoma. J Endourol 2011;25:1323.
54. Strong VE, D'Angelica M, Tang L, et al. Laparoscopic adrenalectomy for isolated adrenal metastasis. Ann Surg Oncol 2007;14:3392.
55. You JY, Lee HY, Son GS, et al. Comparison of robotic adrenalectomy with traditional laparoscopic adrenalectomy with a lateral transperitoneal approach: a single-surgeon experience. Int J Med Robot 2013;9:345.

Robotic-assisted Sacrocolpopexy for Pelvic Organ Prolapse

Wesley M. White, MD[a,*], Ryan B. Pickens, MD[a], Robert F. Elder, MD[b], Farzeen Firoozi, MD[c]

KEYWORDS

• Laparoscopy • Robotics • Outcomes • Pelvic organ prolapse • Incontinence

KEY POINTS

- The demand for surgical correction of pelvic organ prolapse is expected to grow as the aging population remains active and focused on quality of life.
- Definitive correction of pelvic organ prolapse can be accomplished through both vaginal and abdominal approaches.
- The preponderance of data cite the superiority of abdominal sacrocolpopexy in the durable correction of apical prolapse.
- The application of robotics and the pervasive concern regarding the transvaginal placement of synthetic mesh has revitalized and emboldened sacrocolpopexy.

INTRODUCTION

Pelvic organ prolapse (POP) is expected to affect nearly 50% of all women during their lifetimes.[1] POP can be severely lifestyle limiting and is a particularly germane concern given the aging population, the frequency with which prolapse affects this subgroup, and their general emphasis on maintaining an active and robust quality of life.[2] Definitive correction of POP is surgical, and is chiefly accomplished through vaginal-based or abdominal-based reconstruction. The optimal choice of treatment is predicated not only on patient-derived factors including the degree and nature of pelvic relaxation, comorbidities, and the integrity of the individual patient's tissue but also on the experience and expertise of the operating surgeon, and is taken in the context of evidence-based outcomes.

Among those patients with severe apical relaxation and/or multicompartment prolapse with an apical component, the superiority of abdominal sacral colpopexy (ASC) is well established.[3] The principal tenet of surgical correction for pelvic prolapse is the durable restoration of the vaginal apex in a fashion that provides improved urinary, sexual, and bowel function.[4] Sufficient level I evidence exists to suggest that open ASC offers consistently higher objective success rates and lower rates of dyspareunia compared with sacrospinous-based vaginal repair.[3,5] However, these favorable results have traditionally come at the expense of increased short-term morbidity and prolonged convalescence.[3]

The application of laparoscopy and robotics during ASC has dramatically improved the morbidity associated with the procedure while

Disclosures: Coloplast, lecturer and/or consultant (W.M. White); none (R.B. Pickens, R.F. Elder, and F. Firoozi).

[a] Department of Urology, The University of Tennessee Medical Center, 1924 Alcoa Highway, Knoxville, TN 37920, USA; [b] Department of Obstetrics and Gynecology, The University of Tennessee Medical Center, 1924 Alcoa Highway, Knoxville, TN 37920, USA; [c] Center for Female Pelvic Health and Reconstructive Surgery, The Arthur Smith Institute for Urology, Hofstra North Shore-LIJ School of Medicine, 270-05, 76th Avenue, New Hyde Park, NY 11040, USA

* Corresponding author. Department of Urology, The University of Tennessee Medical Center, 1928 Alcoa Highway, Suite B-222, Knoxville, TN 37920.

E-mail address: wwhite@utmck.edu

Urol Clin N Am 41 (2014) 549–557
http://dx.doi.org/10.1016/j.ucl.2014.07.009
0094-0143/14/$ – see front matter

continuing to offer durable and satisfactory outcomes.[6] Coupled with the current litigious climate surrounding mesh-augmented vaginal repair, laparoscopic and, more recently, robotic ASC has become the preferred corrective procedure for POP among many patients and providers.[7] This article focuses on the indications and patient evaluation for robotic ASC, describes its surgical nuances through intraoperative photographs, discusses the economic ramifications of robotic ASC, and addresses the controversy surrounding the application of synthetic mesh.

PATIENT EVALUATION AND PREPARATION

Candidates for robotic ASC include women with symptomatic stage II or greater POP including apical relaxation, those with recurrent prolapse following primary vaginal repair, and/or those with POP and the need for concomitant abdominal surgery. Women with an in situ uterus should be evaluated for postmenopausal or abnormal uterine bleeding, undergo transvaginal ultrasonography as indicated to rule out a suspicious mass, and should have a clearly documented Pap smear history. Based on the aforementioned evaluation, appropriate candidates may be considered for sacrohysteropexy or may elect to undergo concomitant supracervical hysterectomy at the time of sacrocolpopexy (our preferred practice). Prior abdominal surgery is common among this patient population but is not a contraindication. Although patients should be counseled on the risk of a hostile abdomen and the potential need for extensive adhesiolysis or enterotomy, we have encountered few women for whom a minimally invasive approach to ASC was untenable.

Surgical candidates should undergo a thorough but directed history and physical examination. Utmost effort should be made to reconcile the patient's symptoms with their examination findings. The most common presenting symptoms include vaginal pressure or heaviness, the presence of a vaginal bulge, as well as urinary, sexual, and bowel disorders. Women with severe prolapse may report the need for manual reduction and/or the ability to palpate or directly visualize the vaginal apex or uterus. Urinary incontinence is frequently encountered and is typically mixed in nature. Occult stress urinary incontinence should be considered and accounted for. A weeklong voiding log and postvoid residual measurement are recommended, and quality-of-life questionnaires are useful to establish a baseline for later reference. Multichannel urodynamics may be judiciously used, especially among women with high-grade prolapse. In our experience, many women with severe POP have an element of detrusor underactivity owing to prolonged relaxation. Patients should be counseled before surgery on the possibility of persistent and/or de novo postoperative voiding dysfunction or hesitancy, especially in the setting of concomitant midurethral sling. It is critically important to assess the patient's desire for sexual activity and whether the existing prolapse has been a factor in that decision. Dyspareunia should be discussed as a rare but possible adverse event. In addition, many women with multicompartment POP report chronic constipation, and particular attention must be paid to bowel function after surgery to avoid repetitive stress on the integrity of the reconstruction.

Physical examination should be systematic and thorough. A bimanual examination should be performed to assess for the presence and size of a uterus (if present) and the presence of adnexal disorder. We prefer to use a bivalve speculum to assess the vaginal apex and/or cervix. The speculum is then disarticulated to evaluate the anterior and posterior compartments separately. The presence and grade of prolapse in the anterior, apical, and posterior compartments should be quantified using the pelvic organ prolapse quantification (POP-Q) system.[8] Estrogen status and the integrity of the levator musculature and perineal body are likewise assessed.

A cough stress test and/or cotton swab test may be performed in the office to address potential urethral hypermobility and stress urinary incontinence. Likewise, in-office cystoscopy can be selectively performed at the time of vaginal examination to concomitantly assess the degree of POP, the anatomy of the bladder and urethra, and to perform the cough stress test. Although published studies suggest that women without existing complaints of stress incontinence may benefit from midurethral sling owing to the presence of occult leakage, our practice is to individualize our approach to sling placement including intraoperative Credé maneuver.[9]

Informed consent for robotic ASC should include a thorough explanation of the surgical steps of the procedure and well as its surgical risks including, but not limited to, injury to the bladder or ureters, mesh-related complications including erosion or extrusion (approximately 5%), inadvertent vaginal entry, vaginal foreshortening, dyspareunia, postoperative voiding dysfunction including retention, bowel injury, and other imponderables. Selective medical clearance should be performed. A type and screen is not needed. Venous thromboembolism prophylaxis is used with either sequential compression devices or subcutaneous heparin.[10]

ROBOTIC SACROCOLPOPEXY: TECHNIQUE AND NUANCES

Step 1

General endotracheal anesthesia is administered in the supine position and the patient is then converted to the low lithotomy position in Allen stirrups (**Fig. 1**). The patient's arms are tucked and a foam back pad is used to prevent movement while in the Trendelenburg position. The patient's perineum should approach the edge of the bed to facilitate external manipulation of the vagina during the procedure as well as to facilitate access to the vagina for subsequent midurethral sling and/or distal rectocele repair, as needed. A Foley catheter and vaginal manipulator are placed.

Step 2

The relevant pelvic landmarks are identified and an approximately 12-mm incision is made in a periumbilical or supraumbilical fashion. Access to the peritoneum is achieved with either a Veress needle or a Hassan trocar. The abdomen is insufflated with CO_2 gas to a maximum pressure of 15 mm Hg. If a Veress needle is used, it is exchanged for a standard 12-mm operative trocar. We often use a balloon-tipped cannula to prevent inadvertent slippage of the trocar, which is commonly encountered in the very obese or the very petite. The da Vinci robotic 0° camera (Intuitive Surgical, Sunnyvale, CA) is introduced and the abdomen widely inspected. The patient is then placed in steep Trendelenburg position and the table is maximally lowered. Under direct vision, three 8-mm robotic trocars and one 12-mm standard trocar are placed at or below the level of the umbilicus in a standard sawtooth configuration (**Fig. 2**). The robot is then positioned with its base either between the patient's legs (standard docking) or at an acute perpendicular angle near the base of the operative table (side dock). Many urologists are more comfortable with a standard docking approach given its ubiquity during male pelvic surgery. However, side docking, commonly used during benign gynecologic procedures, offers several distinct advantages during ASC, including unfettered access to the vagina for manipulation and anatomic guidance (**Fig. 3**).

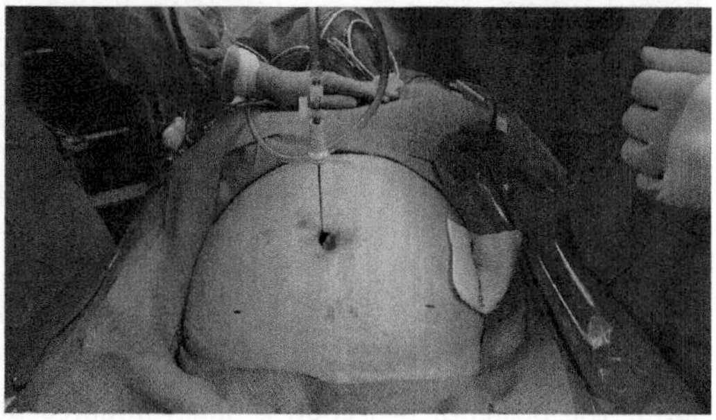

Fig. 1. Patient positioning and representative port placement during robotic sacrocolpopexy. A Veress needle has been placed and insufflation has been initiated.

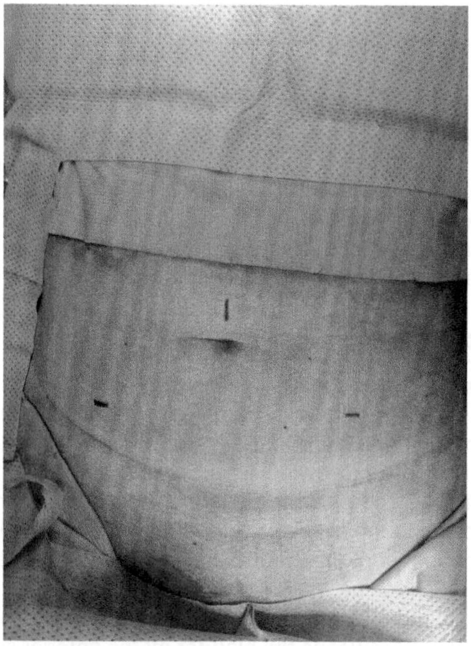

Fig. 2. Representative port placement for robotic sacrocolpopexy.

Step 3

Once the robot has been docked, we insert right-handed 8-mm monopolar shears and left-handed ProGrasp forceps. The accessory (most lateral 8-mm robotic trocar on the left side) robotic port

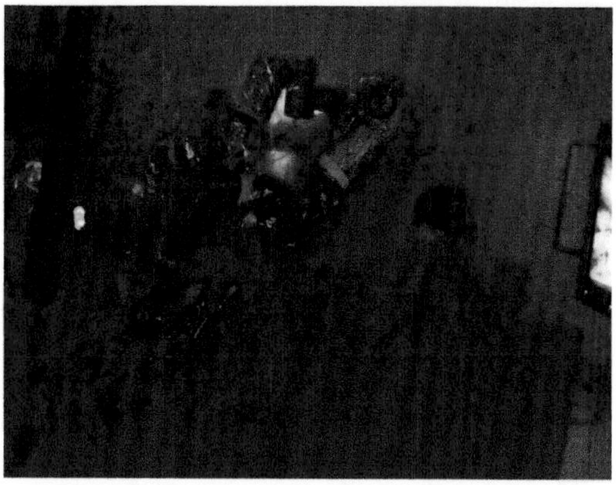

Fig. 3. The robot was side-docked during robotic ASC. The surgical assistant has unencumbered access to the patient's vagina and is able to manipulate the uterus/vagina as dictated by the operating surgeon.

is provided with Cadiere forceps. We prefer Cadiere forceps for manipulation and retraction of the sigmoid mesentery because the closing force/crushing potential of the Cadiere is significantly less than that of the ProGrasp. Identification of relevant pelvic anatomy ensues including adhesiolysis as needed. The Foley catheter is manipulated to clearly demarcate the limits of the bladder and the vaginal manipulator is used to define the apex of the vagina.

Step 4

Dissection is carried onto the anterior surface of the vagina following hysterectomy or continues onto the anterior surface of the cervix and vagina immediately following supracervical hysterectomy (**Fig. 4**). The peritoneum is incised at the vaginal apex and the avascular plane between the posterior aspect of the bladder and the anterior aspect of the vagina is developed. In general, blunt dissection with directed pinpoint monopolar cautery nicely sweeps the bladder off the anterior surface of the vagina. This dissection is carried down to the approximate level of the trigone, which can be identified by manipulating the Foley catheter. In some instances, identification of this plane of dissection can be tedious, especially among those women who have undergone prior hysterectomy or transvaginal prolapse repair. Filling of the bladder through the Foley catheter may help delineate its contours. Inadvertent vaginotomy or cystotomy may occur and should be recognized immediately. Although less than ideal, this type of surgical misadventure may ultimately afford the surgeon a clearer understanding of the patient's anatomy and the limits and contours of the bladder and vagina. These entries should be used to inform the remaining dissection and then closed in multiple layers using absorbable suture. Care should be taken to avoid direct mesh apposition, if possible, at the site of any vaginotomy or cystotomy.

Step 5

The posterior peritoneum is then dissected off the cervical stump/posterior vagina and carried distally toward the rectovaginal pouch. In general, the initial dissection can be indistinct (**Fig. 5**) but, with further progress, a nice areolar plane avails itself down to at least the level of peritoneal reflection and perhaps farther to the presumed level of the perineal body (**Fig. 6**). Again, the bedside assistant can help reconcile the approximate level of posterior dissection.

Step 6

The sacral promontory is then palpated and the retroperitoneum opened to expose the anterior longitudinal ligament (**Fig. 7**). The promontory typically is readily apparent in all but the most obese of patients. A bedside assistant can directly palpate the sacrum using a laparoscopic suction/irrigator to verify its location. However, in our experience, learned tactile feedback with the robot makes identification straightforward.

Step 7

A retroperitoneal tunnel is created from the level of the sacral promontory down the length of the posterior cul-de-sac to meet with the previously created peritoneotomy over the posterior aspect of the vagina (**Figs. 8** and **9**). As an alternative,

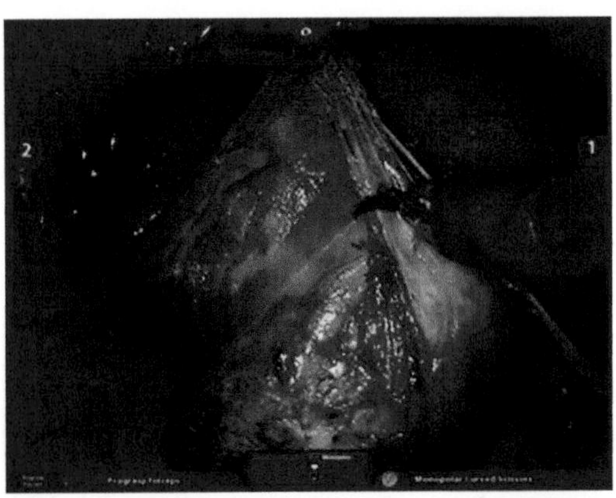

Fig. 4. Dissection is initiated at the vaginal apex. The peritoneum is incised and an areolar dissection plane is developed between the anterior aspect of the vagina and the posterior aspect of the bladder.

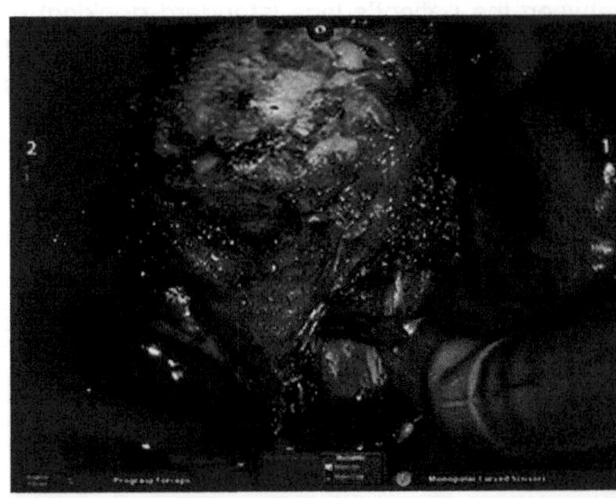

Fig. 5. The posterior dissection is again initiated at the vaginal apex or posterior aspect of the cervical stump. Creation of this plane posteriorly can be challenging and care must be taken to avoid inadvertent vaginotomy or thinning of the peritoneum.

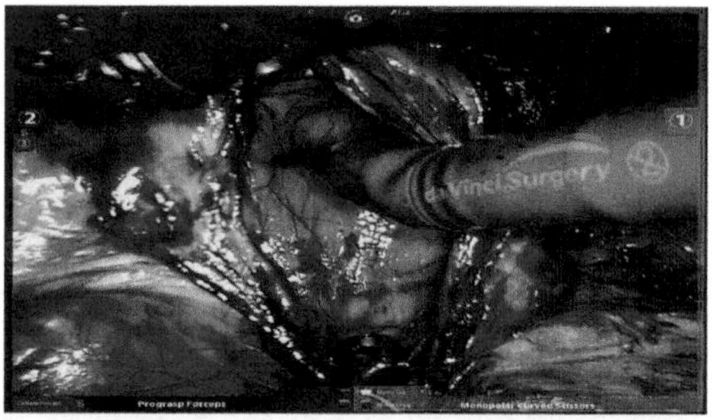

Fig. 6. Similar to the anterior dissection, a clearly visualized areolar plane becomes apparent as the posterior dissection is carried toward the posterior cul-de-sac and perineal body.

the retroperitoneum can be opened down the length of the posterior pelvis. Although creating a retroperitoneal tunnel hastens reconstruction later in the procedure, the availability of barbed suture has made reconstruction of the incised peritoneum straightforward. If a tunnel is not created, clinicians must be cognizant of the right ureter and must avoid its entrapment during closure.

Step 8

A prefashioned, Y-shaped, lightweight (macroporous) polypropylene mesh is trimmed to approximately 6 to 7 cm anteriorly and posteriorly but this length is depends heavily on patient-specific anatomy and must be individualized. The mesh is rolled up and introduced (**Fig. 10**).

Step 9

The Y-shaped graft is unrolled and laid flat over the anterior aspect of the vagina and/or cervical stump and vagina (**Fig. 11**). It is affixed to the anterior aspect of the vagina and/or cervical stump using a series of 0-Vicryl sutures (**Fig. 12**). Six sutures are typically placed both anteriorly and posteriorly in 3 rows of 2 sutures each. We prefer to take full-thickness bites of the vagina/robust bites of the

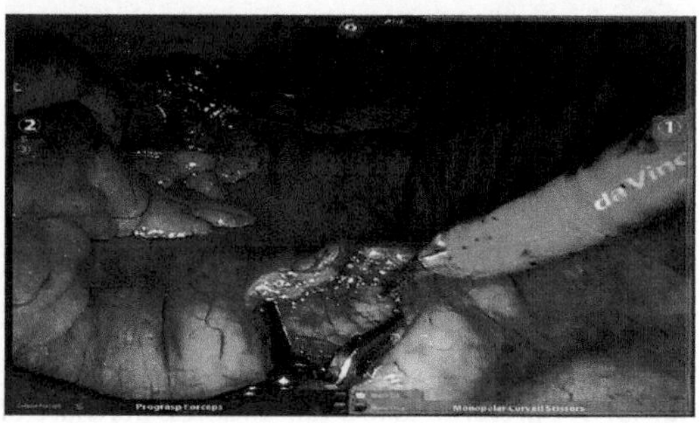

Fig. 7. The sacral promontory is identified and the retroperitoneum incised. The anterior longitudinal ligament is exposed.

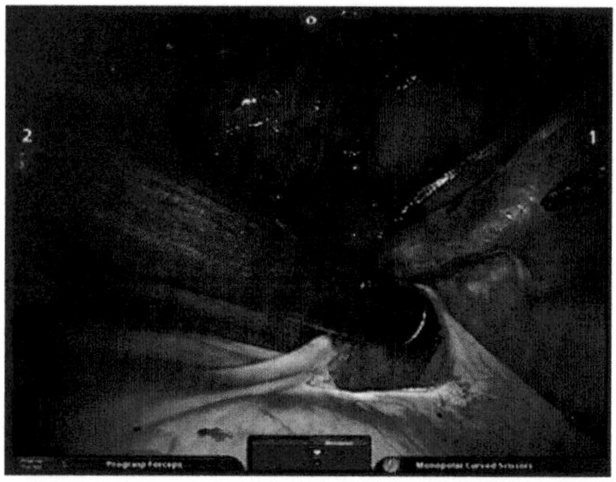

Fig. 8. A retroperitoneal tunnel is created using the blunt tip of the ProGrasp forceps. In some circumstances, a single tunnel cannot be developed and a stepwise approach to creating the tunnel should be adopted. As an alternative, the retroperitoneum may be opened from the level of the promontory down to the posterior cul-de-sac.

cervical stump but not enough to bunch the graft (**Fig. 13**). Suture fixation posteriorly can be tedious and clinicians should be comfortable throwing sutures at a variety of angles to best seat the graft in a flat fashion (**Fig. 14**). We also prefer to use a MegaCut or suture-cut needle driver in the right hand to expedite this step through economy of movement. Clinicians may also consider fixing the graft to the vagina using a barbed suture in a switchback fashion. The flexibility of the barbed suture obviates repetitive suture exchange but may cause transient scalloping of the vaginal mucosa if thrown in a full-thickness fashion.

Step 10

The tail of the graft is brought out through the retroperitoneal tunnel (or up to the level of the promontory if the retroperitoneum was split) (**Fig. 15**). The tail of the graft is affixed to the

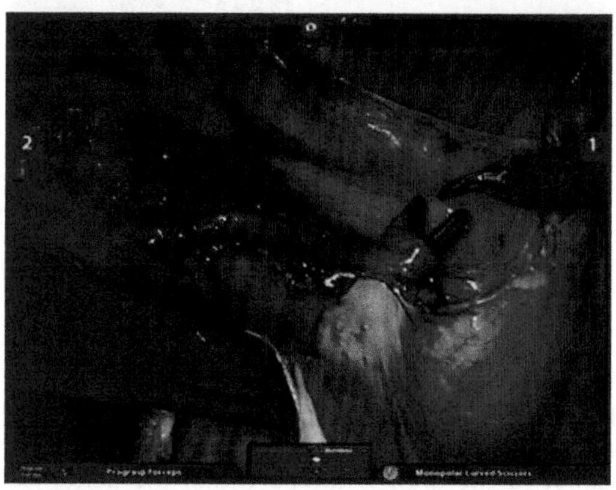

Fig. 9. Creation of the retroperitoneal tunnel.

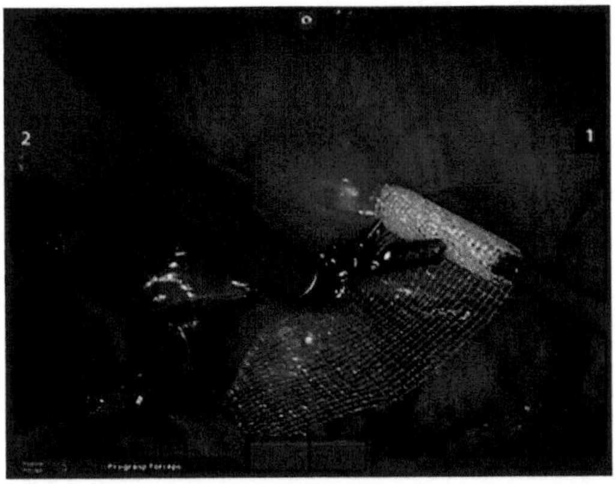

Fig. 10. The Y-shaped polypropylene graft is introduced into the patient's abdomen by rolling the graft around a laparoscopic instrument.

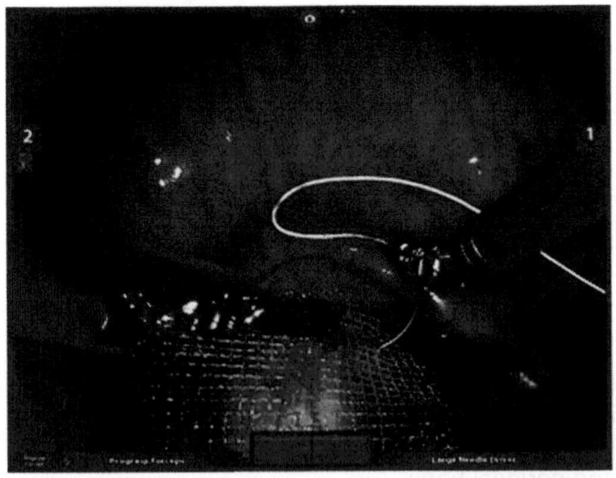

Fig. 12. The anterior leaflet of the graft is affixed to the vagina/cervical stump using interrupted, dyed 0-Vicryl suture on a CT-2 needle.

anterior longitudinal ligament using 2 interrupted 0 Ethibond sutures (**Fig. 16**). We prefer to throw a right forehand, left forehand slipknot stitch that allows the graft to be securely affixed to the ligament. Care must be taken to apply appropriate but not undue tension when reducing the vaginal apex externally. Overtightening of the graft fails to account for inevitable mesh contracture and potential vaginal foreshortening.

Step 11

The retroperitoneum is closed over the vagina and sacrum using a running barbed suture of choice (**Fig. 17**). We find this technique again provides secure and efficient coverage of the graft.

Step 12

The abdomen is desufflated following removal of all ports under direct vision. The midline 12-mm incision is closed using a 0-Vicryl suture in a meticulous fashion. Skin incisions are then closed in a subcuticular fashion.

Step 13

The patient is converted to the exaggerated lithotomy position and a thorough vaginal examination performed to assess for apical support. Often, a distal rectocele has been inadequately addressed abdominally and requires primary vaginal repair at this stage. Cystoscopy is likewise performed to ensure ureteral efflux and integrity of the bladder. If a midurethral sling is planned, it is performed at this time. A Foley catheter is replaced as well as an estrogen-soaked vaginal pack.

COST CONSIDERATIONS OF ROBOTIC SACROCOLPOPEXY

As with any new technology-driven surgical approach or technique, a thorough inquisition of

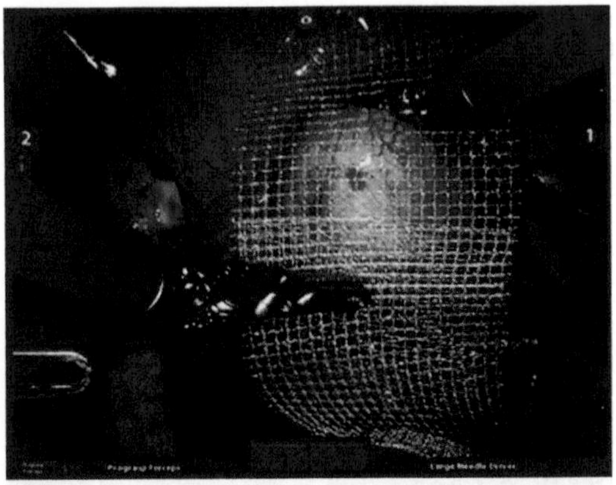

Fig. 11. The graft is laid flat against the anterior aspect of the vagina/cervical stump and the posterior leaflet of the graft is tucked within the peritoneal pocket.

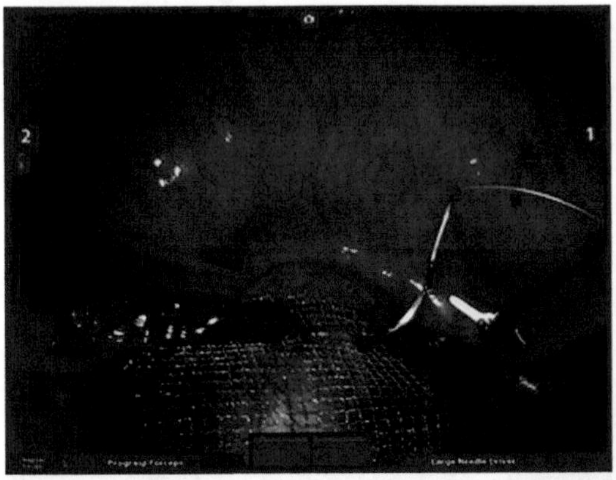

Fig. 13. We prefer to take a full-thickness purchase of the vaginal wall that spans 4 pores on the graft. This technique affords secure fixation of the graft without bunching.

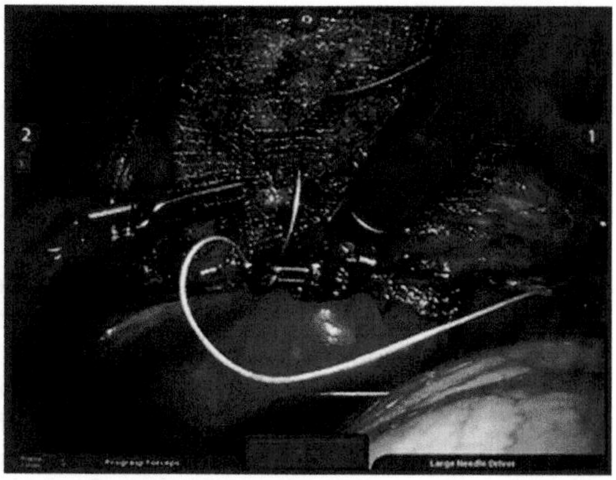

Fig. 14. The posterior leaflet of the graft is affixed in a similar fashion. This intraoperative image shows the surgical flexibility that is needed in obtaining a robust posterior bite. The needle may need to be thrown in a vertical, horizontal, forehand, or backhand fashion to obtain the ideal results.

its safety/morbidity, efficacy, and economics must be performed. Robotic ASC offers the promise of decreased morbidity compared with its open counterpart and, based on multiple published studies, seems to offer comparable durability without discordant risk or surgical complexity.[11–13] Despite its clear ability to be effective in accomplishing its task, it remains uncertain whether robotic ASC can be efficient to that end.

Research on the cost-effectiveness of robotic ASC has thus far largely consisted of retrospective studies and/or cost-minimization analyses.[14–16] Results have been conflicting, with most studies detecting increased costs with the robotic approach compared with either open or laparoscopic ASC. In addition, although the sunk cost of the robot is an expected cost driver, prolonged

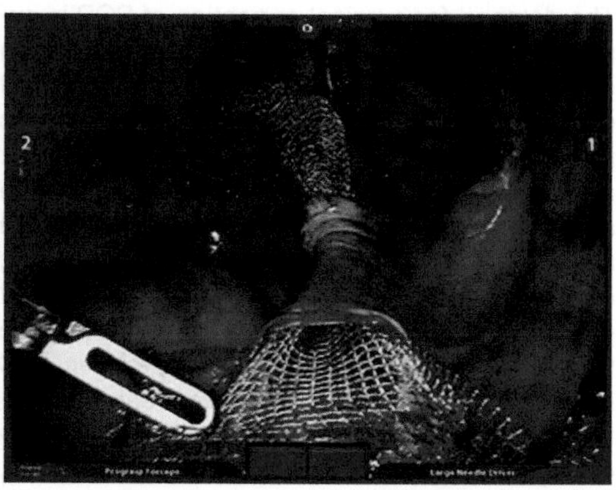

Fig. 15. The tail of the graft is brought up through the retroperitoneal tunnel. The vagina is reduced from below and the graft is tensioned appropriately.

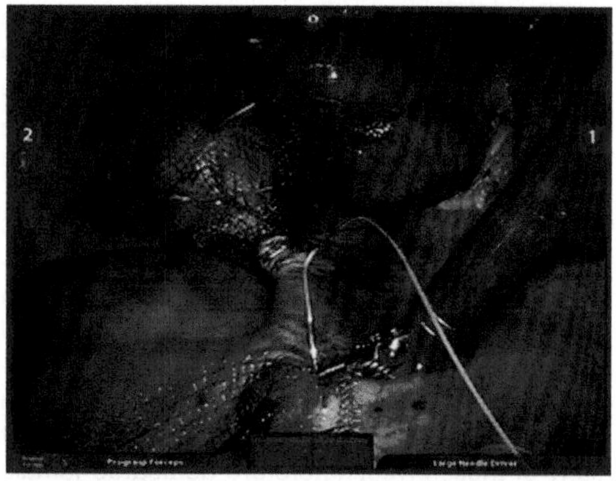

Fig. 16. The graft is affixed to the anterior longitudinal ligament using 2 interrupted 0 Ethibond sutures on an SH needle (tapered). A slipknot stitch affords secure apposition of the graft to the promontory.

operative time and general operating room costs with robotic ASC seem significant as well.[17]

More recently, a randomized controlled trial was conducted specifically to assess outcomes between laparoscopic and robotic ASC.[18] A total of 78 women with symptomatic stage II or greater POP including significant apical support loss were randomized to either laparoscopic (n = 38) or robotic (n = 40) ASC. Primary outcomes focused on cost and readmission rates with secondary outcomes centered on anatomic outcomes and quality of life. No differences were noted in the two groups with respect to these secondary outcomes or readmission rates. Robotic ASC was more expensive than laparoscopic ASC by nearly $1000 ($12,586 vs $11,573) per case, but this difference was not statistically significant. The investigators cited the robot purchase price and maintenance costs as the primary difference makers with respect to cost.

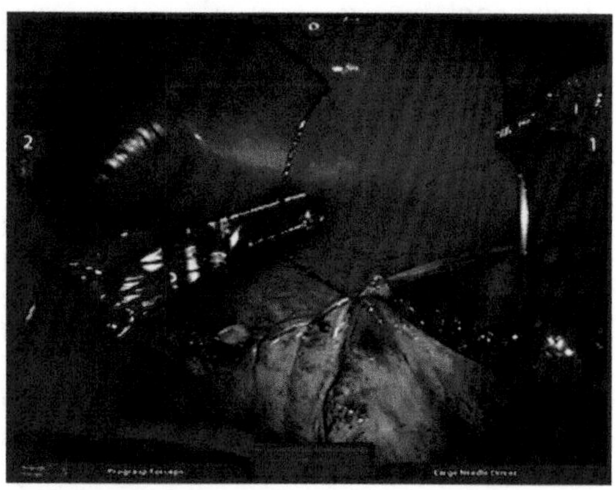

Fig. 17. The peritoneal defect is closed using a running barbed suture.

Critics of these aforementioned studies (both prorobot and prolaparoscopy) cite the difficulty in capturing cost versus charges and the absolute lack of uniformity with which charges are calculated. Still others point out the inherent bias in many of these prospective studies, namely the investigators' lack of experience with robotic ASC compared with laparoscopic ASC. The investigators of many of these studies, many of whom have years of laparoscopic ASC experience and are known to be excellent laparoscopists, regarded a surgeon who had completed more than 10 robotic ASCs as proficient.[17,18] Given that many of these investigators are dedicated female medicine/pelvic floor surgeons who are not otherwise exposed to robotics in general, these costs must be considered in the potential context of inexperience. A surgeon who has only completed 10 robotics cases naturally expends more resources on a per-case basis than a robotic surgeon who performs 10 robotics cases per week. With greater experience comes reduced operative times, reduced disposable waste, the need for fewer robotic surgical instruments (suturing with a MegaCut driver to save disposable scissors and a ProGrasp as opposed to an additional needle driver), and less surgical variability. These surgical refinements translate into reduced costs consistent with the focused factory principle of business.[19] A better study design might compare costs incurred by an experienced laparoscopic ASC surgeon with a surgeon who regularly performs robotic cases, including robotic ASC.

Does robotic ASC ultimately make economic sense? The capital investment of purchasing and maintaining a robot is an undeniable expense, but a recoverable one. With sufficient volume and surgical experience, standardization of disposables, sensible negotiating with industry driven by a value analysis team at the hospital level, and constant vigilance by the surgeon, we think that robotic ASC can offer patients and hospitals mutual benefits.

CLIMATE OF FEAR: SYNTHETIC MESH IN THE TREATMENT OF POP

The resurgence of ASC, brought about in part through robotics, has transpired at a time of great uncertainty in female pelvic medicine. In 2008, owing to growing public concern over a litany of reports focused on mesh-related complications, the US Food and Drug Administration (FDA) issued a public health notice regarding complications associated with the implantation of vaginal polypropylene mesh.[20] In the years that followed, additional investigation by the FDA culminated in a formal public health safety notification and update in 2011 with the following findings[21]:

- The FDA emphasized that complications associated with synthetic mesh are not rare.
- Vaginal shortening, tightening, and/or pain caused by mesh were cited as previously unidentified risks.
- Mesh used during transvaginal pelvic organ prolapse repair introduces risks not present in traditional nonmesh surgery.
- Mesh placed abdominally for pelvic organ prolapse seems to result in lower rates of mesh-related complications compared with transvaginal prolapse repair with mesh.
- Surgeons must fully explain the postoperative risks and complications associated with mesh and the limited long-term data regarding its use.

The aforementioned communications have engendered a punitive and poorly substantiated litigious climate that has invoked concern, bewilderment, and fear among providers and patients regarding the vaginal implantation of synthetic polypropylene mesh. The market for transvaginal mesh has experienced significant contracture as manufacturers have voluntarily withdrawn and/or narrowed its commercial availability. Further, the reclassification of vaginal mesh by the FDA and its attendant regulatory demands are likely to dissuade industry from future entry into the fray. Many providers have abandoned mesh-augmented repairs and are choosing to perform native-tissue transvaginal repairs or abdominal-based reconstruction. It is expected that ASC, particularly laparoscopic and robotic ASC, will experience significant growth.[22]

SUMMARY

The demand for surgical correction of POP is expected to grow rapidly as the general population of the United States ages and remains focused on quality of life. Robotic sacrocolpopexy is poised to become the preferred treatment approach for women with moderate prolapse and an apical component. Aversion to transvaginal mesh repair by patients, coupled with increasing comfort with robotics and abdominal-based reconstruction by providers, is expected to drive this conversion. Although costs with robotic ASC may seem to outpace alternative treatment options, market forces and increased surgical proficiency are likely to render this issue outdated. Clinicians ultimately must seek to offer patients a tailored treatment algorithm that balances consistent and durable effectiveness with fiscal responsibility, minimizes risk to the patient, and marries the goals of the patient to the experience and purview of the surgeon.

REFERENCES

1. Olsen AL, Smith VJ, Bergstrom JO, et al. Epidemiology of surgically managed pelvic organ prolapse and urinary incontinence. Obstet Gynecol 1997;89:501.
2. Adams SR, Dramitinos P, Shapiro A, et al. Do patient goals vary with degree of prolapse? Am J Obstet Gynecol 2011;205:502.
3. Maher C, Feiner B, Baessler K, et al. Surgical management of pelvic organ prolapse in women [review]. Cochrane Database Syst Rev 2013;(4):CD004014.
4. Nygaard IE, McCreery R, Brubaker L, et al. Abdominal sacrocolpopexy: a comprehensive review. Obstet Gynecol 2004;104:805.
5. Mueller ER. Why complex pelvic organ prolapse should be approached abdominally. Curr Opin Urol 2013;23:317.
6. Paraiso MF, Walters MD, Rackley RR, et al. Laparoscopic and abdominal sacral colpopexies: a comparative cohort study. Am J Obstet Gynecol 2005;192:1752.
7. Elterman DS, Chughtai BI, Vertosick E, et al. Changes in pelvic organ prolapse surgery in the last decade among United States urologists. J Urol 2014;191:1022.
8. Bump RC, Mattiasson A, Bo K, et al. The standardization of terminology of female pelvic organ prolapse and pelvic floor dysfunction. Am J Obstet Gynecol 1996;175(1):10.
9. Richardson ML, Elliott CS, Shaw JG, et al. To sling or not to sling at time of abdominal sacrocolpopexy: a cost-effectiveness analysis. J Urol 2013;190:1306.
10. Clarke-Pearson DL, Abaid LN. Prevention of venous thromboembolic events after gynecologic surgery. Obstet Gynecol 2012;199:155.
11. Geller EJ, Parnell BA, Dunivan GC. Robotic vs abdominal sacrocolpopexy: 44-month pelvic floor outcomes. Urology 2012;79:532.
12. Lee RK, Mottrie A, Payne CK, et al. A review of the current status of laparoscopic and robot-assisted sacrocolpopexy for pelvic organ prolapse. Eur Urol 2014;65(6):1128–37.
13. Serati M, Bogani G, Sorice P, et al. Robot-assisted sacrocolpopexy for pelvic organ prolapse: a systematic review and meta-analysis of comparative studies. Eur Urol 2014;66:303.
14. Judd JP, Siddiqui NY, Barnett JC, et al. Cost-minimization analysis of robotic-assisted, laparoscopic, and abdominal sacrocolpopexy. J Minim Invasive Gynecol 2010;17:493.
15. Elliott CS, Hsieh MH, Sokol ER, et al. Robot-assisted versus open sacrocolpopexy: a cost-minimization analysis. J Urol 2012;187:638.
16. Hoyte L, Rabbanifard R, Mezzick J, et al. Cost analysis of open versus robotic-assisted sacrocolpopexy. Female Pelvic Med Reconstr Surg 2012;18:335.
17. Paraiso MF, Jelovsek JE, Frick A, et al. Laparoscopic compared with robotic sacrocolpopexy for vaginal prolapse: a randomized controlled trial. Obstet Gynecol 2011;118:1005.
18. Anger JT, Mueller ER, Tarnay C, et al. Robotic compared with laparoscopic sacrocolpopexy: a randomized controlled trial. Obstet Gynecol 2014;123:5.
19. Skinner W. The focused factory. Harvard Business Review 1974;113.
20. FDA public health notification: serious complications associated with transvaginal placement of surgical mesh in repair of pelvic organ prolapse and stress urinary incontinence. Available at: http://www.fda.gov/medicaldevices/safety/alertsandnotices/publichealthnotifications/ucm061976.htm. Date issued: October 20, 2008. Page last updated: March 09, 2012.
21. FDA safety communication: UPDATE on serious complications associated with transvaginal placement of surgical mesh for pelvic organ prolapse. Available at: http://www.fda.gov/medicaldevices/safety/alertsandnotices/ucm262435.htm. Date issued: July 13, 2011.
22. Rosenblum N. Robotic approaches to prolapse surgery. Curr Opin Urol 2012;22:292.

Robot-Assisted Microsurgery in Male Infertility and Andrology

Ahmet Gudeloglu, MD[a,b], Jamin V. Brahmbhatt, MD[c], Sijo J. Parekattil, MD[c,*]

KEYWORDS

• Robotic • Vasectomy reversal • Varicocelectomy • Denervation • Spermatic cord

KEY POINTS

- The use of robotic assistance for microsurgery is still evolving.
- Early experiences seem to confer some benefits, and more data are developing from many institutions.
- As with any technology, the long-term feasibility and cost-effectiveness will be determined as further evaluation and randomized controlled studies are presented.

INTRODUCTION

The late 1970s witnessed 2 critical innovations in the treatment of infertility: (1) the operative microscope was introduced into male infertility microsurgical procedures, and (2) baby Louise was born as a result of the first use of assisted reproductive technology (ART).[1,2] Since then, several developments have occurred in ART. However, the technology in microsurgical infertility procedures has not really progressed until recently with the use of the da Vinci robotic platform (Intuitive Surgical, Inc, Sunnyvale, CA) for microsurgical vasectomy reversal.[3] Other disciplines, such as plastic surgery and hand surgery, have also explored the use of robotic assistance for microsurgical procedures.

Recent studies have shown that many microsurgical procedures for male infertility can be performed using the da Vinci robot.[4] This article provides the tips and tricks of robotic-assistance for microsurgical procedures in the treatment of male infertility and andrology, and also reviews the latest literature.

ROBOTIC-ASSISTED MICROSURGICAL VASECTOMY REVERSAL

Vasectomy reversal is one of the most technically challenging procedures in urology (especially vasoepididymostomy). The operating microscope significantly improved outcomes of these demanding procedures.[5] However, these techniques require dedicated training, experience and a skilled microsurgical assistant. Robotic-assisted microsurgical approaches with the da Vinci robotic platform can provide some advantages to overcome some of these caveats. Parekattil and colleagues[6] reported comparable outcomes for robotic assisted microsurgical vasectomy reversal (RAVV) compared with the pure microsurgical technique. However, these outcomes were achieved in the robotic group without the need for a skilled microsurgical assistant, and also included the robotic procedures performed during the early learning curve, thus indicating that perhaps the learning curve was shorter with robotic assistance than with the pure microscopic technique.

[a] Department of Urology, Memorial Ankara Hospital, Ankara, Turkey; [b] The PUR Clinic (Personalized Urology & Robotics), Clermont, FL, USA; [c] The PUR Clinic (Personalized Urology & Robotics), South Lake Hospital, 1900 Don Wickham Drive, Clermont, FL 34711, USA
* Corresponding author.
E-mail address: sijojp@gmail.com

Urol Clin N Am 41 (2014) 559–566
http://dx.doi.org/10.1016/j.ucl.2014.07.010
0094-0143/14/$ – see front matter

Recommended Instruments and Materials

- da Vinci Si surgical robotic system
- Zero-degree robotic camera
- VITOM camera system (KARL STORZ GmbH & Co. KG, Tuttlingen, Germany)
- Black Diamond Micro Forceps (Intuitive Surgical, Inc) in left and right arms
- Potts scissors (Intuitive Surgical, Inc) in the fourth arm
- 10-0 nylon sutures (Sharpoint, Surgical Specialties Corporation, Reading, PA)
- 9-0 nylon sutures (Ethilon; Ethicon Endo-Surgery, Inc, Cincinnati, OH)

Technique and Outcomes

Both robotic and pure microsurgical approaches are performed with similar microsurgical principles.[4] The 2 ends of the vas deferens are prepared through a scrotal incision and the proximal (testicular) vas fluid is assessed to see if any sperm are present. Robotic microsurgical vasectomy reversal is performed if sperm are found in the proximal vas deferens. If no sperm are found in the proximal vas deferens, robotic-assisted microsurgical vasoepididymostomy (RMVE) is then performed. The da Vinci robotic platform is docked on the right side with the patient in the supine position. Black Diamond Micro Forceps are used as needle drivers in the left and right arms, and the Potts scissors in the fourth arm is used to cut tied sutures (**Fig. 1**). This configuration allows the surgeon to control 3 instruments, thus obviating the need for a skilled microsurgical assistant.

Suture materials and techniques are similar to those used in standard microsurgery. Eight to ten 9-0 nylon sutures are used for the muscularis anastomosis. Five to six double-arm 10-0 nylon sutures are used for mucosal lumen anastomosis (**Fig. 2**). The two posterior 9-0 sutures are first placed to anastomose the posterior muscularis plate. Two 10-0 posterior sutures are then used to anastomose the posterior mucosal plate. Four to Five 10-0 anterior sutures are placed to complete the mucosal lumen anastomosis. Six to eight 9-0 nylon sutures are used to complete the anterior muscularis anastomosis.

In RMVE, 2 double-arm 10-0 sutures are used for vasal mucosal lumen to epididymal tubule anastomosis (**Fig. 3**) using a longitudinal intussusception technique. The vasal muscularis layer is sutured to the epididymal tunica using six to eight 9-0 nylon sutures.

The 0 degree camera of the da Vinci robotic platform provides up to 12× to 15× magnification. The authors incorporate an additional camera system (VITOM) as a fifth arm to the da Vinci robotic platform to obtain better (up to 16×–20×) magnification (see **Fig. 1**; **Fig. 4**). The TilePro (Intuitive Surgical, Inc) robotic surgical console software system allows viewing of 3 simultaneous real-time images (see **Figs. 2** and **3**). This 5-arm robotic approach enables microsurgeons to perform challenging maneuvers, including ultrafine suture placement and knot tying at 2 different focal lengths (2 different camera views, each at a different magnification), without needing to zoom in and out. The simultaneous viewing capabilities also allow microsurgeons to evaluate seminal fluid or tissues without having to stop operating.

Santomauro and colleagues[7] reported a 93% patency rates in 20 patients undergoing RMVV (18 bilateral RAVV, 2 unilateral RMVV). In this study, surgical residents (novice surgeons) were allowed to perform RMVV on one side, and the staff surgeon (experienced surgeon) performed the anastomosis on the contralateral side. No statistically significant difference in operative times was noted between the experienced and novice surgeons. This study illustrated that the robotic platform could potentially be used to decrease the learning curve for microsurgery.

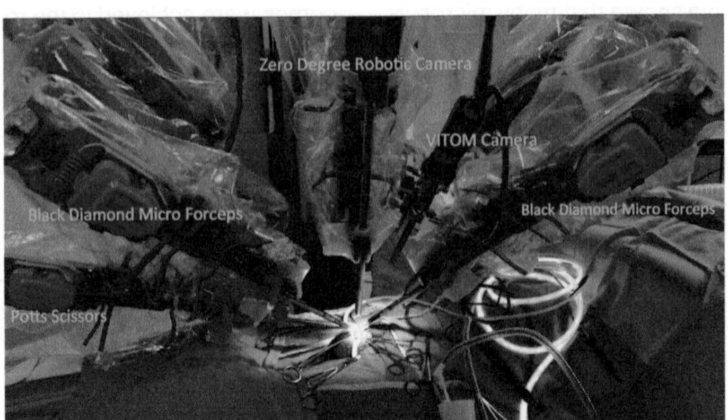

Fig. 1. Operative set up for robotic-assisted microsurgical vasectomy reversal.

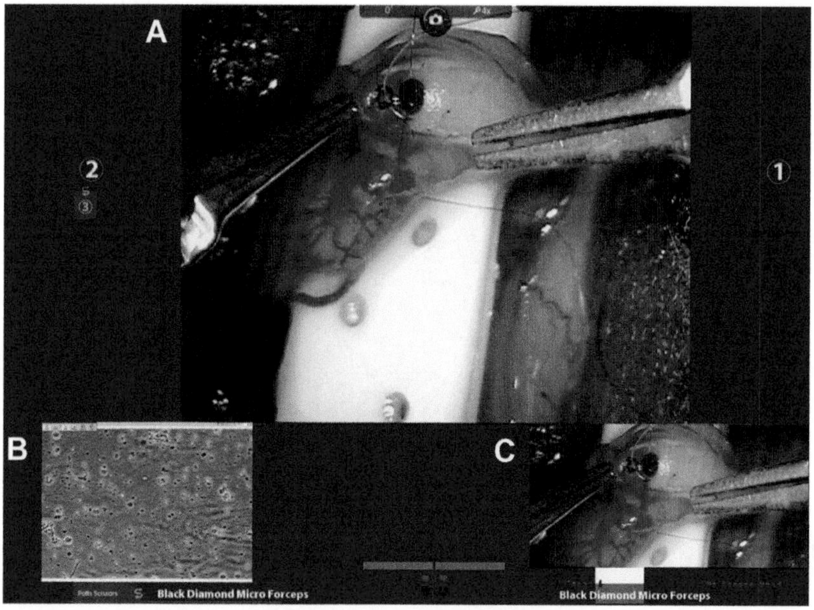

Fig. 2. View from surgeon console during RMVV. (*A*) Main view from the camera system of the da Vinci robotic platform, (*B*) real-time image from the left side with the andrology optical microscope (100×), and (*C*) view from the right side with the VITOM camera view for enhanced magnification.

Gudeloglu and colleagues[8] recently published outcomes for 180 vasectomy reversal procedures (106 RMVV, 74 RMVE). In their series they reported 97% and 55% success rates in RMVV and RMVE procedures, respectively. Median operative durations (skin to skin) were also reasonable, at 120 minutes for RMVV and 150 minutes for RMVE.

Robotic-assisted microsurgery also allows for novel microsurgical approaches; it allows microsurgery to be performed in locations of the body that would otherwise be difficult to access with open and standard microscopic techniques. Trost and colleagues[9] recently described the first bilateral intracorporeal robot-assisted microsurgical vasovasostomy in a patient who had

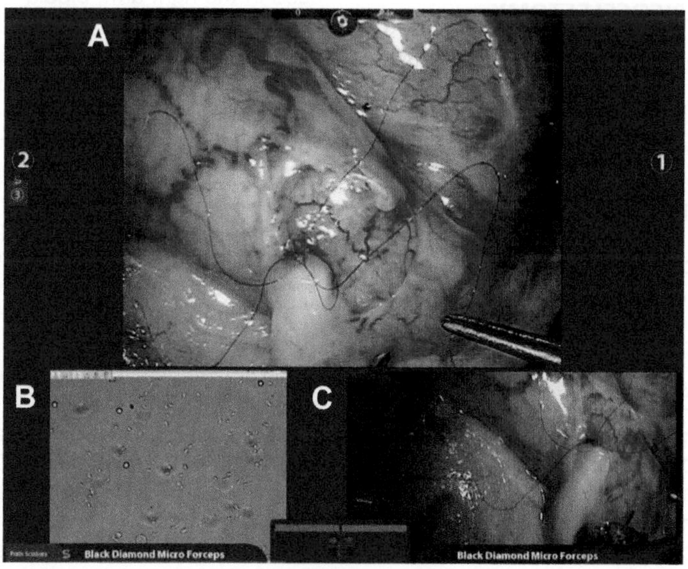

Fig. 3. View from surgeon console during RMVE. (*A*) Main view from the camera system of the da Vinci robotic platform, (*B*) real-time image from the left side with the andrology optical microscope (100×), and (*C*) view from the right side with the VITOM camera view for enhanced magnification.

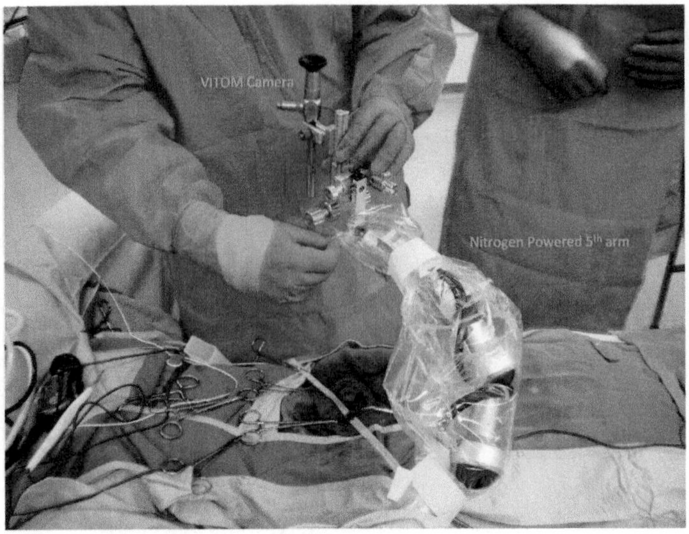

Fig. 4. VITOM camera system is being set up.

bilateral iatrogenic vasal obstruction from prior bilateral inguinal hernia repair. The investigators reported a successful minimally invasive bilateral intracorporeal anastomosis. This procedure would have been very difficult and would have required a very large abdominal incision with standard microsurgical and open approaches. The robotic approach allowed the surgeon to perform this type of reconstruction successfully with only 4 small skin incisions (port sites, <1 cm each).

ROBOTIC-ASSISTED MICROSURGICAL SUBINGUINAL VARICOCELECTOMY

Robotic assistance can also be successfully used for microsurgical subinguinal varicocelectomy procedures.[4,10] In this procedure, dilated veins are extracorporeally tied and ligated with robotic microinstruments through a subinguinal incision. Use of the robotic platform allows microsurgeons to simultaneously use additional instruments, such as a micro-Doppler probe with the fourth robotic arm in real-time during dissection of vessels with the other 2 hands.

Recommended Instruments and Materials

- da Vinci Si surgical robotic system
- Zero-degree robotic camera
- VITOM camera system
- Black Diamond Micro Forceps in the right arm
- Bipolar microforceps (Intuitive Surgical, Inc) in the left arm
- Monopolar curved scissors (Hot Shears; Intuitive Surgical, Inc) in the fourth arm
- Micro-Doppler probes: VTI (Vascular Technology, Inc, Nashua, NH) or Aloka (Hitachi Aloka Medical America, Inc, Tokyo, Japan)
- Two-inch 4-0 silk ties (Ethicon Endo-Surgery, Inc)

Technique and Outcomes

The procedure begins with a 1- to 2-cm subinguinal incision. The spermatic cord is brought up and placed on a tongue-blade platform, and the da Vinci robotic platform is docked from the patient's right side. The Black Diamond Micro Forceps are used in the right arm, bipolar microforceps in the left arm, and curved monopolar scissors in the fourth arm. The cremasteric muscle layer is separated and retracted using snaps on either side of the cord. The dilated veins are carefully dissected within the internal spermatic sheath. To avoid any inadvertent testicular arterial injury, Doppler ultrasound confirmation is performed with micro-Doppler ultrasound probes (**Fig. 5**). Two different micro-Doppler probes are commercially available. The VTI micro-Doppler probe (Vascular Technology Inc) generates audible signals, and the Aloka micro-Doppler probe (Hitachi Aloka) produces a visual image that can be simultaneous seen in the surgeon console via the TilePro software during the surgery. These probes are used to identify the testicular arteries. Once Doppler ultrasound confirmation is performed, the dilated veins are securely ligated with 4-0 silk ties and cut using the robotic curved monopolar scissors.

The authors' group has recently published the outcomes of 238 robotic-assisted microsurgical varicocelectomy.[8] Significant improvement was

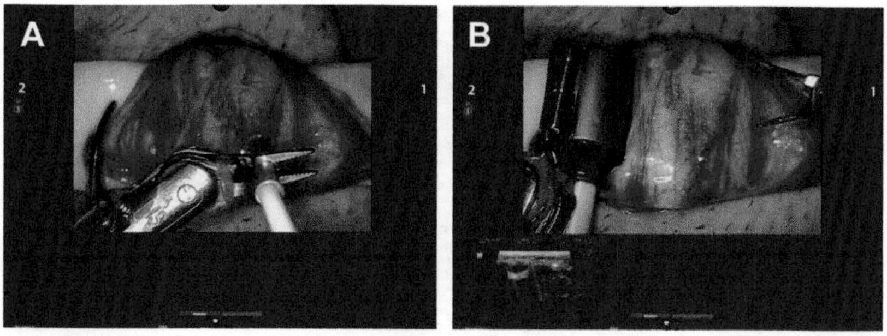

Fig. 5. Doppler evaluation of the spermatic cord vessels. (*A*) VTI audio micro-Doppler probe. (*B*) Aloka visual micro-Doppler probe.

seen in sperm count and/or motility in 76% of the patients who had oligospermia; 28% of patients with preoperative azoospermia were found to have sperm in their ejaculate 6 months postoperatively. Pain scores were also significantly decreased in 92% of patients who had testicular pain preoperatively. Eighty-four percent of these patients with testicular pain had also undergone robotic-assisted targeted microsurgical denervation of the spermatic cord during the varicocelectomy.

Mechlin and McCullough[11] recently also showed comparable outcomes with robotic varicocelectomy. They also found that the robotic approach provided a more controlled training environment for residents and fellows to advance their microsurgical and robotic skills.[11]

ROBOTIC-ASSISTED MICROSURGICAL TESTICULAR SPERM EXTRACTION

Microsurgical testicular sperm extraction (micro-TESE) has the highest sperm retrieval rates among various sperm retrieval techniques in patients with nonobstructive azoospermia.[12] The use of robotic assistance for micro-TESE provides the surgeon with real-time simultaneous imaging of the testicular tissue evaluation by the embryologist while the surgeon is operating. This capability is helpful for identifying areas or tubules that may be more likely to harbor sperm. As future sperm imaging detection techniques evolve (such as probe-based confocal laser endomicroscopy and multiphoton microscopy), integration of this technology will likely be easier in the robotic platform compared with standard microsurgery.

Recommended Instruments and Materials

- da Vinci Si surgical robotic system
- Zero-degree robotic camera
- VITOM camera system
- Black Diamond Micro Forceps in the right arm
- Bipolar microforceps in the left arm
- Potts scissors in the fourth arm

Technique and Outcomes

The procedure is performed with the patient in the supine position. The testicles are delivered through a midline scrotal incision and the da Vinci robotic platform is docked from the patient's right side after the testicular tunica is incised. Black Diamond Micro Forceps, bipolar microforceps, and the Potts scissors are loaded into the right, left, and the fourth arms, respectively. The surgeon view on the robotic console is seen in **Fig. 6**. The microsurgeon can easily identify dilated seminiferous tubules with the da Vinci 3-dimensional camera and the extramagnified VITOM image, and simultaneously evaluate the tissues sampled by the embryologist using the 100× phase-contrast microscope.

New imaging technology is being developed that may better identify tubules that harbor sperm during micro-TESE.[13,14] The robotic platform would provide an ideal platform for the integration of these types of adjunctive tools.

ROBOTIC-ASSISTED MICROSURGICAL TARGETED DENERVATION OF THE SPERMATIC CORD

Microsurgical denervation of the spermatic cord (MDSC) is a viable surgical treatment option for chronic groin or scrotal content pain (CGSCP). Chronic groin or scrotal content pain can be defined as pain that is unilateral or bilateral, intermittent or constant, and lasts longer than 3 months in the groin area or scrotal area (inguinal canal, spermatic cord, testis, or scrotum).[15,16] The authors' group has established a potential anatomic basis for MDSC.[17] They found structural abnormalities in 3 nerve fiber areas in the spermatic cord: (1) the cremasteric muscle, (2) the perivasal sheath, and (3) the posterior lipomatous and posterior arterial tissues. Microsurgical denervation of the spermatic cord is based on targeting these 3 nerve areas, and the authors focus on ligating these specific tissues.

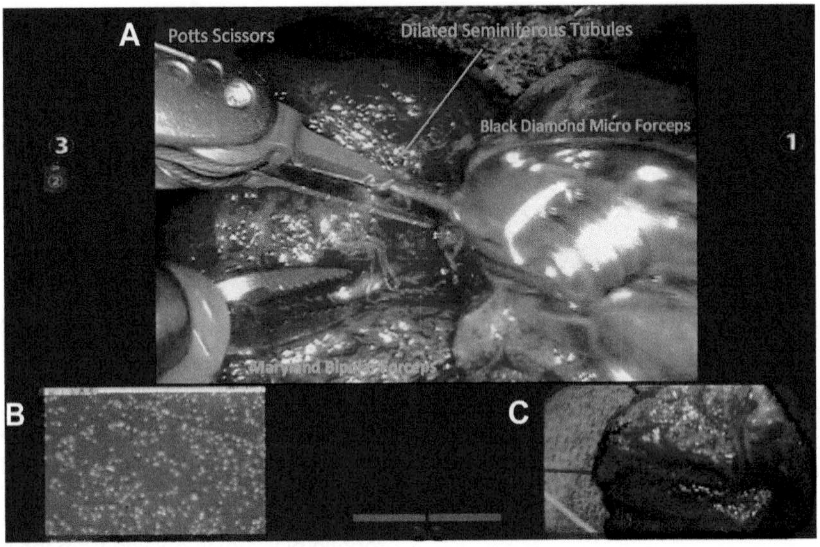

Fig. 6. View from surgeon console during robotic micro-TESE. (*A*) Main view from robotic camera. (*B*) Real-time image from andrology laboratory microscope. (*C*) VITOM camera view for enhanced magnification.

Recommended Instruments and Materials

- da Vinci Si surgical robotic system
- Zero-degree robotic camera
- VITOM camera system
- Black Diamond Micro Forceps in the right arm
- Bipolar microforceps in the left arm
- Curved monopolar scissors in the fourth arm
- FlexGuide carbon dioxide (CO_2) laser fiber (OmniGuide Inc, Cambridge, MA)
- ERBEJET2 hydrodissector (ERBE Inc, Tuebingen, Germany).
- AxoGuard bio-inert matrix (Axogen Inc, Gainesville, FL)

Technique and Outcomes

The spermatic cord is brought out via a small 1- to 2-cm subinguinal incision, similar to with the varicocelectomy procedure. The branches of the ilioinguinal and genitofemoral nerves at the external inguinal ring level are carefully cauterized medial, posterior, and lateral to the spermatic cord. The da Vinci robotic platform is docked from the right side of the patient. The Black Diamond Micro Forceps, bipolar microforceps, and curved monopolar scissors are used on the right, left, and fourth arms, respectively. In this targeted approach, the authors ligate the spermatic cord tissues more selectively than in the standard MDSC technique.[17,18] In standard or traditional MDSC, all tissues in the spermatic cord are ligated except for 1 to 2 arteries, 1 vein, and a few lymphatics. This targeted technique only involves the selective ligation of 3 specific areas in the spermatic cord based on the authors' anatomy study[17]: (1) the cremasteric muscle, (2) the perivasal sheath, and (3) the posterior lipomatous tissues. The entire internal spermatic sheath, the vas deferens, and most of the cord are preserved.

The authors compared peripheral tissue thermal injury from monopolar energy versus CO_2 laser energy in a cadaver study[19] and found significantly less peripheral thermal injury when the CO_2 laser was used. Thus, they use the flexible fiberoptic CO_2 laser fiber for ligation of all tissues to create the least amount of peripheral thermal injury (**Fig. 7**).

A recent study illustrated that targeted MDSC can be safely performed without any adverse testicular effects in an animal model.[20] The authors' group has also shown that use of a high-pressure water jet on the vas deferens can significantly reduce the number of residual nerve fibers without vascular compromise.[21] Thus, once ligation of the perivasal tissue is completed, the vas deferens are washed with a high-pressure waterjet (ERBEJET2 hydrodissector) to ablate any residual nerve fibers.

Finally, the spermatic cord is wrapped with a noncellular bioinert matrix material (Axoguard). This procedure is performed to reduce neuroma formation and decrease scar formation and irritation of the transected nerve endings.

Chronic groin or scrotal content pain can significantly impact a patient's quality of life. It can be caused by prior vasectomy, varicocele, trauma, any type of inguinal or scrotal surgery, hernia repair, or abdominal surgery, or it can be idiopathic.[22–25] The authors use a validated pain assessment tool (PIQ-6; QualityMetric Inc, Lincoln, RI) to assess preoperative and postoperative pain.

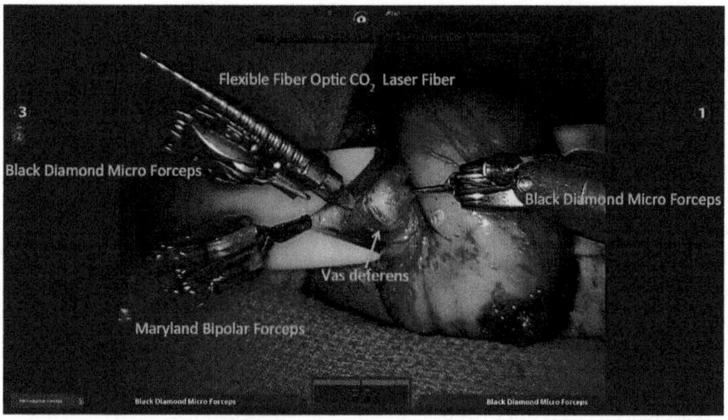

Fig. 7. View from surgeon console during robotic MDSC. Perivasal sheath is being ligated with CO_2 laser without compromising vas deferens.

Their recent analysis showed that robotic-assisted MDSC significantly relieved pain in 84.8% of patients with CGSCP (463/546).[8] Complete pain resolution was achieved in 70.5% of the patients, and more than 50% reduction in the pain score was obtained in 14.3% of patients.

The use of robotic assistance for MDSC allows surgeons to use several instruments simultaneously, eliminates physiologic tremor, and provides a stable ergonomic microsurgical platform and enhanced multiview magnification.

SUMMARY

The use of robotic assistance for microsurgery is still evolving. The early experiences seem to confer some benefits, and more data are developing from many institutions. As with any technology, the long-term feasibility and cost-effectiveness will be determined as further evaluation and randomized controlled studies are presented. The future looks promising.

REFERENCES

1. Silber SJ. Microsurgery in clinical urology. Urology 1975;6(2):150–3.
2. Steptoe PC, Edwards RG. Birth after the reimplantation of a human embryo. Lancet 1978;2(8085):366.
3. Fleming C. Robot-assisted vasovasostomy. Urol Clin North Am 2004;31(4):769–72.
4. Parekattil SJ, Gudeloglu A. Robotic assisted andrological surgery. Asian J Androl 2013;15(1):67–74.
5. Silber SJ, Grotjan HE. Microscopic vasectomy reversal 30 years later: a summary of 4010 cases by the same surgeon. J Androl 2004;25(6):845–59.
6. Parekattil SJ, Gudeloglu A, Brahmbhatt J, et al. Robotic assisted versus pure microsurgical vasectomy reversal: technique and prospective database control trial. J Reconstr Microsurg 2012;28(7):435–44.
7. Santomauro MG, Choe CH, James O, et al. Robotic vasovasostomy: description of technique and review of initial results. J Robot Surg 2012;6(3):217–21.
8. Gudeloglu A, Brahmbhatt JV, Parekattil SJ. Robotic microsurgery in male infertility and urology—taking robotics to the next level. Transl Androl Urol 2014;3(1):102–12.
9. Trost L, Parekattil S, Wang J, et al. Intracorporeal robot-assisted microsurgical vasovasostomy for the treatment of bilateral vasal obstruction occurring following bilateral inguinal hernia repairs with mesh placement. J Urol 2014;191(4):1120–5.
10. Shu T, Taghechian S, Wang R. Initial experience with robot-assisted varicocelectomy. Asian J Androl 2008;10(1):146–8.
11. Mechlin C, McCullough A. V1590 robotic microsurgical varicocele repair: initial experience and surgical outcomes from a single academic center. J Urol 2013;189(4):e652–3.
12. Schlegel PN. Nonobstructive azoospermia: a revolutionary surgical approach and results. Semin Reprod Med 2009;27(2):165–70.
13. Trottmann M, Liedl B, Becker A, et al. 847 Probe-based confocal laser endomicroscopy (pCLE): a new imaging technique for in situ localization of vital spermatozoa. Eur Urol Suppl 2013;12(1):e847.
14. Najari BB, Ramasamy R, Sterling J, et al. Pilot study of the correlation of multiphoton tomography of ex vivo human testis with histology. J Urol 2012;188(2):538–43.
15. Davis BE, Noble MJ, Weigel JW, et al. Analysis and management of chronic testicular pain. J Urol 1990;143(5):936–9.
16. Levine L. Chronic orchialgia: evaluation and discussion of treatment options. Ther Adv Urol 2010;2(5–6):209–14.
17. Parekattil SJ, Gudeloglu A, Brahmbhatt JV, et al. Trifecta nerve complex: potential anatomic basis for microsurgical denervation of the spermatic cord for chronic orchialgia. J Urol 2013;190:265–70.

18. Levine LA. Microsurgical denervation of the spermatic cord. J Sex Med 2008;5(3):526–9.
19. Gudeloglu A, Brahmbhatt J, Parekattil S. Prospective comparison of flexible fiberoptic CO2 laser and standard monopolar cautery for robotic microsurgical denervation of the spermatic cord procedure. Fertil Steril 2013;100(3):S123–4.
20. Laudano MA, Osterberg EC, Sheth S, et al. Microsurgical denervation of rat spermatic cord: safety and efficacy data. BJU Int 2014;113:795–800.
21. Gudeloglu A, Iqbal Z, Parekattil SJ, et al. Hydrodissection for improved microsurgical denervation of the spermatic cord: prospective blinded randomized control trial in a rat model. Fertil Steril 2011;96(Suppl 3):S87–8.
22. Tandon S, Sabanegh E Jr. Chronic pain after vasectomy: a diagnostic and treatment dilemma. BJU Int 2008;102(2):166–9.
23. Granitsiotis P, Kirk D. Chronic testicular pain: an overview. Eur Urol 2004;45(4):430–6.
24. Alfieri S, Amid PK, Campanelli G, et al. International guidelines for prevention and management of postoperative chronic pain following inguinal hernia surgery. Hernia 2011;15(3):239–49.
25. Larsen SM, Benson JS, Levine LA. Microdenervation of the spermatic cord for chronic scrotal content pain: single institution review analyzing success rate after prior attempts at surgical correction. J Urol 2013;189(2):554–8.

Image-Guided Surgery and Emerging Molecular Imaging

Advances to Complement Minimally Invasive Surgery

Christopher R. Mitchell, MD, S. Duke Herrell, MD*

KEYWORDS

• Image guidance • Robotics • Surgical navigation • Molecular imaging • Urologic surgery

KEY POINTS

- Image-guided surgery and molecular imaging remain areas of intense basic science and clinical research.
- Image-guided surgery technologies have become standards of surgical care in other specialties, including neurosurgery and orthopedics, but remains in its infancy in urologic and other soft tissue–based surgical specialties.
- Current research endeavors into the combined application of image-guided surgery and robotic urologic surgery presents the unique challenges of soft tissue registration, tissue deformation, operative navigation, and incorporation into the surgical work flow.
- Although progress has been made, continued collaboration between engineers and surgeons is required to achieve the ultimate goals of improved ease and accuracy of performing surgery leading to improved patient outcomes.
- The incorporation of molecular imaging into minimally invasive surgery remains in the early stages of development, however, is likely to continue to increase in importance with development of molecular markers specific to urologic malignancies.

INTRODUCTION

With recent advances in imaging and surgical instrumentation, there has been transition away from traditional open surgery toward new minimally invasive approaches. Open surgery has its distinct advantages in providing the surgeon with unrestricted visual, force, and tactile feedback, often at the expense of large incisions and surgical trauma. The emergence of robotic surgery with mechatronically enhanced or robotic-assisted instruments has significantly improved the capabilities of the minimally invasive surgeon, allowing surgical procedures to be carried out with unprecedented accuracy and efficiency. However, one of the drawbacks of minimally invasive surgery is the lack of haptic sensing and feedback to assist with tissue discrimination. Accordingly, extensive work is being done in the area of image guidance to thereby integrate enhanced visual information to improve ease, accuracy, and surgeon comfort with performing complex robotic surgeries.

Department of Urologic Surgery, Vanderbilt University Medical Center, A1302 Medical Center North, Nashville, TN 37232-2765, USA
* Corresponding author.
E-mail address: duke.herrell@vanderbilt.edu

Urol Clin N Am 41 (2014) 567–580
http://dx.doi.org/10.1016/j.ucl.2014.07.011
0094-0143/14/$ – see front matter

Traditional approaches to surgery, both open and robotic, are planned preoperatively using high-fidelity axial medical imaging, such as computed tomography (CT) and magnetic resonance imaging (MRI). These images are typically reviewed off-line and often only as a 2-dimensional (2D) display of the 3-dimensional (3D) anatomy. The surgeon then uses innate knowledge of human anatomy combined with the ability of the human brain to align objects in 3D space in what is referred to as *mental coregistration* of the imaging onto the body and organs. This, in essence, serves as a road map of anatomic relationships to facilitate the proposed surgery. Conversely, image-guided surgery (IGS) provides in situ, real time covisualization of either preoperative or intraoperative data along with the actual anatomy, and the imaging is displayed in a spatially accurate manner coordinated (registered) to the actual anatomy. Thus, the overall goals of IGS are to provide a fully planned procedure before its execution, integrate either real-time intraoperative imaging or preoperative imaging for enhanced accuracy, and to track anatomic changes and tissue deformation during surgery.[1] In the most simplistic form, image guidance is used to improve the surgeon's awareness of both the anatomy of the target organ and its relationship with surrounding structures. This review explores recent advances in IGS and emerging molecular imaging technologies aimed to improve accuracy, precision, safety, and surgeon confidence during urologic robotic surgery.

GENERAL PRINCIPLES OF IGS

IGS can be divided into 2 broad categories, which either utilize preoperatively obtained images or intraoperative, real-time imaging. In the first method, preoperatively obtained images for a specific patient are actively integrated into the workflow and visual display for the operation. Therefore, the images are used to map surgical position and orientation rather than functioning simply as a reference atlas. The second method involves active intraoperative imaging with real-time production of imaging (ie, fluoroscopy, ultrasound, CT, MRI) and requires operating room–based imaging modalities, special instrumentation, and ancillary personnel. With intraoperative CT or MRI, the obvious drawbacks of increased cost and personnel and the limited availability of these imaging modalities within the operating room setting, will likely restrict development and widespread adoption of techniques within this realm of IGS. Thus, most research has focused on using preoperative imaging to create an augmented reality with these images superimposed onto the surgical field of view. Imaging is registered with the patient's intraoperative anatomy to actively display organ, instrumentation, and vital structure location. This type of surgical navigation presents a unique set of challenges to overcome, which primarily involves concepts such as image registration, tracking, and deformation adjustment.

Registration

Central to any IGS system is the process of registration, that is, determining the mathematical relationship between objects in the preoperative images and their physical locations in the operating room. Basic registration is premised on aligning imaging and anatomy in a 3D coordinate space system.[2] A 3D-rendered surface allows for easier understanding of the spatial relationship between a surgical target and other structures the surgeon may wish to avoid. Registration may be done based on anatomic landmarks (points) or markers (fiducials) inserted before image acquisition that can be seen precisely on the imaging study and also identified within the patient in the operating room. Using high-speed computer algorithms, rigid 3D point-to-point alignment is performed. Thus, subsurface anatomy and location of important surrounding structures can be displayed to the surgeon on a video screen or as a virtual overlay on to the patient (ie, augmented virtual reality). The most common example of rigid fiducial-based registration is found with image-guided brain and spine interventions, in which the bony structure's relationships to the vital other structures is available to the surgeon before bringing the patient to the operating room. However, abdominal organs pose a particular challenge, as they are not accessible preoperatively for placement of fiducials and also lack easily identifiable landmarks that can function as points. Therefore, most work with registration for soft tissue applications has been based on surface registration, whereby a captured topographic surface (physical space) is then matched to a surface that has been extracted from preoperative images (image space). With this technique, large numbers of surface point coordinates are captured by sweeping a tracked tool over the surface of the target organ or assembling a surface using a reflected laser beam geometry captured from a laser range scanner.

Localization and Tracking Techniques

Localization is the process by which the surgeon is able to identify and display surgical tool tip locations within the viewing field and in relationship to the registered imaging and vital structures, which are commonly not yet encountered. This requires accurate tracking of the 3D tool, which is most commonly performed with either of 2 methods, optical or electromagnetic tracking. Optical tracking uses a specialized camera system, which can repetitively determine the tool tip position using the recording of geometric alignment of special trackers (geometrically arranged optical sources or optical reflectors) placed on the proximal end of the tool. These systems have submillimeter accuracy but require line of sight between the camera and trackers, which can be difficult to obtain because of constraints of the operating room environment. Electromagnetic tracking uses a magnetic field sensor device and a wire-based electromagnetic tracker on the patient and instruments, allowing tracking actively by the system. Advantages of this method are no requirement for direct line of sight and good accuracy; however, variations in the electromagnetic field strength and presence of large metallic objects, such as the robot or the operating table, can result in error.

Registration Error and Tissue Deformation

A target is a point with known locations in both real and virtual space that is not used in the creation of the transformation matrix. The difference between the transformed location and its actual location in real space is the target registration error (TRE).[3] This serves as the true assessment of registration quality. However, to be able to obtain this metric, the points must be definitively identified in both spaces, which can be challenging given issues with exposure of the target, tissue deformation, and validation. The most significant barrier to real-time image overlay is that of tissue deformation, which can occur from a variety of sources, including respiratory and patient motion, changes to perfusion, and surgical manipulation. When considering that for many procedures, millimeter or even submillimeter precision is required for safe and effective performance, the ability to account for tissue change (deformation) is essential, especially for image-guided tumor resection. Naturally, the process of surgical manipulation, dissection, and resection results in significant changes to the target tissue, which must be taken into account to ensure accuracy and reduce error.

Intraoperative Imaging

Real-time intraoperative imaging presents a strategy for avoiding issues related to tissue deformation, as the information being obtained is live and dynamic. Examples of intraoperative imaging techniques are MRI, fluoroscopy, CT, cone-beam CT, and ultrasound scan (US); however, to date, no single modality has proven to be the answer to IGS. Intraoperative MRI is costly, slow, and a major intrusion into the surgical process. Fluoroscopy and CT involve significant radiation and accompanied risk to the patient and operating room staff. Cone-beam CT based on flat panel digital detector technology is a modified technique to allow for use in the operating room. X-rays are delivered in a cone rather than the conventional fan shape used in helical scanners. This allows for acquisition of a large area in a single pass of the C-arm using a digital flat panel detector. This modality is not without significant limitations, as it is expensive and not widely available at most hospitals and also produces images of a lower quality than customarily obtained with conventional CT scan. US is mostly a 2D imaging modality that lacks clear tissue discrimination and results in overall poor image quality compared with axial 3D imaging, thereby limiting its utility in IGS. However, in the future, by combining real-time intraoperative imaging with high-resolution axial 3D preoperative images, the strengths of both can be preserved and the weaknesses mitigated.

IMAGE-GUIDED PARTIAL NEPHRECTOMY

To date, most work and progress toward true image guidance in the urologic field has occurred during robotic-assisted laparoscopic partial nephrectomy. Given the nature of the surgery, partial nephrectomy seems ideally suited for potential improvements with image guidance. First, image guidance may facilitate more facile and accurate identification of important landmark structures, such as the renal hilum and subsequent major blood vessels and their respective relationship to the target. Furthermore, image guidance may improve the precision of tumor resection to ensure complete tumor resection, while achieving maximal nephron sparing. Finally, IGS for partial nephrectomy may increase surgeon comfort with this complex operation, thereby potentially increasing the application of nephron-sparing surgeries.

Initial work on image-guided partial nephrectomy focused on the simplest form of registration, whereby 3D reconstructions were manually overlaid to the best fit of the operative view by the surgeon using knowledge of human anatomy.[4,5] Manual registration overlay, although an improvement over surgeon mental coregistration, falls short of true IGS and does not allow error calculation. Therefore, fiducial-based registration has been explored by several groups. Teber and colleagues[4] used 3D cone-beam imaging with fiducial markers to create 3D reconstructions of the organ that were subsequently registered to the real time image. This technique produced a high level of accuracy with TRE of 0.5 mm in ex vivo studies (**Fig. 1**). Although the fiducial insertion technique used is valid in the laboratory, insertion of barbed fiducials and the need for intraoperative scanning have limited clinical application of this technique.

Considerable work has been done using surface-based registration for robotic partial nephrectomy. In surface-based methods, digitization and capture of a patch or cloud of the surface anatomy is accomplished through a stylus or a range scanner. This extracted surface is then fit to a surface segmented from preoperative images. Registered preoperative images are displayed using the IGS software application, as multiplanar reformatted slices or as a rendered volume. These visualizations allow surgeons to see their current surgical position in addition to presenting a predicted map based on preoperative imaging of vital anatomy beneath the organ surface or beyond the optically visualized field.

Most research from our laboratory initially used surface-based registration via tracked da Vinci robotic instrument as a topography-defining stylus to create an intraoperative model of the surface anatomy of the kidney (**Fig. 2**).[6,7] To perform this, accurate knowledge of the location of the instrument tip in 3D space is required and can either be obtained via intrinsic or extrinsic tracking. The intrinsic method uses the kinematic chain and tracking capabilities inherent to the da Vinci surgical system (**Fig. 3**A). This approach is limited by

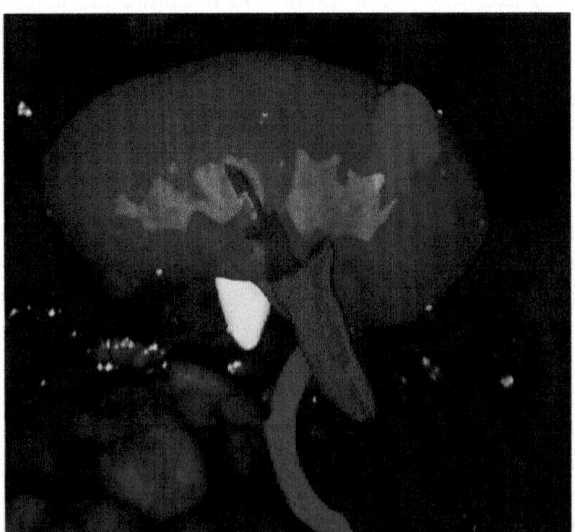

Fig. 1. With the guidance of augmented reality, the renal tumor was identified through the surrounding fat. (*From* Teber D, Guven S, Simpfendörfer T, et al. Augmented reality: a new tool to improve surgical accuracy during laparoscopic partial nephrectomy? Preliminary in vitro and in vivo results. Eur Urol 2009;56(2):335; with permission.)

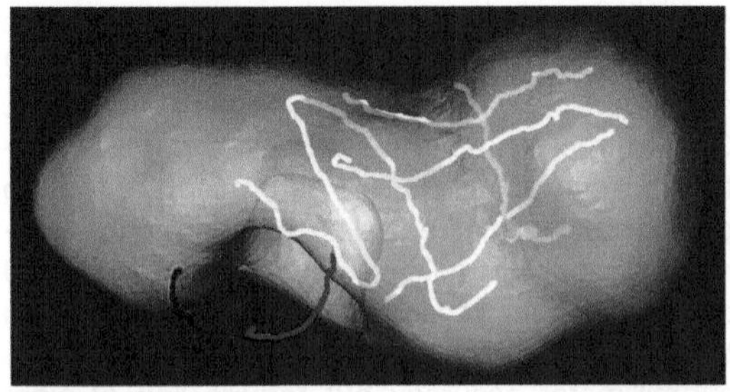

Fig. 2. Surface capture of the kidney registered to segmented CT of the kidney and mass. White lines represent surface tracking done with tracked da Vinci tool. Blue and red lines represent hilar structures. Gray surface model represents segmented kidney surface from preoperative CT scan, including large lower pole tumor (right side of figure). (*From* Herrell SD, Galloway RL, Su LM. Image-guided robotic surgery: update on research and potential applications in urologic surgery. Curr Opin Urol 2012;22(1):50; with permission.)

inaccuracy of measurements of the da Vinci passive and active robotic joint positions, which have been found to exceed 10 mm.[8] Extrinsic tracking uses commercially available magnetic or optical tracking systems to ascertain the positions of the surgical instrument (see **Fig. 3**B). We developed[7] a hybrid approach combining both intrinsic and extrinsic tracking (optical tracking, Polaris Spectra), which significantly decreased the tracking error to less than 2 mm (see **Fig. 3**C). Although surface registration through a tracked tool is feasible, error and lack of rapid ability to recapture and reregister remained limitations. Laser range finders present an alternative approach, which has been used with success in open surgery (**Fig. 4**). However, to date, no suitable laparoscopic laser range finder has yet to undergo trial for renal surgery.[6]

The stereoscopic camera used in the da Vinci Robotic Surgical System offers a platform for 3D-to-3D registration of preoperative cross-sectional imaging with a live intraoperative view. Potential advantages of this approach include no requirements for preplacement of fiducials, markers, or external tracking devices, while still offering the ability to account for organ movement with rapid image update. Su and colleagues[9] published the initial report of the theory and postprocedure display on using robotic vision–based image-guided renal surgery by creating an augmented reality overlay for partial nephrectomy. They used reconstructed, segmented preoperative 3D CT data and posthoc manual registration to previously recorded video feeds from the binocular robotic endoscope. Next, a 3D reconstructed

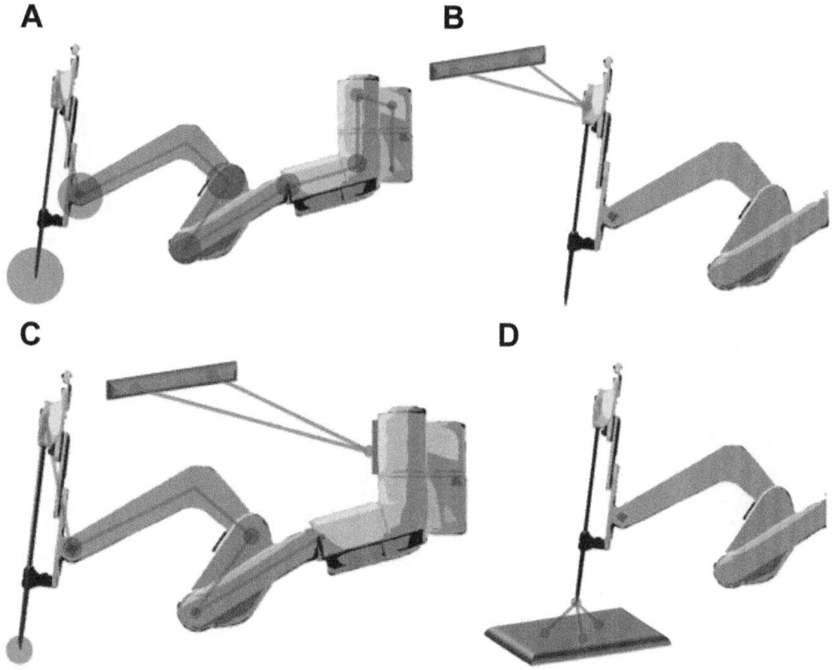

Fig. 3. (*A*) Intrinsic tracking using the joint positions of the da Vinci robotic arms. (*B*) Optical tracking of robotic instrument requires a continuous direct line of sight. (*C*) Hybrid tracking system uses optical tracking to ascertain the position of the passive joints, thereby reducing error at the instrument tip. (*D*) Electromagnetic tracking. (*From* Hughes-Hallett A, Mayer EK, Marcus HJ, et al. Augmented reality partial nephrectomy: examining the current status and future perspectives. Urology 2014;83(2):269; with permission.)

mesh model was manually aligned to the video image of the kidney with edges in the mesh model and anchored in the algorithm to identifiable kidney surface points on the video allowing for repetitive tracking of the overlay with the kidney during camera and kidney motion (**Fig. 5**). Although this initial work was encouraging, the inability to assess a true accuracy of the registration and lack of further development does not allow for a formal assessment of the accuracy or potential.

IMAGE-GUIDED MINIMALLY INVASIVE RADICAL PROSTATECTOMY

Robotic assisted laparoscopic prostatectomy (RALP) has emerged as the most commonly

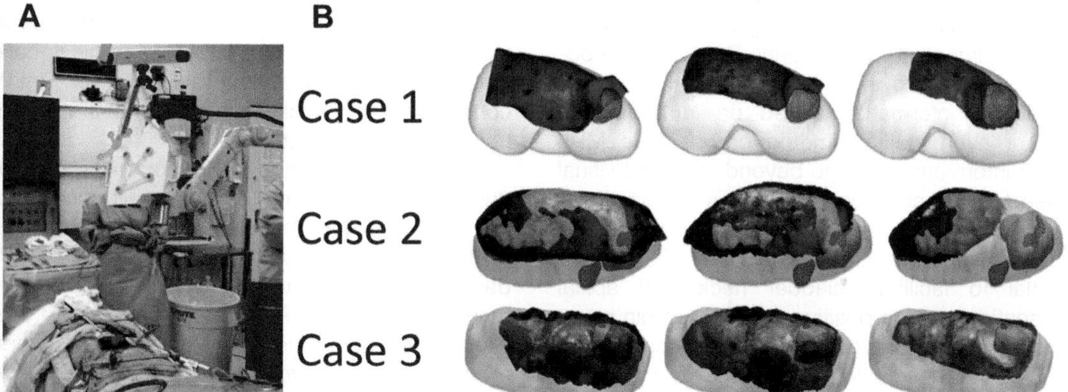

Fig. 4. (*A*) Laser range scanner capturing kidney surface during open partial nephrectomy. (*B*) Posthoc-registered laser range scanner surfaces (*red*) shown over corresponding preoperative segmented CT surfaces (*white*). (*From* Herrell SD, Galloway RL, Su LM. Image-guided robotic surgery: update on research and potential applications in urologic surgery. Curr Opin Urol 2012;22(1):50; with permission.)

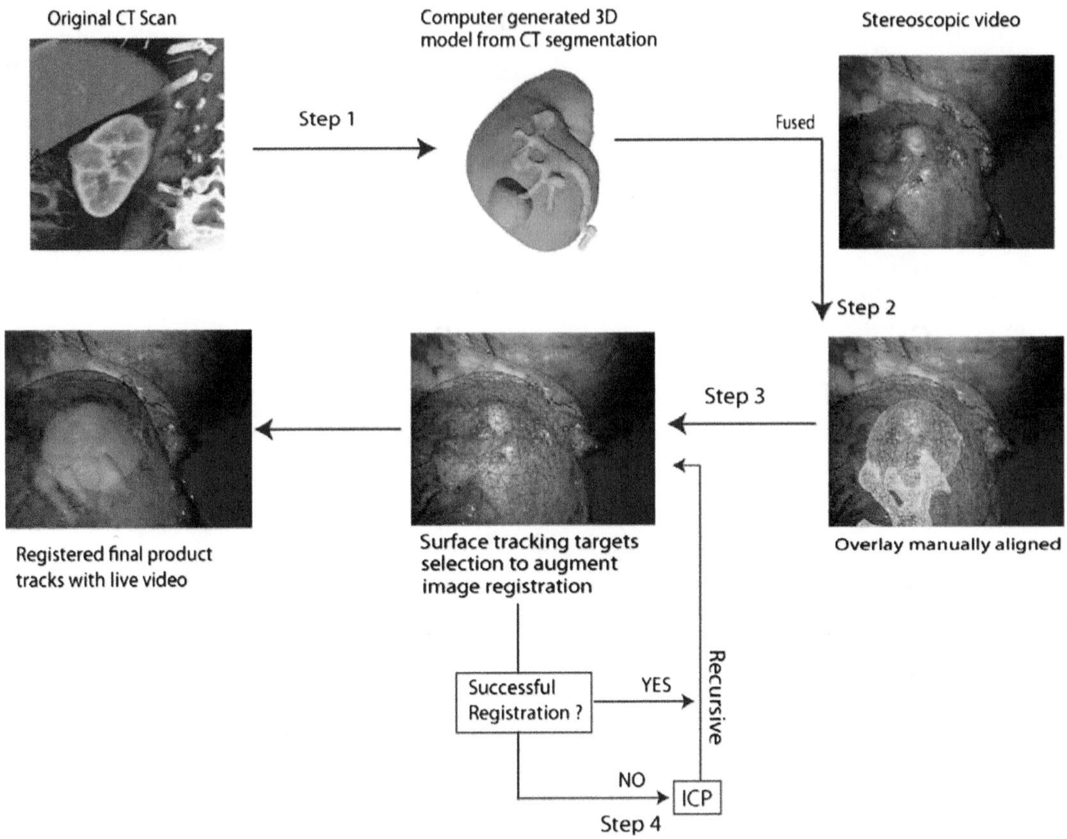

Fig. 5. Stereoscopic video overlay registration algorithm. Flow chart displays intermediary steps needed to achieve successful 3D manual registration of preoperative CT image to live stereoscopic video. (*From* Su LM, Vagvolgyi BP, Agarwal R, et al. Augmented reality during robot-assisted laparoscopic partial nephrectomy: toward real-time 3D-CT to stereoscopic video registration. Urology 2009;73(4):898; with permission.)

performed surgical treatment for prostate cancer.[10] The robotic platform offers capability for integration of image guidance into the surgical procedure and, therefore, has the potential to improve functional and oncologic outcomes. Specifically, image guidance during RALP has the potential to improve the surgery by providing additional information based on intraoperative US or even multiparametric preoperative MRI. Such information may go beyond standard visual cues to locating critical structures including the neurovascular bundles, urethra, capsule, and extracapsular tumor(s). In turn, this may offer the potential to facilitate bladder neck and apical dissection, reduce positive surgical margin rates, and increase neurovascular bundle preservation.

The initial description of real-time intraoperative transrectal US (TRUS) guidance as an adjunct to laparoscopic prostatectomy was made by Ukimura and Gill.[11] The authors reported improved accuracy in performing various steps in the procedure, most notably dissection of the neurovascular bundles, with vascular flow being used as a surrogate for bundle preservation. This technique was able to yield lower rates of positive surgical margins.[12] Similarly, van der Poel and colleagues[13] reported that a robotic novice surgeon achieved a reduction in the number of positive surgical margins during the initial learning curve of RALP compared with a similarly inexperienced surgeon not using TRUS guidance.

Routine incorporation of intraoperative TRUS during RALP was limited by the requirement of a human assistant for manipulation of the US probe. To circumvent this problem, Han and colleagues[14] developed a novel, robotic transrectal US probe manipulator (TRUS Robot) compatible for use with the daVinci Surgical Robot, in a tandem robot-assisted laparoscopic radical prostatectomy (**Fig. 6**). The robotic arm supports and manipulates the transrectal US probe under the joystick control of surgeon, while positional tracking and reconstruction software allows for 3D reconstructions to be viewed on the display

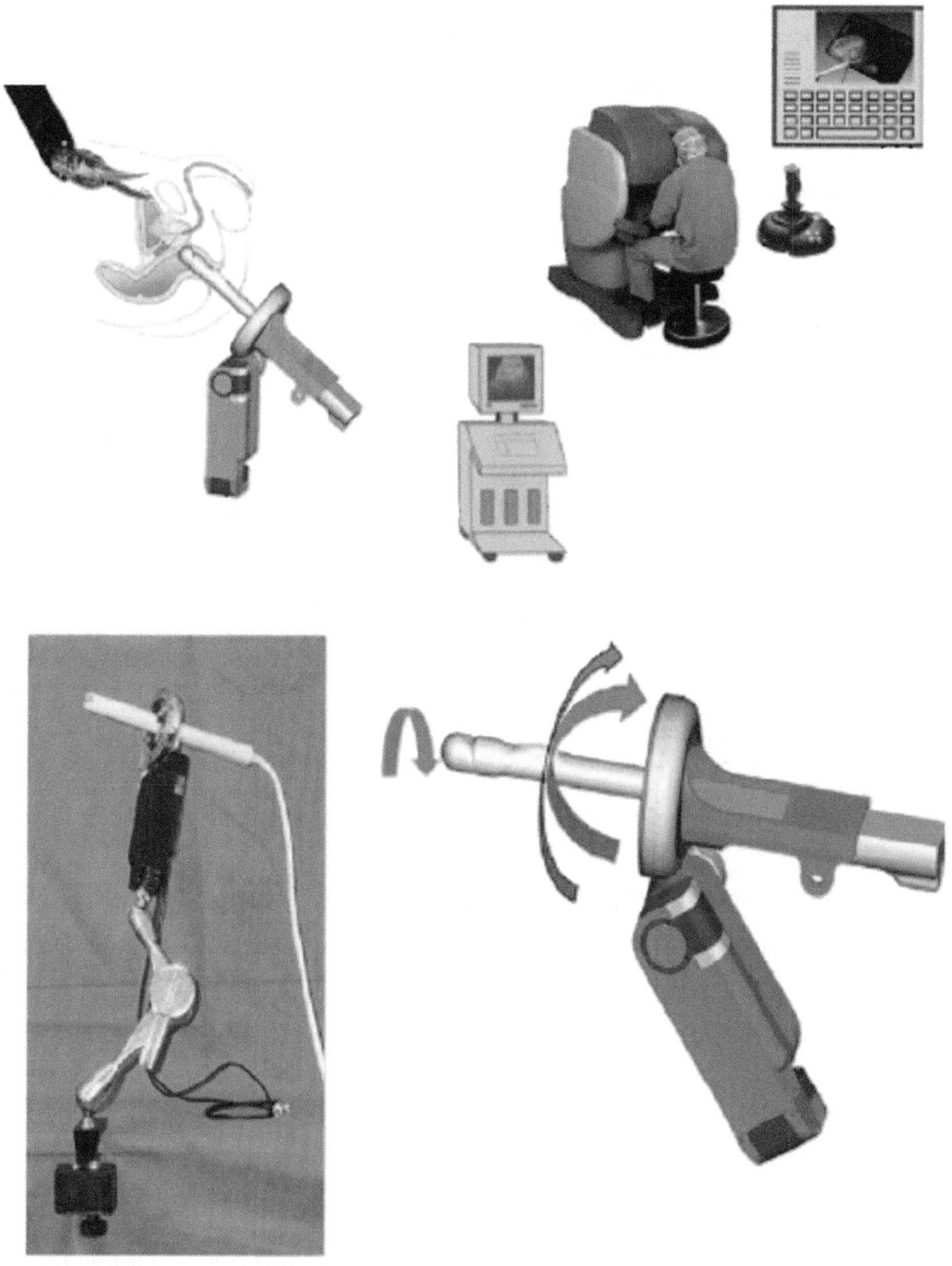

Fig. 6. Tandem robot-assisted robotic prostatectomy schematic and TRUS robot. The TRUS probe is robotically controlled by a manipulator robot with multidirectional control. (*From* Han M, Kim C, Mozer P, et al. Tandem-robot assisted laparoscopic radical prostatectomy to improve the neurovascular bundle visualization: a feasibility study. Urology 2011;77(2):503; with permission.)

within the da Vinci surgeon console. An additional robotic TRUS-manipulated system, the ViKY robot has been used with noted improvements in positive surgical margin rates and good surgeon feedback while performing RALP.[15,16] The most obvious limitation, the inability of US to provide precise anatomic detail, especially as it relates to identifying the neurovascular bundles, remains problematic, thus, has curbed widespread adoption of this technology.

Accurate and reliable imaging of the location and relevance in preservation of urinary and sexual function of critical structures in and around the prostate remains a developing field. The ability to use such preoperative functional anatomic information intraoperatively would be the ultimate goal but would require registration and organ tracking. To that end, Simpfendorfer and colleagues[17] proposed a system in which fiducial markers are inserted into the prostate during laparoscopic prostatectomy, which can be visualized on both TRUS imaging and a live endoscopic video. The system traces the navigation aids in real time and computes a registration between TRUS image and laparoscopic video based on the 2D-3D point correspondences.

Many researchers remain skeptical about the requirement of fiducial(s) placement within the target organ and have sought alternative solutions, using modeling of the bony pelvis as the basis for registration and tracking.[18,19] Gao and colleagues[18] found that bony pelvis can be accurately and robustly segmented using a combination of statistical deformation and modeling using multiatlas techniques to provide accurate registration (TRE, 1.33 mm) and tracking (average position error, 0.13 mm). However, currently, segmentation schemes are extremely time consuming to run and currently cannot realistically be applied to the current operative environment. Although steps in right direction, the currently proposed methods remain limited by the ability to deform preoperative images to mimic intraoperative tissue deformation, thus, the search for a clinical applicable IGS system for minimally invasive prostatectomy continues.

MOLECULAR IMAGING FOR UROLOGIC SURGERY

Molecular imaging (MI) represents the visualization, characterization, and measurement of biologic processes at the molecular and cellular level in humans and other living systems. MI uses probes known as *biomarkers*, which target specific molecular pathways that are fundamentally involved in disease processes. Therefore, molecular imaging evaluates changes in cellular physiology and function, rather than anatomy, potentially leading to earlier and more sensitive manifestations of the disease. Recent advances in MI technology have permitted translation from bench research to valuable clinically applicable imaging studies. The most well-established molecular imaging modality, positron emission tomography uses positron-emitting radioisotopes as molecular probes.[20] Various positron emission tomography imaging modalities have recently been shown to be useful in certain circumstances for urologic malignancies including testicular cancer,[21,22] prostate cancer,[23,24] and bladder cancer.[25] Importantly, continued work has led to an expansion of MI technologies to include various forms of fluorescent and optical imaging techniques to aid in disease identification and treatment. However, translating these technologies into real-time information available to the operating surgeon remains a challenging obstacle. Ideally, in the future interventional molecular image-guided technologies will be routinely incorporated into the operative flow to allow for better detection and treatment of tumors and facilitate improved surgical outcomes.

MOLECULAR IMAGING DURING PROSTATECTOMY

MI has been sought to improve both functional and oncologic outcomes of surgically managed prostate cancer. Specifically, attempts have been made to use fluorescent imaging to accurately identify the neurovascular bundles to facilitate nerve sparing prostatectomy. Davila and colleagues[26] evaluated whether fluorescent tracers could be used to label the neurovascular bundles and major pelvic ganglion to assist with nerve-sparing radical prostatectomy. In this study, male Sprague-Dawley rats received injections of deionized water, Flouro-Gold, Fast Blue, Flouro-Ruby, or green fluorescent pseudorabies virus (**Fig. 7**). They found that injection of Flouro-Gold into the rat penis 2 to 3 days before surgery might help with identification of the neurovascular bundles during surgery. Although considered a breakthrough, this technology has not been trialed on humans and remains investigational.

Other efforts to use MI during prostatectomy have focused on improving oncologic resection margins. It has been proposed that by labeling the cancerous portions of the prostate to be identified intraoperatively, improvements in rates of positive surgical margins can be obtained. Previous studies have found selective enhancement of 5-aminolevulinic acid (5-ALA) in human prostate cancer after oral administration.[27] Therefore, Adam and colleagues[28] sought to investigate the feasibility of intraoperative identification of positive surgical margins during open or laparoscopic radical prostatectomy. In this prospective study, 39 patients were given oral 5-ALA and subsequently underwent radical prostatectomy (either open or laparoscopically) with a photodynamic

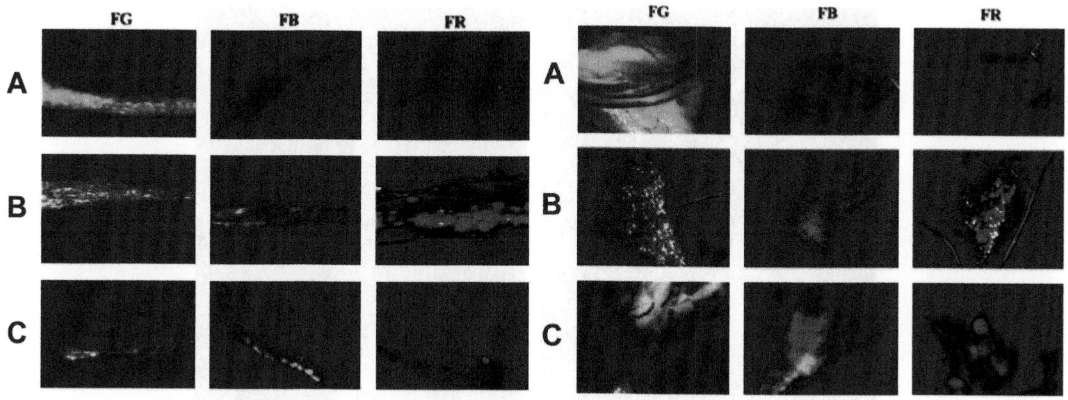

Fig. 7. Identification of the neurovascular bundles (*left*) and major pelvic ganglion (*right*) at (*A*) 2 days, (*B*) 3 days, and (*C*) 12 days after injection with Flouro-Gold (FG), Fast Blue (FB), and Flouro-Ruby (FR). Only FG was considered to have significant ($P<.05$) positive staining compared with the other groups. (*From* Davila HH, Mamcarz M, Nadelhaft I, et al. Visualization of the neurovascular bundles and major pelvic ganglion with fluorescent tracers after penile injection in the rat. BJU Int 2008;101(8):1050; with permission.)

diagnosis (PDD)-suitable camera used to perform fluorescence imaging (**Fig. 8**). They found that there were more false-negative cases in the open group and more false-positive cases in the laparoscopic group. Nonetheless, they concluded that PDD with 5-ALA during radical prostatectomy was feasible and might be an effective method for reducing positive surgical margins.

Another potential application of MI is identification of the lymph nodes draining directly from the primary tumor (ie, sentinel lymph nodes) to facilitate lymph node dissection.[29–31] Practically, this can be performed by intraprostatic or intratumoral injection of a pharmaceutical agent, which then migrates into lymphatic channels and ultimately coalesces into the sentinel lymph node region. The signals generated can then be detected intraoperatively by a γ probe, fluorescence camera, or a combination of both. Initial work in this area by van der Poel and colleagues,[31] utilized an indocyanine green (ICG)-technetium Tc99 conjugate, which was injected into the prostate of men at increased risk of nodal metastasis, via TRUS 3 hours before prostatectomy. The sentinel lymph nodes were localized with lymphoscintigraphy and single-photon emission computerized tomography (SPECT)/CT and then surgically dissected, guided by a laparoscopic γ probe and a fluorescence laparoscope. This initial report was viewed as highly successful; however, others have sought to simplify and improve the technique.

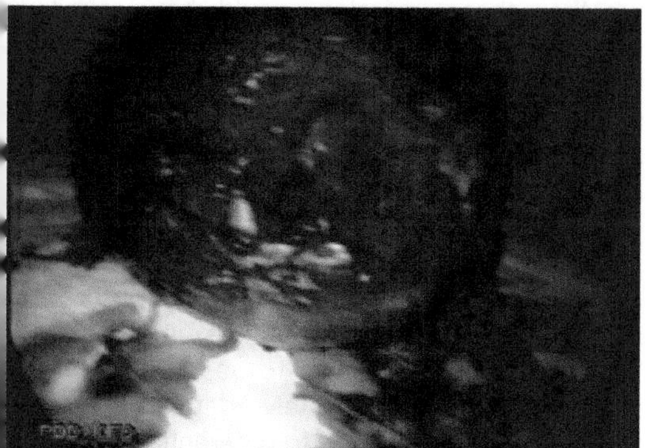

Fig. 8. Resected prostate viewed using PDD. (*From* Adam C, Salomon G, Walther S, et al. Photodynamic diagnosis using 5-aminolevulinic acid for the detection of positive surgical margins during radical prostatectomy in patients with carcinoma of the prostate: a multicentre, prospective, phase 2 trial of a diagnostic procedure. Eur Urol 2009;55(6):1286; with permission.)

More recently, Manny and colleagues,[30] reported on their initial series of fluorescence-enhanced robotic radical prostatectomy using real-time injection of ICG for tissue marking and identification of sentinel lymphatic drainage. In this study, ICG was injected into each lobe of the prostate using a robotically guided percutaneous needle. After ICG was allowed to travel through the pelvic lymphatic channels, lymphadenectomy was performed under the near-infrared visualization system of the da Vinci Si surgical robot (**Fig. 9**). They found that using this technique, sentinel lymph nodes were identified in 76% of patients at a mean time of 30 minutes after injection and had 100% sensitivity, 75.4% specificity, 14.6% positive predictive value, and 100% negative predictive value for detection of nodal metastasis. Thus, they concluded that ICG sentinel nodes are highly sensitive, but nonspecific for the detection of nodal metastasis, likely as a result of

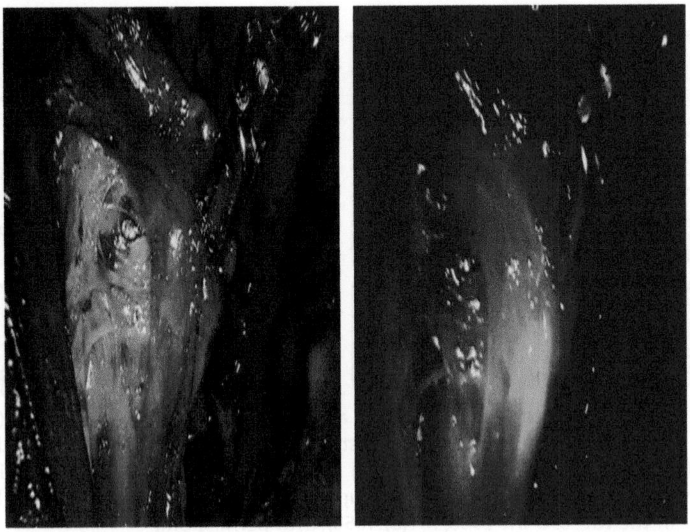

Fig. 9. Sentinel prostatic lymph node drainage identified during fluorescence-enhanced, robotic radical prostatectomy. Here the left external iliac lymph node packet is seen under white light (*left*) and near infrared fluorescence (*right*) containing fluorescent nodes. (*From* Manny TB, Patel M, Hemal AK. Fluorescence-enhanced robotic radical prostatectomy using real-time lymphangiography and tissue marking with percutaneous injection of unconjugated indocyanine green: the initial clinical experience in 50 patients. Eur Urol 2014;65(6):1165; with permission.)

ICG not being biochemically prostate specific. Future work will likely center on intratumoral injection of tracer to more accurate identify tumor drainage, rather than prostate drainage, and development of hybrid prostate cancer–specific fluorescent markers.

Additionally, Brouwer and colleagues[32] reported on an intraoperative surgical navigation system based on preoperative 3D scintigraphic images that improved the efficacy of a hybrid endoscopic radioactive and fluorescence tracer-guided surgery for prostate cancer. This study successfully showed the feasibility of combined rigid navigation based on preoperative SPECT/CT images and intraoperative fluorescence imaging for soft tissue navigation. Use of this technique using hybrid (radioactive and fluorescent) tracers allows for preoperative surgical planning and intraoperative navigation toward the lesions using the radioactive signal, whereas accurate target localization and visualization can take place using the fluorescent signature (**Fig. 10**). Navigation systems such as this remain complicated and have not shown any breakthrough clinical application and thus remain limited to the experimental realm.

FLUORESCENCE DURING RENAL SURGERY

The application of fluorescence to improve surgical outcomes and decrease positive surgical margins has also been investigated for renal surgery.[33–36] The initial reports using this technology examined the use of PDD after administration of oral 5-ALA to assess tumor type and surgical margins during partial nephrectomy.[33] They found that this adjunct therapy was able to predict the type of lesion (malignant vs nonmalignant) with accuracy of 94% and was able to detect both cases of a positive surgical margin intraoperatively, both of which were confirmed histologically. However, it remains unclear whether these margins would have similarly been identified visually alone. Nonetheless, this interesting study has failed to produce widespread acceptance and use of this technology as an adjunct during minimally invasive partial nephrectomy.

Other studies have examined the use of near infrared fluorescence (NIRF) with ICG in patients undergoing both open and robotic partial nephrectomy.[34,36,37] Intraoperative imaging with ICG and NIRF were found to be safe and effective methods to accurately identify the renal vasculature (**Fig. 11**) and to differentiate renal tumors from surrounding normal parenchyma (**Fig. 12**). This technology provides small advantages in reduction of warm ischemia times, without any clinically significant improvement in preserved renal function and has also allowed for safe selective hilar clamping.[34,38,39] Although it was hoped that this technology would

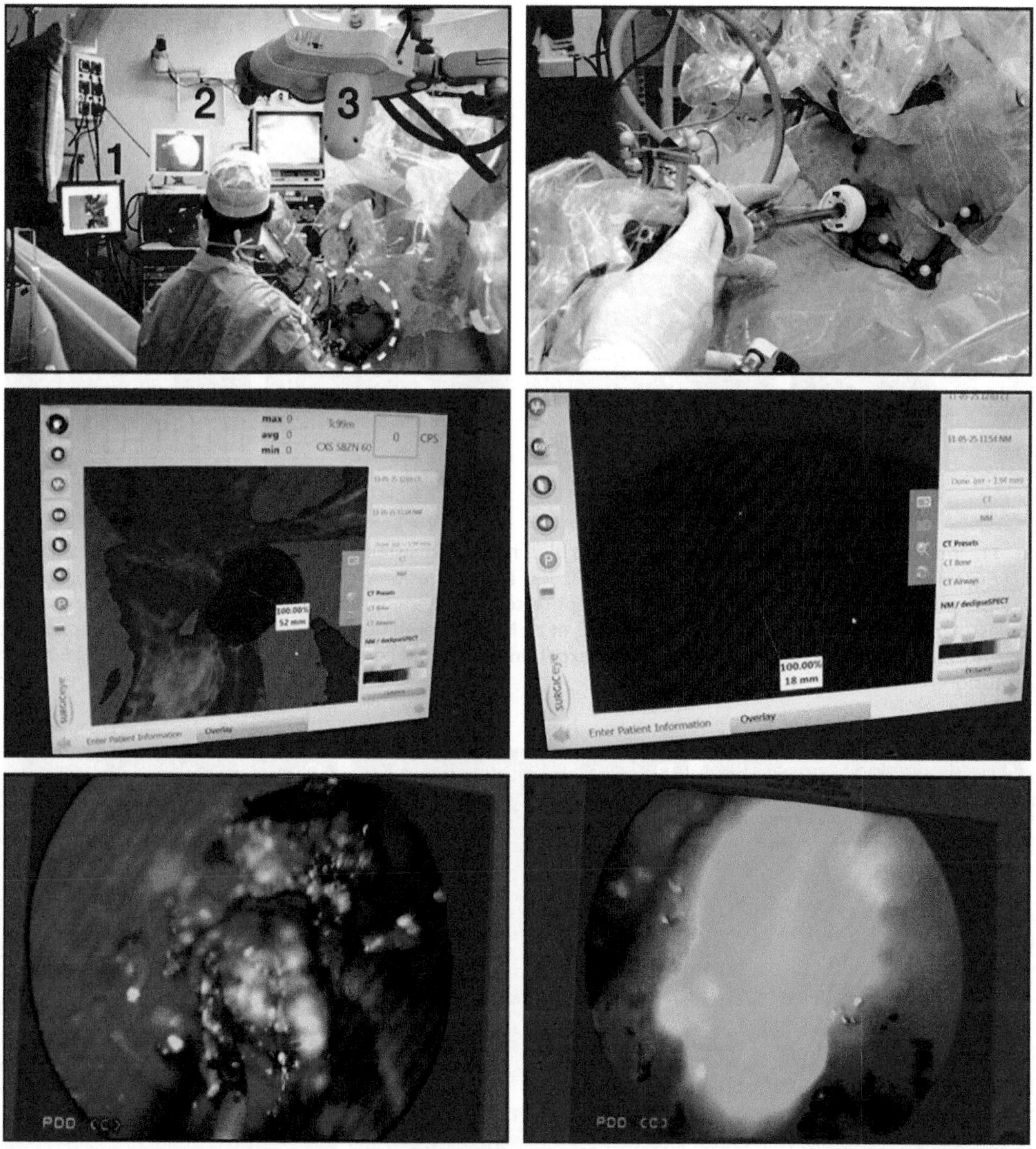

Fig. 10. Laparoscopic navigation toward the prostate in a patient undergoing robot-assisted prostatectomy. Intraoperative setup of surgical robot system with navigation system, the fluorescence camera system, and the optical tracking system are shown. Based on the preoperative SPECT/CT, navigation of the tracked fluorescence endoscope toward the target identified on SPECT/CT resulted in real-time gradual visualization of the fluorescent signal in the prostate, thus, providing an intraoperative confirmation of the navigation accuracy. (*From* Brouwer OR, Buckle T, Bunschoten A, et al. Image navigation as a means to expand the boundaries of fluorescence-guided surgery. Phys Med Biol 2012;57(10):3123–3. © Institute of Physics and Engineering in Medicine. Reproduced by permission of IOP Publishing. All rights reserved.)

maximize oncologic and renal functional outcomes of partial nephrectomy, no definitive advantages in improvement of positive surgical margin rates or change in renal function have yet been found in clinical studies. Furthermore, although many have observed that in general, renal tumors exhibit hypofluorescence compared with normal parenchyma, ICG fluorescence is unable to reliably predict malignant versus benign lesions.[35] Overall, ICG fluorescence with NIRF is an emerging technology that is increasingly being incorporated into robotic partial nephrectomy; however, more rigorous clinically studies are warranted to assess whether this will translate into any clinically significant improvements in outcomes.

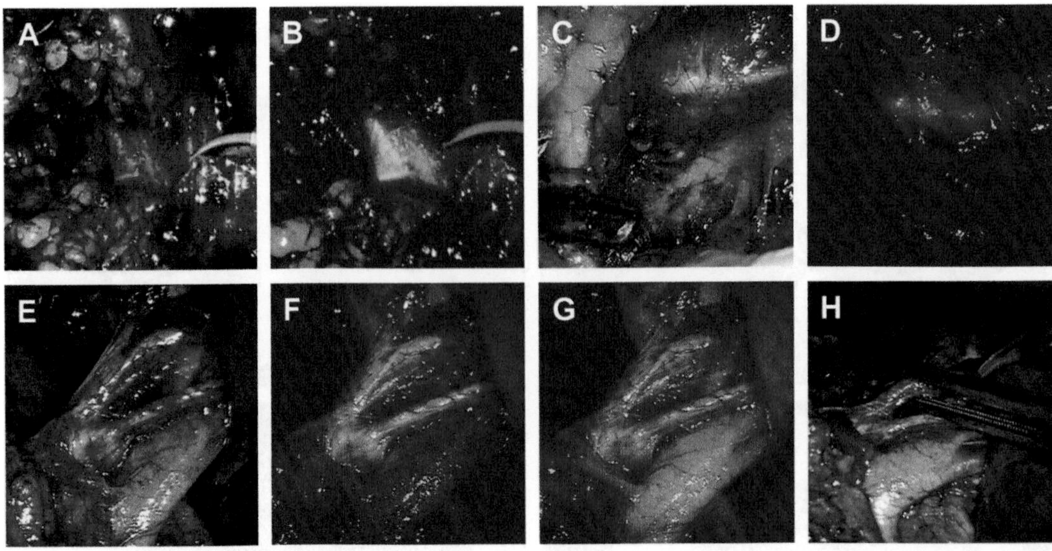

Fig. 11. Intraoperative identification of renal vasculature. NIRF assisted with identification of the renal hilum (*B,D,F,G*) when compared with white light (*A,C,E,H*). ICG administration with NIRF allowed for selective clamping of upper pole arterial branch (*H*) during partial nephrectomy, preserving flow to remainder of kidney and avoiding vascular injury. (*From* Tobis S, Knopf J, Silvers C, et al. Near infrared fluorescence imaging with robotic assisted laparoscopic partial nephrectomy: initial clinical experience for renal cortical tumors. J Urol 2011;186(1):50; with permission.)

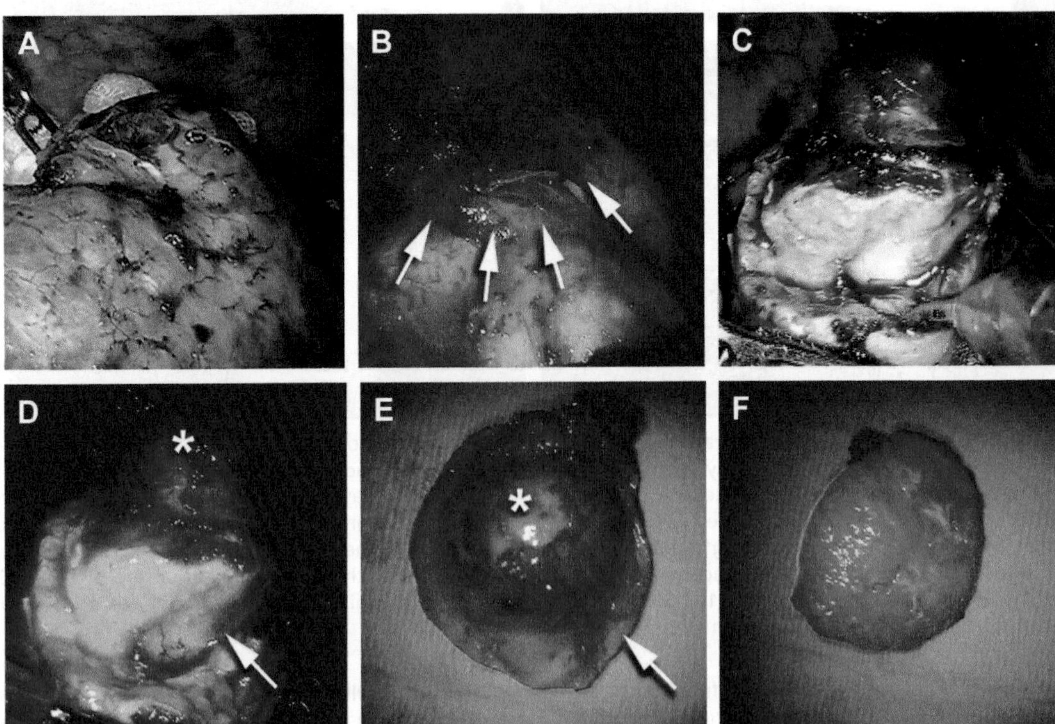

Fig. 12. Renal lesion identification. Use of ICG with NIRF is accurately able to show between normal and malignant tissue. (*A*) and (*C*) show the kidney and tumor under white light. Administration of ICG helped obtain negative margin during resection of endophytic portion of tumor, which was seen with NIRF before and after resection (*B,D,E,F*). Note the tumor is hypofluorescent (*asterisk*) compared with the fluorescent parenchyma (*arrow*). (*From* Tobis S, Knopf J, Silvers C, et al. Near infrared fluorescence imaging with robotic assisted laparoscopic partial nephrectomy: initial clinical experience for renal cortical tumors. J Urol 2011;186(1):51; with permission.)

SUMMARY

IGS and MI remain areas of intense basic science and clinical research. IGS technologies have become standards of surgical care in other specialties, including neurosurgery and orthopedics, but remain in their infancy in urologic and other soft tissue–based surgical specialties. Current research endeavors into the combined application of IGS and robotic urologic surgery present the unique challenges of soft tissue registration, tissue deformation, operative navigation, and incorporation into the surgical work flow. Although progress has been made, continued collaboration between engineers and surgeons is required to achieve the ultimate goals of improved ease and accuracy of performing surgery leading to improved patient outcomes. Lastly, the incorporation of molecular imaging into minimally invasive surgery remains in the early stages of development; however, is likely to continue to increase in importance with development of molecular markers specific to urologic malignancies.

REFERENCES

1. Lee SL, Lerotic M, Vitiello V, et al. From medical images to minimally invasive intervention: computer assistance for robotic surgery. Comput Med Imaging Graph 2010;34(1):33–45.
2. Galloway RL Jr. The process and development of image-guided procedures. Annu Rev Biomed Eng 2001;3:83–108.
3. West JB, Fitzpatrick JM, Toms SA, et al. Fiducial point placement and the accuracy of point-based, rigid body registration. Neurosurgery 2001;48(4):810–6 [discussion: 816–7].
4. Teber D, Guven S, Simpfendorfer T, et al. Augmented reality: a new tool to improve surgical accuracy during laparoscopic partial nephrectomy? Preliminary in vitro and in vivo results. Eur Urol 2009; 56(2):332–8.
5. Ukimura O, Gill IS. Imaging-assisted endoscopic surgery: cleveland clinic experience. J Endourol 2008;22(4):803–10.
6. Altamar HO, Ong RE, Glisson CL, et al. Kidney deformation and intraprocedural registration: a study of elements of image-guided kidney surgery. J Endourol 2011;25(3):511–7.
7. Herrell SD, Kwartowitz DM, Milhoua PM, et al. Toward image guided robotic surgery: system validation. J Urol 2009;181(2):783–9 [discussion: 789–90].
8. Kwartowitz DM, Miga MI, Herrell SD, et al. Towards image guided robotic surgery: multi-arm tracking through hybrid localization. Int J Comput Assist Radiol Surg 2009;4(3):281–6.
9. Su LM, Vagvolgyi BP, Agarwal R, et al. Augmented reality during robot-assisted laparoscopic partial nephrectomy: toward real-time 3D-CT to stereoscopic video registration. Urology 2009;73(4):896–900.
10. Trinh QD, Sammon J, Sun M, et al. Perioperative outcomes of robot-assisted radical prostatectomy compared with open radical prostatectomy: results from the nationwide inpatient sample. Eur Urol 2012;61(4):679–85.
11. Ukimura O, Gill IS. Real-time transrectal ultrasound guidance during nerve sparing laparoscopic radical prostatectomy: pictorial essay. J Urol 2006;175(4): 1311–9.
12. Ukimura O, Magi-Galluzzi C, Gill IS. Real-time transrectal ultrasound guidance during laparoscopic radical prostatectomy: impact on surgical margins. J Urol 2006;175(4):1304–10.
13. van der Poel HG, de Blok W, Bex A, et al. Peroperative transrectal ultrasonography-guided bladder neck dissection eases the learning of robot-assisted laparoscopic prostatectomy. BJU Int 2008;102(7):849–52.
14. Han M, Kim C, Mozer P, et al. Tandem-robot assisted laparoscopic radical prostatectomy to improve the neurovascular bundle visualization: a feasibility study. Urology 2011;77(2):502–6.
15. Hung AJ, Abreu AL, Shoji S, et al. Robotic transrectal ultrasonography during robot-assisted radical prostatectomy. Eur Urol 2012;62(2):341–8.
16. Long JA, Lee BH, Guillotreau J, et al. Real-time robotic transrectal ultrasound navigation during robotic radical prostatectomy: initial clinical experience. Urology 2012;80(3):608–13.
17. Simpfendorfer T, Baumhauer M, Muller M, et al. Augmented reality visualization during laparoscopic radical prostatectomy. J Endourol 2011;25(12): 1841–5.
18. Gao Q, Chang PL, Rueckert D, et al. Modeling of the bony pelvis from MRI using a multi-atlas AE-SDM for registration and tracking in image-guided robotic prostatectomy. Comput Med Imaging Graph 2013; 37(2):183–94.
19. Thompson S, Penney G, Billia M, et al. Design and evaluation of an image-guidance system for robot-assisted radical prostatectomy. BJU Int 2013; 111(7):1081–90.
20. Phelps ME. Positron emission tomography provides molecular imaging of biological processes. Proc Natl Acad Sci U S A 2000;97(16):9226–33.
21. De Santis M, Becherer A, Bokemeyer C, et al. 2-18fluoro-deoxy-D-glucose positron emission tomography is a reliable predictor for viable tumor in postchemotherapy seminoma: an update of the prospective multicentric SEMPET trial. J Clin Oncol 2004;22(6):1034–9.
22. Hinz S, Schrader M, Kempkensteffen C, et al. The role of positron emission tomography in the

evaluation of residual masses after chemotherapy for advanced stage seminoma. J Urol 2008;179(3): 936–40 [discussion: 940].
23. Giovacchini G, Picchio M, Coradeschi E, et al. Predictive factors of [(11)C]choline PET/CT in patients with biochemical failure after radical prostatectomy. Eur J Nucl Med Mol Imaging 2010;37(2):301–9.
24. Mitchell CR, Lowe VJ, Rangel LJ, et al. Operational characteristics of (11)c-choline positron emission tomography/computerized tomography for prostate cancer with biochemical recurrence after initial treatment. J Urol 2013;189(4):1308–13.
25. Kibel AS, Dehdashti F, Katz MD, et al. Prospective study of [18F]fluorodeoxyglucose positron emission tomography/computed tomography for staging of muscle-invasive bladder carcinoma. J Clin Oncol 2009;27(26):4314–20.
26. Davila HH, Mamcarz M, Nadelhaft I, et al. Visualization of the neurovascular bundles and major pelvic ganglion with fluorescent tracers after penile injection in the rat. BJU Int 2008;101(8):1048–51.
27. Zaak D, Sroka R, Khoder W, et al. Photodynamic diagnosis of prostate cancer using 5-aminolevulinic acid–first clinical experiences. Urology 2008;72(2):345–8.
28. Adam C, Salomon G, Walther S, et al. Photodynamic diagnosis using 5-aminolevulinic acid for the detection of positive surgical margins during radical prostatectomy in patients with carcinoma of the prostate: a multicentre, prospective, phase 2 trial of a diagnostic procedure. Eur Urol 2009;55(6):1281–8.
29. Jeschke S, Lusuardi L, Myatt A, et al. Visualisation of the lymph node pathway in real time by laparoscopic radioisotope- and fluorescence-guided sentinel lymph node dissection in prostate cancer staging. Urology 2012; 80(5):1080–6.
30. Manny TB, Patel M, Hemal AK. Fluorescence-enhanced robotic radical prostatectomy using real-time lymphangiography and tissue marking with percutaneous injection of unconjugated indocyanine green: the initial clinical experience in 50 patients. Eur Urol 2014;65(6):1162–8.
31. van der Poel HG, Buckle T, Brouwer OR, et al. Intraoperative laparoscopic fluorescence guidance to the sentinel lymph node in prostate cancer patients: clinical proof of concept of an integrated functional imaging approach using a multimodal tracer. Eur Urol 2011;60(4):826–33.
32. Brouwer OR, Buckle T, Bunschoten A, et al. Image navigation as a means to expand the boundaries of fluorescence-guided surgery. Phys Med Biol 2012;57(10):3123–36.
33. Hoda MR, Popken G. Surgical outcomes of fluorescence-guided laparoscopic partial nephrectomy using 5-aminolevulinic acid-induced protoporphyrin IX. J Surg Res 2009;154(2):220–5.
34. Krane LS, Manny TB, Hemal AK. Is near infrared fluorescence imaging using indocyanine green dye useful in robotic partial nephrectomy: a prospective comparative study of 94 patients. Urology 2012; 80(1):110–6.
35. Manny TB, Krane LS, Hemal AK. Indocyanine green cannot predict malignancy in partial nephrectomy: histopathologic correlation with fluorescence pattern in 100 patients. J Endourol 2013;27(7):918–21.
36. Tobis S, Knopf J, Silvers C, et al. Near infrared fluorescence imaging with robotic assisted laparoscopic partial nephrectomy: initial clinical experience for renal cortical tumors. J Urol 2011;186(1): 47–52.
37. Tobis S, Knopf JK, Silvers CR, et al. Near infrared fluorescence imaging after intravenous indocyanine green: initial clinical experience with open partial nephrectomy for renal cortical tumors. Urology 2012; 79(4):958–64.
38. Tobis S, Knopf JK, Silvers C, et al. Robot-assisted and laparoscopic partial nephrectomy with near infrared fluorescence imaging. J Endourol 2012; 26(7):797–802.
39. Borofsky MS, Gill IS, Hemal AK, et al. Near-infrared fluorescence imaging to facilitate super-selective arterial clamping during zero-ischaemia robotic partial nephrectomy. BJU Int 2013;111(4):604–10.

Training in Robotic Surgery

Simulators, Surgery, and Credentialing

Clinton D. Bahler, MD, Chandru P. Sundaram, MD*

KEYWORDS

• Computer simulation • Curriculum • Teaching • Robotics • Credentialing

KEY POINTS

- Recently, increased attention has been given to reports of adverse events related to robotic surgery, which has put an emphasis on robotic training and credentialing.
- Robotic training should include cognitive, psychomotor, and teamwork/communication skills.
- Simulation should be an integral part of a robotic surgical curriculum and could use inanimate models, animal models, or virtual reality simulators.
- Assessments for credentialing and certification should not be based only on number of surgeries performed but also on proven proficiency.

INTRODUCTION

As technology brings new tools to the operating room, there is increasing pressure to ensure patient safety and cost-effectiveness. The Halstedian motto of "see one, do one, teach one" is inadequate as new complex tools such as robot-assisted surgery are adopted.[1] On the other hand, the even older motto of *primum non nocere* or "above all, do no harm" remains a guiding principle for the adoption of new tools.[2]

Since its approval by the US Food and Drug Administration (FDA) in 2000, the use of robot-assisted laparoscopic surgery has surpassed that of pure laparoscopy for not only radical prostatectomy but also dismembered pyeloplasty and partial nephrectomy.[3,4] Between 2007 and 2011, the annual number of total robotics cases according to Intuitive Surgical increased by nearly 400% in the United States (**Fig. 1**).[5,6] Despite numerous institutional and surgical societal efforts to define a standardized curriculum for training and certification of robotic surgeons, no unifying pathway exists. Thus, robotics residency training is heterogeneous and certification requirements vary by hospital, as was reported in a recent FDA survey.[7]

Adverse Events in Robotic Surgery

In 2013, public awareness of complications related to robotic surgery increased through information released by the FDA and other media outlets. The FDA updated their Web site on computer-assisted surgical systems to note that an increasing number of medical device reports were being filed.[8] The FDA stated that it was not clear whether this increase represented worse complication rates or was the result of the increasing number of overall procedures and improved reporting. More recently, a report by Alemzadeh and colleagues[9] on 5374 adverse robotic events (86 deaths and 455 injuries) reported to the FDA between 2000 and 2012 noted conflicting trends. Although the overall likelihood of adverse events reported has been decreasing, the

Disclosure statement: nothing to disclose (C.D. Bahler); received grant (T145023) from Intuitive Surgical for simulation study (C.P. Sundaram).
Department of Urology, Indiana University, 535 North Barnhill Drive, STE 420, Indianapolis, IN 46202, USA
* Corresponding author.
E-mail address: sundaram@iupui.edu

Urol Clin N Am 41 (2014) 581–589
http://dx.doi.org/10.1016/j.ucl.2014.07.012

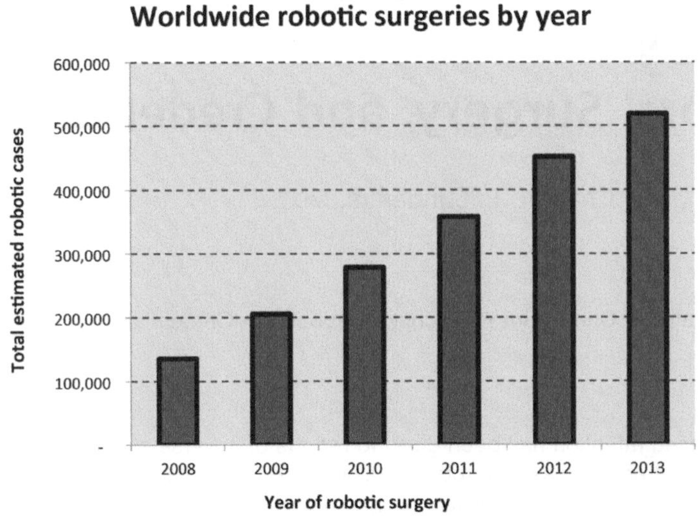

Fig. 1. Estimated number of robot-assisted cases worldwide. (*Data from* Intuitive Surgical investor presentation, 2014. Available at: http://investor.intuitivesurgical.com/phoenix.zhtml?c=122359&p=irol-irhome. Accessed April 21, 2014.)

trend of significant events (injury or death) increased from 12.8 events per 100,000 in 2004 to 35 events per 100,000 in 2012. The report noted that lower-risk urologic and gynecologic procedures had a lower rate of injury or death than higher risk cardiothoracic surgeries.

Also in 2013, a study compared reports of robotic complications in an FDA database with reports found in the Public Access to Court Electronic Records and LexisNexis. Finding that 8 of 253 (3%) complications were improperly reported to the FDA, the study[10] questioned whether the true incidence of robotic complications is known. This question prompted editorials and articles[5,11] in prominent publications to question the safety of robotic surgery and the training methods used. That same year, the Massachusetts Board of Registration in Medicine[12] made recommendations on training, patient selection, and credentialing in response to an increasing number of reports of patient complications related to robotic surgery.

This review focuses on the progress toward creating a unified curriculum for training and credentialing in robotic surgery. The following topics are addressed:

- Available cognitive resources
- Efforts to validate and incorporate surgical simulation
- Examples of currently used institutional curricula
- The Fundamentals of Robotic Surgery (FRS): a 14-society consensus template of outcomes measures and curriculum development
- Credentialing models

COGNITIVE RESOURCES

The American Urological Association (AUA)[13] recommends that residency program directors document satisfactory training and competence of residents to independently perform robotic surgery. Although simulators are not specifically addressed, recommendations are made regarding online curriculum and case participation. The AUA has included a section on robotics in their core curriculum (*The Basics of Urologic Laparoscopy and Robotics*) and also have separate e-learning modules.[14] The e-learning site has both a general module (*Fundamentals of Urologic Robotic Surgery*) and multiple procedure specific modules. The AUA recommends 80% or higher on the module posttests to show proficiency. These modules are also recommended for practicing urologists who have no formal training in robotic surgery.

The AUA also recommends completing online modules provided by Intuitive Surgical. The da Vinci Online Community offers technical modules and evaluations on topics such as operating room setup, docking, draping, safety features, and troubleshooting. Platform-specific modules for each generation of the robot are also provided.

SURGICAL SIMULATION

Simulation is a critical component of avoiding patient harm and adopting complex surgical technologies. Operating room time is viewed as both a limited and expensive commodity. Surveys of program directors in both the United Kingdom and the

United States showed a unanimous conclusion that simulators play a role in improving the quality of resident training.[15,16] Furthermore, reports from other surgical fields such as plastic surgery, neurosurgery, and gynecology support the integration of simulation into surgical training.[17–19]

Surgical simulation refers to multiple methods of training, including inanimate (box trainer), animal laboratories, and virtual reality (computer-assisted). Simulators can be categorized as either physical (inanimate or animal laboratory) or virtual reality (computer-assisted). In addition, the simulators can be further subdivided as either low or high fidelity. Low fidelity describes simple tasks and skills and is represented by virtual reality exercises involving rings and cones and inanimate exercises such as placing letters on a checkerboard. High-fidelity or full-scale simulation attempts to simulate procedural steps (**Table 1**).

An example of a high-fidelity simulator is using a tumor mimic model in a porcine laboratory to simulate partial nephrectomy. A report in 2008 showed the ability to create pseudotumors in a porcine model using bulking materials such as gelatin and psyllium.[20] The tumor mimic model was used as a simulator for tumor biopsy, partial nephrectomy, nephrectomy, and renal vein thrombectomy.

Another example of a high-fidelity simulator is a recently reported inanimate simulator of a pyeloplasty model. Studies using the model at the 2011 and 2012 AUA mentored renal laparoscopy courses showed construct, face, and content validity.[21] Cadaver simulation has been used for procedural training and specifically for experts during the design of novel procedures.[22,23] The FRS curriculum supports low fidelity for training, but recommends only high-fidelity simulator exercises for examination of psychomotor skills for credentialing.[24]

Validity

A challenge of surgical simulation is verifying the conversion of simulator skills to the operating room. There are few studies showing a direct association between simulator and operating room robotic skills regardless of simulator type. Initial simulator studies[25] attempted to confirm validity by comparing expert surgeons and novices (construct validity). Surveying of simulator participants has also been completed to determine how well the simulator mimicked the real procedure or task (face validity) or how useful (content validity) the task was.[26] Two other forms of validity

Table 1
Comparing low-fidelity and high-fidelity surgical simulators

Low vs High Fidelity	Type of Simulation	Examples/Materials
Low fidelity		
Console controls, spatial skills, basic surgical skills	Virtual reality/inanimate	String running Checkerboard Pattern cutting Suturing Pegboard[26,49]
High fidelity		
Urethrovesical anastomosis	Chicken (dead) Chicken (dead) Inanimate Porcine Virtual reality	Esophagostomach junction[52] Chicken skin[53] Latex model[54] Urethrovesical anastomosis[54] Augmented reality (Robotic Surgery Simulator)[55]
Prostatectomy	Canine	Prostatectomy and reconstruction[56]
Ureteral reimplant	Inanimate	Water-based hydrogel[57]
Pyeloplasty	Inanimate	Organosilicate: Black Light Assessment of Surgical Technique[21]
Partial nephrectomy, tumor mimic	Porcine Porcine Virtual reality	Agarose[58] Psyllium and gelatin[20] Augmented reality (Mimic)[59]
Nephrectomy	Virtual reality[a] Porcine	Procedicus MIST (Mentice)[60]

[a] Available only as a pure laparoscopic simulator.

testing are assessing whether simulator performance predicts future performance (predictive validity) and comparing the simulator with the gold standard for teaching surgical skills (concurrent validity).[27]

Only 2 studies have attempted to associate simulator time or performance to intraoperative performance on the robot. Syan and colleagues[28,29] reported on a small group (n = 9) of residents and fellows who performed 6 exercises on the da Vinci simulator and were then graded on taking down the bladder during a robotic prostatectomy using the Global Evaluative Assessment of Robotic Skills. Overall scores did not correlate, although the score for controller clutching efficiency was associated with the time required to drop bladder. The investigators concluded that low-fidelity simulation is important for basic robotic skills, but that high-fidelity simulation is needed to improve advanced steps of robotic surgery.

Culligan and colleagues[30] reported that a simulation protocol improved operative times during robotic hysterectomy. Twenty hours of virtual reality simulation (time to reach expert level simulator scores) was followed by a porcine animal laboratory for credentialed gynecologic surgeons naive to robotics. The trainees then performed their first robotic hysterectomy, and their operative time was comparable with expert surgeons and better than controls with no simulator training.

Commercially Available Virtual Reality Simulators

At least 3 robotic virtual reality simulators that incorporate a three-dimensional display have been reported in the literature (**Fig. 2**). Mimic produced the first prototype for testing in 2007.[26] Validation studies have been performed for each simulator, but few comparative studies have been performed. Details of virtual reality simulators can be found in **Table 2**. Lerner and colleagues[31] evaluated concurrent validity by comparing virtual reality simulation on the dV Trainer (Mimic Technologies) to inanimate simulation on the da Vinci robot. These investigators found that the dV Trainer provided similar improvements to the inanimate training and concluded that virtual reality simulation is helpful for junior trainees. Similarly, Korets and colleagues[32] evaluated the dV Trainer by randomizing trainees to virtual reality training on the dV Trainer, inanimate training on the da Vinci robot, or no training. These investigators found significant improvements for both the virtual reality and inanimate exercises, but none for the no training group.

Validation studies for the Robotic Surgery Simulator (RoSS) and the da Vinci Skills Simulator have shown beneficial results. Stegemann and colleagues[33] randomized junior trainees to a structured virtual reality curriculum versus no training. These investigators found that the RoSS simulator curriculum significantly improved

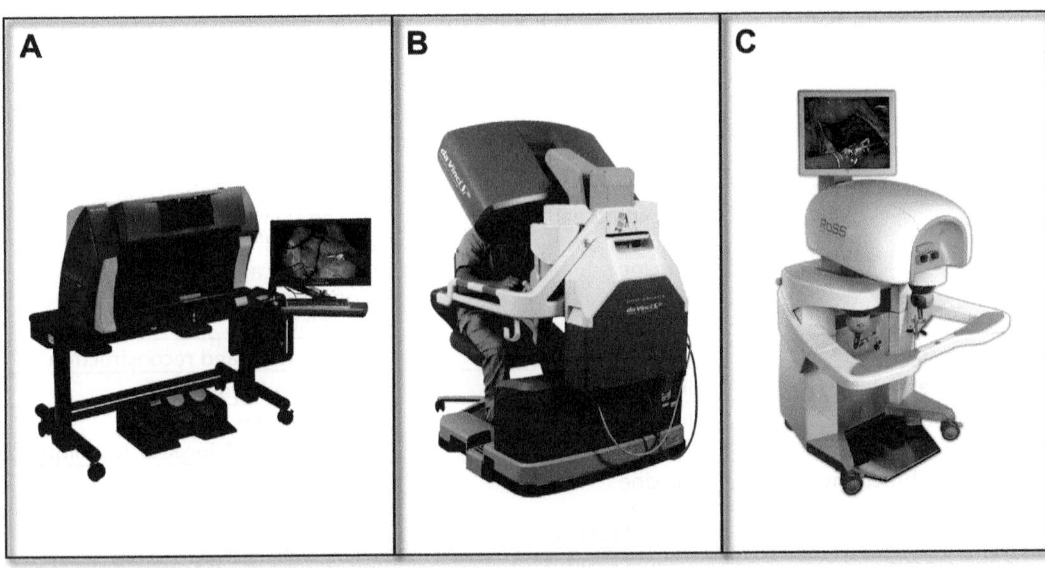

Fig. 2. Three commercially available virtual reality simulator platforms. (*A*) dV Trainer. (*B*) da Vinci Skills Simulator. (*C*) Robotic Surgery Simulator. (*Courtesy of* [*A*] Mimic Technologies, Seattle, WA, with permission; and [*B*] Intuitive Surgical, Sunnyvale, CA, with permission; [*C*] Simulated Surgical Systems, LLC, Williamsville, NY, with permission.)

Table 2
Three-dimensional virtual reality simulators

Simulator	Details
dV Trainer (Mimic Technologies)	First dedicated robotic simulator (2007)[26] Stand-alone unit Augmented reality is available[59]
da Vinci Skills Simulator (Intuitive Surgical)	Uses da Vinci console Uses Mimic software
Robotic Surgery Simulator (RoSS, Simulated Surgical Systems, LLC)	Stand-alone unit Augmented reality available (hands-on surgical training): uses haptics to guide the user's hands through the operative steps[55]

multiple inanimate exercises on the da Vinci robot. Finnegan and colleagues[34] enrolled 39 surgeons and grouped them based on how many robotic cases each had completed to assess for construct validity. Each surgeon completed 24 virtual reality exercises on the da Vinci Skills Simulator and found that overall and time-specific scores were significantly better for the more experienced groups in a linear fashion.

Validity in Pure Laparoscopy Simulation

Several studies have found the use of simulation to improve performance in pure laparoscopy. Grantcharov and colleagues[35] reported a study in which 16 surgical trainees performed a laparoscopic cholecystectomy and were then randomized to simulation versus no simulation. Those randomized to the simulator showed greater improvement in error, operative time, and economy of motion on a subsequent laparoscopic cholecystectomy. A Cochrane review[36] of randomized trials that studied the association of virtual reality simulators to performance during human or animal surgery found that skills in laparoscopic surgery can be increased by simulation. The study claimed substantial evidence (grade IA–IIB) for the use of simulators in laparoscopic training.

Warm-Up Exercises

Virtual reality and box trainer simulation have both been found to improve surgical performance when used as a warm-up before pure laparoscopic surgery. Lee and colleagues[37] pointed out that if warm-ups are beneficial for athletes and musicians, they might also be for surgeons. These investigators randomized surgical trainees between box trainer exercises for warm-up before surgery versus no warm-up. They found that warm-up exercises improved cognitive, psychomotor, and technical scores on subsequent laparoscopic renal surgeries. Similar benefits to warm-up exercises have been found in general and gynecologic surgery.[38,39]

Cost

The cost associated with animal laboratories and virtual reality simulation is significant and controversial. Rehman and colleagues[40] surveyed the time that urology residents spent on the RoSS over the span of 1 year and found that 105 trainees spent 361 hours. This time was equated to 72 robotic-assisted prostatectomies and 72 animal laboratories for a combined estimated cost of $600,000. Because the cost of the simulator was near $100,000, it was concluded that simulation was cost-effective. However, these investigators did not justify their assumption that 1 minute on the simulator was equivalent to 1 minute in the operating room. Also, traditional inanimate simulation provides the advantage of increased familiarity with the da Vinci robot and adds essentially no additional cost. Of course, inanimate simulation is often limited to nights and weekends when the robot is not being used for surgery. Comparative studies are few and generally find inanimate, animal, and virtual reality simulations to all be helpful.[41]

EXAMPLE CURRICULA

Fundamentals of Laparoscopic Surgery

The Fundaments of Laparoscopic Surgery (FLS) is a combined cognitive and psychomotor curriculum, which has been validated for training and credentialing of pure laparoscopic surgery. In 2003, the Society of American Gastrointestinal Endoscopic Surgeons and the American College of Surgeons combined the McGill Inanimate System for Testing and Evaluation of Laparoscopic Skills with a 10-chapter cognitive component.[42,43] The American Board of Surgery mandated the successful completion of the FLS program for certification in 2009 in addition to Advanced Cardiac Life Support and Advanced Trauma Life Support.[44] Okrainec and colleagues[45] published data in 2011 on the first 5 years of FLS certification testing and found widespread acceptance of the program, with an 88% overall pass rate for 2689 participants.

Robotic Training Curriculum

There is not a standardized curriculum for robotic training and credentialing, although institution-specific curricula have been described. Dulan and colleagues[46] described a comprehensive, proficiency-based curriculum used at University of Texas Southwestern Medical Center. Their content domain contains 23 specific skill sets, and their curriculum consists of 3 parts:

- Online tutorial
- Half-day interactive session
- Nine inanimate exercises with objective metrics

Initial studies showed face and content validity.[47] Arain and colleagues[48] reported on 55 participants in the course who showed improvement in simulator scores and concluded that the course was feasible, with high reliability. They found that the total time to complete the curriculum ranged from 9 to 17 hours, and inanimate simulation proficiency was reached by an average of 72 repetitions, taking an average of 5 hours.

Lucas and colleagues[49] described a second curriculum that is used at Indiana University School of Medicine. Participants complete both the Intuitive da Vinci Online Community technical modules and the AUA e-learning modules as part of the cognitive component. Participants then sign up for at least four 1-hour weekend training sessions, consisting of 5 inanimate robotic exercises, which are scored for time and accuracy:

- Pegboard
- Checkerboard
- String running
- Pattern cutting
- Suturing

Additional high-fidelity simulations such as a urethrovesical anastomosis model are available as participants acquire basic skills. After obtaining adequate time as a bedside assistant, the participants are allowed to proceed to console time during live surgeries. Participation in live surgeries follows a customized and graduated process based on evidence of proficiency. Lucas and colleagues[49] found that pegboard, checkerboard, cutting, and suturing scores were all improved for 16 participants who completed the program. Average time to complete the curriculum was 14 months, and participants noted that it was easy to attend, useful, and improved robotic skills.

FRS

In 2011, a group of 14 surgical societies convened 3 consensus conferences with the stated goal to:

> *Create and develop a validated multi-specialty, technical skills competency based curriculum for surgeons to safely and efficiently perform basic robotic-assisted surgery.*

Using the modified Delphi method, the participants identified 25 outcomes measures that represented the minimal skills needed to safely perform robotic surgery regardless of specialty.[24] Consensus conferences also focused on building a curriculum to address each of the outcomes measures. The resultant curriculum was divided into 3 components:

- Cognitive skills
- Psychomotor skills
- Team training and communication skills

Guiding principles for psychomotor skills included three-dimensional simulation, cost-effectiveness, low-fidelity and high-fidelity simulation for training, and high fidelity for examination.

Team training and communication skills have been recognized as an important component of technical errors. Rogers and colleagues[50] reported on 444 malpractice claims from insurers, which represented more than 20,000 physicians. These investigators found that 75% of surgeon-related errors occurred intraoperatively, with the leading causes being inexperience or lack of technical competence (41%) and communication (24%). Cases with technical errors were more likely to include multiple phases of care and multiple personnel, which argues for the importance of teamwork and communication during surgical care. Principles for team training and communication skills included inclusion, empowerment, person specific, and ownership.

CREDENTIALING

In contrast to the FLS requirement for pure laparoscopic credentialing by the American Board of Surgery, there are no curriculum requirements to perform robotic surgery in the United States. Recommendations for credentialing exist, but individual institutions have the responsibility for defining requirements. Therefore, unless the local hospital has taken steps in advance to provide privileging guidelines, a urologist may schedule a robot-assisted case with no verification of competence.

The AUA[13] recommends that the residency program director must document satisfactory training and confirm competence to independently perform robotic surgery. The AUA also recommends that trainees are involved in a total of 20 cases and 10 cases in which they have console time during a key portion of the case.

For practicing urologists with no formal robotic training, a structured program including online modules from Intuitive Surgical and the AUA is recommended. Other recommendations by the AUA include:

- Hands-on training with an instructor, including case observation and video review of cases
- A written report from a proctor confirming robotic skills
- Review of surgical outcomes after the surgeon's initial experience by an unbiased group

Society-based guidelines require evidence of competence for credentialing. For example, the FRS[24] recommends a competency-based curriculum, in which a trainee continues to practice until curriculum scores equivalent to experienced surgeons are reached. Also, the Society of Urologic Robotic Surgeons[51] recommends that, in addition to existing training tools and guidelines, competence of robotic skills should be confirmed through a period of proctoring. Specifically, the society recommends that a proctor report confirming robotic skills be required before full privileges are granted.

SUMMARY

The use of robot-assisted laparoscopic surgery has increased rapidly, and with it, the need to better define a structured curriculum and credentialing process. Numerous efforts have been made by surgical societies to define the requisite skills for robotic surgeons, but in the United States, individual institutions have the responsibility for granting privileges. Recently, efforts have focused on creating a standardized curriculum with competency-based assessments. A competency-based approach offers a better hope of honoring the principle of "above all, do no harm" and obtaining continued acceptance of new operative technologies such as robot-assisted surgery.

REFERENCES

1. Halsted WS. The training of the surgeon. Bull Johns Hop Hosp 1904;XV:8.
2. Smith CM. Origin and uses of primum non nocere–above all, do no harm! J Clin Pharmacol 2005;45(4):371–7.
3. Monn MF, Bahler CD, Schneider EB, et al. Emerging trends in robotic pyeloplasty for the management of ureteropelvic junction obstruction in adults. J Urol 2013;189(4):1352–7.
4. Yu HY, Hevelone ND, Lipsitz SR, et al. Use, costs and comparative effectiveness of robotic assisted, laparoscopic and open urological surgery. J Urol 2012;187(4):1392–8.
5. Pinkerton S. The pros and cons of robotic surgery. In: The Wall Street Journal. 2013. Available at: http://online.wsj.com/news/articles/SB10001424052702304655104579163430371597334. Accessed April 8, 2014.
6. Investor presentation. Intuitive Surgical; 2014. Available at: http://phx.corporate-ir.net/phoenix.zhtml?c=122359&p=irol-irhome. Accessed April 21, 2014.
7. Small Sample Survey–Final report. Topic: da Vinci Surgical System. US Food and Drug Administration, Centers for Devices and Radiological Health; 2013. Available at: http://www.fda.gov/downloads/medicaldevices/productsandmedicalprocedures/surgeryandlifesupport/computerassistedroboticsurgicalsystems/ucm374095.pdf. Accessed April 8, 2014.
8. Computer-assisted (robotic) surgical systems. US Food and Drug Administration; 2013. Available at: http://www.fda.gov/MedicalDevices/ProductsandMedicalProcedures/SurgeryandLifeSupport/ComputerAssistedRoboticSurgicalSystems/default.htm. Accessed April 8, 2014.
9. Alemzadeh H, Iyer RK, Raman J. Safety implications of robotic surgery: analysis of recalls and adverse event reports of da Vinci surgical systems. In: The Society of Thoracic Surgeons Annual Meeting, January 25–29. Orlando (FL): 2014. p. 68–9.
10. Cooper MA, Ibrahim A, Lyu H, et al. Underreporting of robotic surgery complications. J Healthc Qual 2013. [Epub ahead of print].
11. Caryn Rabin R. New concerns on robotic surgeries. In: The New York Times. 2013. Available at: http://well.blogs.nytimes.com/2013/09/09/new-concerns-on-robotic-surgeries/?_php=true&_type=blogs&_r=0. Accessed April 8, 2014.
12. Advisory on robotic-assisted surgery. Massachusetts Board of Registration in Medicine; 2013. Available at: http://www.mass.gov/eohhs/docs/borim/physicians/pca-notifications/robot-assisted-surgery.pdf. Accessed April 8, 2014.
13. Standard operating practices for urologic robotic surgery. American Urological Association; 2013. Available at: http://www.auanet.org/common/pdf/about/SOP-Urologic-Robotic-Surgery.pdf. Accessed April 7, 2014.
14. E-Learning: urologic robotic surgery course. The American Urological Association Education and Research; 2012. Available at: http://www.auanet.org/education/modules/robotic-surgery/. Accessed April 8, 2014.
15. Forster JA, Browning AJ, Paul AB, et al. Surgical simulators in urological training–views of UK Training Programme Directors. BJU Int 2012;110(6):776–8.

16. Le CQ, Lightner DJ, VanderLei L, et al. The current role of medical simulation in American Urological Residency training programs: an assessment by program directors. J Urol 2007;177(1):288–91.
17. Schreuder HW, Wolswijk R, Zweemer RP, et al. Training and learning robotic surgery, time for a more structured approach: a systematic review. BJOG 2012;119(2):137–49.
18. Rosen JM, Long SA, McGrath DM, et al. Simulation in plastic surgery training and education: the path forward. Plast Reconstr Surg 2009;123(2):729–38 [discussion: 739–40].
19. Malone HR, Syed ON, Downes MS, et al. Simulation in neurosurgery: a review of computer-based simulation environments and their surgical applications. Neurosurgery 2010;67(4):1105–16.
20. Eun D, Bhandari A, Boris R, et al. A novel technique for creating solid renal pseudotumors and renal vein-inferior vena caval pseudothrombus in a porcine and cadaveric model. J Urol 2008;180(4):1510–4.
21. Poniatowski LH, Wolf JS Jr, Nakada SY, et al. Validity and acceptability of a high-fidelity physical simulation model for training of laparoscopic pyeloplasty. J Endourol 2014;28(4):393–8.
22. Humphreys MR, Krambeck AE, Andrews PE, et al. Natural orifice translumenal endoscopic surgical radical prostatectomy: proof of concept. J Endourol 2009;23(4):669–75.
23. Menon M, Abaza R, Sood A, et al. Robotic kidney transplantation with regional hypothermia: evolution of a novel procedure utilizing the IDEAL guidelines (IDEAL phase 0 and 1). Eur Urol 2014;65(5):1001–9.
24. Smith R, Patel V, Satava R. Fundamentals of robotic surgery: a course of basic robotic surgery skills based upon a 14-society consensus template of outcomes measures and curriculum development. Int J Med Robot 2013. [Epub ahead of print].
25. McDougall EM. Validation of surgical simulators. J Endourol 2007;21(3):244–7.
26. Sethi AS, Peine WJ, Mohammadi Y, et al. Validation of a novel virtual reality robotic simulator. J Endourol 2009;23(3):503–8.
27. Vlaovic PD, McDougall EM. New age teaching: beyond didactics. ScientificWorldJournal 2006;6:2370–80.
28. Goh AC, Goldfarb DW, Sander JC, et al. Global evaluative assessment of robotic skills: validation of a clinical assessment tool to measure robotic surgical skills. J Urol 2012;187(1):247–52.
29. Syan S, Ramos P, Gill IS, et al. Does virtual performance correlate with clinical skills in robotics? Investigating concurrent validity of da Vinci simulation with clinical performance. J Urol 2013;189(4):e643.
30. Culligan P, Gurshumov E, Lewis C, et al. Predictive validity of a training protocol using a robotic surgery simulator. Female Pelvic Med Reconstr Surg 2014;20(1):48–51.
31. Lerner MA, Ayalew M, Peine WJ, et al. Does training on a virtual reality robotic simulator improve performance on the da Vinci surgical system? J Endourol 2010;24(3):467–72.
32. Korets R, Mues AC, Graversen JA, et al. Validating the use of the Mimic dV-trainer for robotic surgery skill acquisition among urology residents. Urology 2011;78(6):1326–30.
33. Stegemann AP, Ahmed K, Syed JR, et al. Fundamental skills of robotic surgery: a multi-institutional randomized controlled trial for validation of a simulation-based curriculum. Urology 2013;81(4):767–74.
34. Finnegan KT, Meraney AM, Staff I, et al. da Vinci Skills Simulator construct validation study: correlation of prior robotic experience with overall score and time score simulator performance. Urology 2012;80(2):330–5.
35. Grantcharov TP, Kristiansen VB, Bendix J, et al. Randomized clinical trial of virtual reality simulation for laparoscopic skills training. Br J Surg 2004;91(2):146–50.
36. Larsen CR, Oestergaard J, Ottesen BS, et al. The efficacy of virtual reality simulation training in laparoscopy: a systematic review of randomized trials. Acta Obstet Gynecol Scand 2012;91(9):1015–28.
37. Lee JY, Mucksavage P, Kerbl DC, et al. Laparoscopic warm-up exercises improve performance of senior-level trainees during laparoscopic renal surgery. J Endourol 2012;26(5):545–50.
38. Calatayud D, Arora S, Aggarwal R, et al. Warm-up in a virtual reality environment improves performance in the operating room. Ann Surg 2010;251(6):1181–5.
39. Do AT, Cabbad MF, Kerr A, et al. A warm-up laparoscopic exercise improves the subsequent laparoscopic performance of ob-gyn residents: a low-cost laparoscopic trainer. JSLS 2006;10(3):297–301.
40. Rehman S, Raza SJ, Stegemann AP, et al. Simulation-based robot-assisted surgical training: a health economic evaluation. Int J Surg 2013;11(9):841–6.
41. Hung AJ, Jayaratna IS, Teruya K, et al. Comparative assessment of three standardized robotic surgery training methods. BJU Int 2013;112(6):864–71.
42. Peters JH, Fried GM, Swanstrom LL, et al. Development and validation of a comprehensive program of education and assessment of the basic fundamentals of laparoscopic surgery. Surgery 2004;135(1):21–7.
43. Derossis AM, Bothwell J, Sigman HH, et al. The effect of practice on performance in a laparoscopic simulator. Surg Endosc 1998;12(9):1117–20.
44. ABS to require ACLS, ATLS and FLS for general surgery certification. American Board of Surgery; 2008. Available at: http://www.absurgery.org/default.jsp?news_newreqs. Accessed April 13, 2014.
45. Okrainec A, Soper NJ, Swanstrom LL, et al. Trends and results of the first 5 years of Fundamentals of

Laparoscopic Surgery (FLS) certification testing. Surg Endosc 2011;25(4):1192–8.
46. Dulan G, Rege RV, Hogg DC, et al. Developing a comprehensive, proficiency-based training program for robotic surgery. Surgery 2012;152(3):477–88.
47. Dulan G, Rege RV, Hogg DC, et al. Content and face validity of a comprehensive robotic skills training program for general surgery, urology, and gynecology. Am J Surg 2012;203(4):535–9.
48. Arain NA, Dulan G, Hogg DC, et al. Comprehensive proficiency-based inanimate training for robotic surgery: reliability, feasibility, and educational benefit. Surg Endosc 2012;26(10):2740–5.
49. Lucas SM, Gilley DA, Joshi SS, et al. Robotics training program: evaluation of the satisfaction and the factors that influence success of skills training in a resident robotics curriculum. J Endourol 2011;25(10):1669–74.
50. Rogers SO Jr, Gawande AA, Kwaan M, et al. Analysis of surgical errors in closed malpractice claims at 4 liability insurers. Surgery 2006;140(1):25–33.
51. Zorn KC, Gautam G, Shalhav AL, et al. Training, credentialing, proctoring and medicolegal risks of robotic urological surgery: recommendations of the Society of Urologic Robotic Surgeons. J Urol 2009;182(3):1126–32.
52. Laguna MP, Arce-Alcazar A, Mochtar CA, et al. Construct validity of the chicken model in the simulation of laparoscopic radical prostatectomy suture. J Endourol 2006;20(1):69–73.
53. Yang RM, Bellman GC. Laparoscopic urethrovesical anastomosis: a model to assess surgical competency. J Endourol 2006;20(9):679–82.
54. Sabbagh R, Chatterjee S, Chawla A, et al. Transfer of laparoscopic radical prostatectomy skills from bench model to animal model: a prospective, single-blind, randomized, controlled study. J Urol 2012;187(5):1861–6.
55. Chowriappa A, Raza SJ, Fazili A, et al. Augmented reality based skill training for robot-assisted urethro-vesical anastamosis: a multi-institutional randomized controlled trial. BJU Int 2014. [Epub ahead of print].
56. Price DT, Chari RS, Neighbors JD Jr, et al. Laparoscopic radical prostatectomy in the canine model. J Laparoendosc Surg 1996;6(6):405–12.
57. Tunitsky E, Murphy A, Barber MD, et al. Development and validation of a ureteral anastomosis simulation model for surgical training. Female Pelvic Med Reconstr Surg 2013;19(6):346–51.
58. Taylor GD, Johnson DB, Hogg DC, et al. Development of a renal tumor mimic model for learning minimally invasive nephron sparing surgical techniques. J Urol 2004;172(1):382–5.
59. Hung A, Ramos P, Montez J, et al. Novel augmented reality video simulation for robotic partial nephrectomy surgery training. J Urol 2013;189(4):e643–4.
60. Brewin J, Nedas T, Challacombe B, et al. Face, content and construct validation of the first virtual reality laparoscopic nephrectomy simulator. BJU Int 2010;106(6):850–4.

Economics of Robotic Surgery

Does It Make Sense and for Whom?

Stephen B. Williams, MD[a], Kris Prado, MD[b], Jim C. Hu, MD, MPH[b,*]

KEYWORDS

• Treatments • Utilization • Costs • Robotic • Surgery

KEY POINTS

- There has been a rapid adoption of robotic-assisted laparoscopic surgery (RALS) in the absence of high-level evidence showing its superiority to conventional approaches.
- The authors' systematic literature research revealed that only a few studies compared direct costs of different approaches.
- Despite the heterogeneous nature of cost comparison studies, they demonstrate that RALS is associated with greater direct costs.
- To date, RALS, and in particular robotic-assisted laparoscopic prostatectomy (RALP), has not been found to be cost-effective from a health economic standpoint.
- Although the demand for RALS by surgeons and patients is high, spiraling health care costs and strained health care systems will demand more comprehensive study designs for the inevitable adoption of costly new technologies such as RALS.

INTRODUCTION

Robotic-assisted laparoscopic surgery (RALS) has evolved since its inception in 1985 to its current state in the form of the da Vinci surgical system (Intuitive Surgical, Sunnyvale, California). Following receipt of US Food and Drug Administration approval in 2000 for adult and pediatric surgeries, utilization has increased ahead of empirical evidence demonstrating superiority over conventional surgical approaches. The technology offers advantages of a 3-dimensional view of the operative field, absence of a fulcrum effect, 7° versus 4° of freedom of movement compared with conventional laparoscopy with 'wristed' instruments that facilitate intracorporeal suturing, elimination of surgeon tremor, and ergonomic benefits,[1] hastening the learning curve for open surgeons transitioning to minimally invasive surgery.[2–4] Additional advantages over open surgery include smaller incisions, reduced intraoperative blood loss due to carbon dioxide insufflation, decreased postoperative pain, and shorter hospital lengths of stay (LOS) and convalescence.[4–6] Disadvantages of RALS include relatively longer operative times, absence of tactile feedback, and instrument collisions when traversing broader operative fields.[3,7,8]

Since the introduction of the da Vinci system, most cases are now dedicated toward urology and urologic oncology procedures. With more than 1400 robotic surgical systems installed in US hospitals, with some having up to 5 systems, and the number of robotic systems in other countries doubling from 200 to 400 between 2007 and 2009,[9] RALS

[a] Department of Urology, The University of Texas MD Anderson Cancer Center, 1515 Holcombe Boulevard, Unit 1373, Houston, TX 77030, USA; [b] Department of Urology, David Geffen School of Medicine at UCLA, 924 Westwood, Boulevard, STE 1000, Los Angeles, CA 90024, USA

* Corresponding author. Department of Urology, David Geffen School of Medicine at UCLA, 924 Westwood Boulevard, STE 1000, Los Angeles, CA 90024.

E-mail address: jimhumd@gmail.com

Urol Clin N Am 41 (2014) 591–596
http://dx.doi.org/10.1016/j.ucl.2014.07.013
0094-0143/14/$ – see front matter

has been rapidly adopted in the absence of overwhelming evidence demonstrating superior outcomes compared with laparoscopic and open surgery.[1,10] Further, direct-to-consumer advertising has resulted in heightened patient demand for RALS,[11] particularly for radical prostatectomy. However, men who underwent radical prostatectomy with RALS versus open surgery were more likely to be diagnosed with incontinence and erectile dysfunction, and more likely to experience treatment regret.[10,12] Regarding utilization of pharmacotherapy for erectile dysfunction following treatment for localized prostate cancer, men undergoing minimally invasive surgery including RALS were more likely to use pharmacotherapy after treatment.[13] Moreover, patients were more likely to be regretful and dissatisfied, possibly because of greater expectation of an innovative procedure with less counseling on adverse effects.[12] It has been suggested that urologists carefully portray the risks and benefits of new technologies during preoperative counseling to minimize regret and maximize satisfaction.[12] However, more recent analysis demonstrates that robotic-assisted versus open radical prostatectomy is associated with fewer positive surgical margins and less use of radiation or androgen deprivation therapy within 2 years of surgery, suggesting better cancer control outcomes.[14] As such, further comparative effectiveness research is needed to identify determinants of appropriate dissemination of robotic surgery.

CONSEQUENCES OF RAPID ADOPTION OF ROBOTIC SURGERY

Many patients intuitively perceived minimally invasive approaches as reducing complications compared with conventional surgery. Patients prefer these approaches, especially RALS, because of smaller incisions requiring fewer analgesics and shorter hospital stays, even at a greater cost to the health system.[15] The cosmetic appeal of multiple small incisions versus a single incision is one of personal preference. With rapid adoption, prolonged learning curves, and varying hospital accreditation practices for attaining RALS privileges, there may come unforeseen risks. For example, the rapid adoption of laparoscopic cholecystectomy in the 1990s resulted in a spike in biliary tract injuries from 1500 to 4000 per year.[16] Well-designed studies comparing surgical approaches are sparse, and most studies are comprised of single-surgeon series that may not be generalizable to other practice settings.

RALS was rapidly adopted for radical prostatectomy, and hospital acquisition led to the expansion of RALS for other procedures.[17] A consequence of the rapid adoption of RALS resulted in certain professional organizations recommending against RALS as a preferred treatment option.[18] For instance, robotic hysterectomy has become increasingly utilized with increased complications and costs over open surgery, so much that the American Society of Obstetrics and Gynecology no longer recommends RALS as a first-line surgical option.[18]

A recent population-based comparative effectiveness study of RALS utilization, patterns of care, and costs resulted in several important findings that may provide some insight into lessons learned from the rapid adoption of RALS.[1] First, racial, geographic, and hospital-based variations exist in patients undergoing RALS, with limited access to care for nonwhite patients. Several other studies have demonstrated similar heterogeneity in access to newer technology and therefore limit generalizability of outcomes.[19–21] Second, higher-volume hospitals are more likely to offer RALS for procedures such as radical prostatectomy; however, they are less likely to offer it for other procedures such as cystectomy, owing to likely increased complexity of the latter procedure. Outcomes of robotic cystectomy are comparable to the open approach; however, prior comparative analyses are derived from high-volume open and robotic surgeons.[22] Interestingly, robotic partial nephrectomy has become increasingly adopted over conventional laparoscopy, which had a prolonged learning curve and technical complexity that precluded universal adoption.[1,23,24] A recent population-based study found robotic partial nephrectomy to result in fewer complications and shorter length of stay than either the laparoscopic or open approach.[1] As newer technologies such as RALS become further adapted to more complex procedures, it is critical to understand the consequences of rapid adoption of RALS in order to avoid potential future pitfalls. Some been suggested that state-based certificates of need should be implemented to control RALS utilization and limit costs as they pertain to prostate cancer.[25] However, state-based regulations were ineffective in constraining robotic surgery adoption and intensity-modulated radiation therapy, another controversial, high-cost prostate cancer treatment modality.[26] As health care reform gets underway, one may expect similar constructs to be implemented in order to control RALS and health care costs while striving to improve patient outcomes.

THE COSTS OF ROBOTIC SURGERY

RALS has been consistently shown to be more costly than conventional laparoscopic or open surgery. Others have demonstrated RALS to be $1065 to $2315 higher in direct costs for radical prostatectomy and $535 to $1651 more for partial nephrectomy, despite purported cost savings associated with shorter LOS.[21,27] In regards to radical cystectomy, where there has been conflicting evidence regarding LOS benefit, RALS was $3797 more costly, with $4326 higher 90-day median direct costs than open surgery.[28,29] One study estimated that the incremental cost (without factoring in the purchase of the robotic surgical system) of RALS averages approximately $1600, or an additional 6% per case more than open surgery.[9] Lower costs have been associated with higher RALS volume for radical prostatectomy compared with other procedures, consistent with a study demonstrating 68% lower charges for high- versus low-volume minimally invasive radical prostatectomy surgeons.[30] When analyzing RALS costs as related to radical prostatectomy, the incremental cost when compared to open surgery doubles when factoring in the $1.75 million capital acquisition cost of the robotic surgical system.[9] This projects to $2.5 billion in annual US health care expenditures if RALS universally replaces conventional surgical approaches.[9] Considering medical devices are not subject to the same level of scrutiny compared with pharmaceuticals in demonstrating clinical effectiveness,[1,31] the rapid adoption of new medical technologies such as RALS significantly contributes to spiraling health care costs.[32] Pearson and Bach proposed a tiered payment system,[33] whereby full reimbursement be rendered for therapies demonstrating superior outcomes to existing standards. Under this paradigm, in the absence of demonstrable cost-effectiveness, fiscal responsibility for the incremental cost of RALS shifts from insurers to patients, and may thus attenuate demand.

PROVIDER FACTORS ASSOCIATED WITH COSTS: ROOM TO IMPROVE

High-risk surgical procedures such as pancreatectomy[34] and esophagectomy[35] have decreased morbidity and mortality when performed in high-volume hospitals. Similarly, higher hospital volume is associated with decreased morbidity for colon[36] and breast[37] cancer surgeries. Additionally, hospital volume is inversely related to in-hospital mortality and LOS after radical prostatectomy.[38] However, surgeon rather than hospital volume has been shown to be the primary determinant of radical prostatectomy outcomes, as intensive care admissions and lengths of hospitalization have declined over the past 20 years.[39,40] Taking into account the previously mentioned changes in radical prostatectomy trends and outcomes, hospital and surgeon volumes have been analyzed to assess whether centralization may be beneficial to minimize morbidity, mortality, and health care costs.[38,41,42] Given that most radical prostatectomies are performed by surgeons performing fewer than 10 cases a year,[43] selective referral of radical prostatectomies to high-volume surgeons may be lead to significant cost savings, particularly with the reality of accountable care organizations looming on the horizon.

Several studies have analyzed radical prostatectomy provider effects on costs. Higher surgeon and hospital volumes have been associated with a reduction in radical prostatectomy costs.[44] It has even been suggested that selective referral to high-volume surgeons at intermediate- and high-volume hospitals nationally would reduce health care costs by more than $28.7 million.[44] This amount exceeds the $19 million the National Cancer Institute allocated to funding surgery-related research in 2010 for prostate cancer.[45] Others have shown that higher surgeon volume is associated with lower hospital charges,[46] suggesting that as radical prostatectomy surgeons gain experience, they become more efficient, and have better outcomes with lower costs.[41,47]

Lastly, it has been documented that higher surgeon volume is associated with better perioperative outcomes,[41,42] which may be the more important determinant to offset costs. Higher-volume hospitals tend to be academic medical centers with the mission of furthering research, education, and clinical care, accepting patients regardless of clinical presentation and financial risk.[48] Thus, higher-volume hospitals may have better information technology, documentation, and compliance with reimbursement guidelines to offset potential financial risks.

COSTS: LESSONS LEARNED FROM RAPID ADOPTION OF ROBOTIC PROSTATECTOMY

Mouraviev and colleagues[49] presented the first study comparing actual direct costs associated with robotic-assisted laparoscopic prostatectomy (RALP) versus radical retropubic prostatectomy (RPP) and found RALP to be less cost-effective. In another study, Bolenz and colleagues[21] compared minimally invasive prostatectomy (laparoscopic and robotic) with open surgery, and when considering purchase and maintenance costs, the incremental cost was $2698 per RALP. This was predominantly due to higher costs of surgical supplies and operating room costs. A study performed in accordance with internationally standardized criteria for health economic evaluations confirmed that RALP is significantly more expensive than RRP.[50] Finally, Rebuck and colleagues[51] confirmed higher direct RALP costs, mainly because of high operating room and surgical supply costs. Compounding costs for RALS are utilization of fluorescence imaging, dual consoles, simulation, and additional upgrades, which further contribute to the higher cost of robotic surgery versus conventional approaches.[52] Although modification of the previously mentioned factors, such as faster turnover times and dedicated surgical teams, have been evaluated, these measures did not compensate for the added expenditure for RALP.[53]

Current comparative and cost-effectiveness studies on RALS have several limitations, because different methods were used in assessing health care costs. Cost components may differ between studies, with costs of the procedures not only varying between institutions and different health care systems, but also between different geographic regions.[54] Therefore, cost values are not directly comparable in the literature. The costs for RALP are influenced by hospital characteristics (eg, provider [surgeon/hospital] case volume, academic vs nonacademic center, hospital ownership). It has been shown that costs and surgeon fees for procedures performed in a county government hospital may be less than in a private academic medical center.[53] Other highly variable parameters are hospital charges; cost of hospitalization; purchase and maintenance costs of the robot, which depend on case volume and amortization rates; surgeon experience (ie, operative time and complications); academic or private or community setting; convalescence; long-term oncologic outcomes; and salvage treatment.[52] It is also important to note that in many centers, the learning curve of robotic surgeons is ongoing, and contemporary series may underestimate actual costs. Many studies comparing the costs of RALP and open RRP addressed mainly the costs of the procedure, and initial hospital stay was primarily assessed from a hospital perspective.[53,55] Available studies presented only limited follow-up data, and there is only little evidence from studies using established methods for the economic evaluation of health care programs. There is limited evidence for other cost advantages of RALP, such as earlier return to work,[52] which may contribute to greater value for RALP from a societal perspective.[56] There is also a potential bias that many centers may perform primarily RALP and reserve open RRP for difficult cases that are thought to be difficult with RALS. However, with the rapid adoption of RALP, even the most challenging cases are now being done robotically.[57]

SUMMARY

There has been a rapid adoption of RALS in the absence of high-level evidence showing its superiority to conventional approaches. The authors' systematic literature research revealed that only a few studies compared direct costs of different approaches. Despite the heterogeneous nature of cost comparison studies, they demonstrate that RALS is associated with greater direct costs. To date, RALS, and in particular RALP, has not been found to be cost-effective from a health economic standpoint. Although the demand for RALS by surgeons and patients is high, spiraling health care costs and strained health care systems will demand more comprehensive study designs for the inevitable adoption of costly new technologies such as RALS.

REFERENCES

1. Yu HY, Hevelone ND, Lipsitz SR, et al. Use, costs and comparative effectiveness of robotic assisted, laparoscopic and open urological surgery. J Urol 2012;187:1392–8.
2. Sanchez BR, Mohr CJ, Morton JM, et al. Comparison of totally robotic laparoscopic Roux-en-Y gastric bypass and traditional laparoscopic Roux-en-Y gastric bypass. Surg Obes Relat Dis 2005;1: 549–54.
3. Lim PC, Kang E, Park do H. Learning curve and surgical outcome for robotic-assisted hysterectomy with lymphadenectomy: case-matched controlled comparison with laparoscopy and laparotomy for treatment of endometrial cancer. J Minim Invasive Gynecol 2010;17:739–48.
4. Smith JA Jr, Herrell SD. Robotic-assisted laparoscopic prostatectomy: do minimally invasive approaches offer significant advantages? J Clin Oncol 2005;23:8170–5.
5. Rudich SM, Marcovich R, Magee JC, et al. Hand-assisted laparoscopic donor nephrectomy: comparable donor/recipient outcomes, costs, and decreased convalescence as compared to open donor nephrectomy. Transplant Proc 2001;33: 1106–7.
6. Menon M, Tewari A, Baize B, et al. Prospective comparison of radical retropubic prostatectomy and robot-assisted anatomic prostatectomy: the Vattikuti Urology Institute experience. Urology 2002;60:864–8.
7. Schaeffer EM, Loeb S, Walsh PC. The case for open radical prostatectomy. Urol Clin North Am 2010;37:49–55. Table of Contents.
8. Swanson SJ, Miller DL, McKenna RJ Jr, et al. Comparing robot-assisted thoracic surgical lobectomy with conventional video-assisted thoracic

surgical lobectomy and wedge resection: results from a multihospital database (Premier). J Thorac Cardiovasc Surg 2014;147(3):929–37.
9. Barbash GI, Glied SA. New technology and health care costs—the case of robot-assisted surgery. N Engl J Med 2010;363:701–4.
10. Hu JC, Wang Q, Pashos CL, et al. Utilization and outcomes of minimally invasive radical prostatectomy. J Clin Oncol 2008;26:2278–84.
11. Mulhall JP, Rojaz-Cruz C, Muller A. An analysis of sexual health information on radical prostatectomy websites. BJU Int 2010;105:68–72.
12. Schroeck FR, Krupski TL, Sun L, et al. Satisfaction and regret after open retropubic or robot-assisted laparoscopic radical prostatectomy. Eur Urol 2008;54:785–93.
13. Prasad MM, Prasad SM, Hevelone ND, et al. Utilization of pharmacotherapy for erectile dysfunction following treatment for prostate cancer. J Sex Med 2010;7:1062–73.
14. Hu JC, Gandaglia G, Karakiewicz PI, et al. Comparative effectiveness of robotic-assisted versus open radical prostatectomy cancer control. Eur Urol 2014. [Epub ahead of print].
15. Pappas TN, Jacobs DO. Laparoscopic resection for colon cancer—the end of the beginning? N Engl J Med 2004;350:2091–2.
16. Strasberg SM, Hertl M, Soper NJ. An analysis of the problem of biliary injury during laparoscopic cholecystectomy. J Am Coll Surg 1995; 180:101–25.
17. Ficarra V, Novara G, Artibani W, et al. Retropubic, laparoscopic, and robot-assisted radical prostatectomy: a systematic review and cumulative analysis of comparative studies. Eur Urol 2009;55: 1037–63.
18. Breeden JT. Statement on robotic surgery. vol. 2013. American College of Obstetricians and Gynecologists; 2013. Available at: http://www.acog.org/About-ACOG/News-Room/News-Releases/2013/Statement-on-Robotic-Surgery. Accessed on December 15, 2013.
19. Nguyen PL, Gu X, Lipsitz SR, et al. Cost implications of the rapid adoption of newer technologies for treating prostate cancer. J Clin Oncol 2011; 29(12):1517–24.
20. Hu JC, Gu X, Lipsitz SR, et al. Comparative effectiveness of minimally invasive vs open radical prostatectomy. JAMA 2009;302:1557–64.
21. Bolenz C, Gupta A, Hotze T, et al. Cost comparison of robotic, laparoscopic, and open radical prostatectomy for prostate cancer. Eur Urol 2010;57: 453–8.
22. Orvieto MA, DeCastro GJ, Trinh QD, et al. Oncological and functional outcomes after robot-assisted radical cystectomy: critical review of current status. Urology 2011;78:977–84.
23. Gill IS, Kavoussi LR, Lane BR, et al. Comparison of 1,800 laparoscopic and open partial nephrectomies for single renal tumors. J Urol 2007;178:41–6.
24. Benway BM, Bhayani SB, Rogers CG, et al. Robot assisted partial nephrectomy versus laparoscopic partial nephrectomy for renal tumors: a multi-institutional analysis of perioperative outcomes. J Urol 2009;182:866–72.
25. Jacobs BL, Zhang Y, Skolarus TA, et al. Certificate of need legislation and the dissemination of robotic surgery for prostate cancer. J Urol 2013;189:80–5.
26. Khanna A, Hu JC, Gu X, et al. Certificate of need programs, intensity modulated radiation therapy use and the cost of prostate cancer care. J Urol 2013;189:75–9.
27. Mir SA, Cadeddu JA, Sleeper JP, et al. Cost comparison of robotic, laparoscopic, and open partial nephrectomy. J Endourol 2011;25:447–53.
28. Yu HY, Hevelone ND, Lipsitz SR, et al. Comparative analysis of outcomes and costs following open radical cystectomy versus robot-assisted laparoscopic radical cystectomy: results from the US Nationwide Inpatient Sample. Eur Urol 2012;61: 1239–44.
29. Leow JJ, Reese SW, Jiang W, et al. Propensity-matched comparison of morbidity and costs of open and robot-assisted radical cystectomies: a contemporary population-based analysis in the United States. Eur Urol 2014;16(3):569–76.
30. Budaus L, Abdollah F, Sun M, et al. The impact of surgical experience on total hospital charges for minimally invasive prostatectomy: a population-based study. BJU Int 2011;108:888–93.
31. Garber AM, Sox HC. The role of costs in comparative effectiveness research. Health Aff (Millwood) 2010;29:1805–11.
32. Maxwell S, Zuckerman S, Berenson RA. Use of physicians' services under Medicare's resource-based payments. N Engl J Med 2007;356:1853–61.
33. Pearson SD, Bach PB. How Medicare could use comparative effectiveness research in deciding on new coverage and reimbursement. Health Aff (Millwood) 2010;29:1796–804.
34. Birkmeyer JD, Finlayson SR, Tosteson AN, et al. Effect of hospital volume on in-hospital mortality with pancreaticoduodenectomy. Surgery 1999;125: 250–6.
35. Patti MG, Corvera CU, Glasgow RE, et al. A hospital's annual rate of esophagectomy influences the operative mortality rate. J Gastrointest Surg 1998;2:186–92.
36. Schrag D, Cramer LD, Bach PB, et al. Influence of hospital procedure volume on outcomes following surgery for colon cancer. JAMA 2000;284:3028–35.
37. Roohan PJ, Bickell NA, Baptiste MS, et al. Hospital volume differences and five-year survival from breast cancer. Am J Public Health 1998;88:454–7.

38. Ellison LM, Heaney JA, Birkmeyer JD. The effect of hospital volume on mortality and resource use after radical prostatectomy. J Urol 2000;163:867–9.
39. Hu JC, Gold KF, Pashos CL, et al. Role of surgeon volume in radical prostatectomy outcomes. J Clin Oncol 2003;21:401–5.
40. Hu JC, Gold KF, Pashos CL, et al. Temporal trends in radical prostatectomy complications from 1991 to 1998. J Urol 2003;169:1443–8.
41. Wilt TJ, Shamliyan TA, Taylor BC, et al. Association between hospital and surgeon radical prostatectomy volume and patient outcomes: a systematic review. J Urol 2008;180:820–8 [discussion: 828–9].
42. Barocas DA, Mitchell R, Chang SS, et al. Impact of surgeon and hospital volume on outcomes of radical prostatectomy. Urol Oncol 2010;28:243–50.
43. Savage CJ, Vickers AJ. Low annual caseloads of United States surgeons conducting radical prostatectomy. J Urol 2009;182:2677–9.
44. Williams SB, Amarasekera CA, Gu X, et al. Influence of surgeon and hospital volume on radical prostatectomy costs. J Urol 2012;188:2198–202.
45. Nowroozi MR, Pisters LL. The current status of gene therapy for prostate cancer. Cancer Control 1998;5:522–31.
46. Ramirez A, Benayoun S, Briganti A, et al. High radical prostatectomy surgical volume is related to lower radical prostatectomy total hospital charges. Eur Urol 2006;50:58–62 [discussion: 62–3].
47. Begg CB, Riedel ER, Bach PB, et al. Variations in morbidity after radical prostatectomy. N Engl J Med 2002;346:1138–44.
48. Taheri PA, Butz DA, Dechert R, et al. How DRGs hurt academic health systems. J Am Coll Surg 2001;193:1–8 [discussion: 8–11].
49. Mouraviev V, Nosnik I, Sun L, et al. Financial comparative analysis of minimally invasive surgery to open surgery for localized prostate cancer: a single-institution experience. Urology 2007;69:311–4.
50. Hohwu L, Borre M, Ehlers L, et al. A short-term cost-effectiveness study comparing robot-assisted laparoscopic and open retropubic radical prostatectomy. J Med Econ 2011;14:403–9.
51. Rebuck DA, Zhao LC, Helfand BT, et al. Simple modifications in operating room processes to reduce the times and costs associated with robot-assisted laparoscopic radical prostatectomy. J Endourol 2011;25:955–60.
52. Bolenz C, Freedland SJ, Hollenbeck BK, et al. Costs of radical prostatectomy for prostate cancer: a systematic review. Eur Urol 2014;65(2):316–24.
53. Lotan Y, Cadeddu JA, Gettman MT. The new economics of radical prostatectomy: cost comparison of open, laparoscopic and robot assisted techniques. J Urol 2004;172:1431–5.
54. Makarov DV, Loeb S, Landman AB, et al. Regional variation in total cost per radical prostatectomy in the healthcare cost and utilization project nationwide inpatient sample database. J Urol 2010;183:1504–9.
55. Scales CD Jr, Jones PJ, Eisenstein EL, et al. Local cost structures and the economics of robot assisted radical prostatectomy. J Urol 2005;174:2323–9.
56. Hohwu L, Akre O, Pedersen KV, et al. Open retropubic prostatectomy versus robot-assisted laparoscopic prostatectomy: a comparison of length of sick leave. Scand J Urol Nephrol 2009;43:259–64.
57. Huang AC, Kowalczyk KJ, Hevelone ND, et al. The impact of prostate size, median lobe, and prior benign prostatic hyperplasia intervention on robot-assisted laparoscopic prostatectomy: technique and outcomes. Eur Urol 2011;59:595–603.

Models of Assessment of Comparative Outcomes of Robot-Assisted Surgery

Best Evidence Regarding the Superiority or Inferiority of Robot-Assisted Radical Prostatectomy

Giorgio Gandaglia, MD[a,*], Quoc-Dien Trinh, MD[b]

KEYWORDS

- Radical prostatectomy • Prostate cancer • Robot-assisted radical prostatectomy
- Comparative effectiveness • Models of assessment

KEY POINTS

- The best evidence comparing the effectiveness of robot-assisted radical prostatectomy (RARP) with open radical prostatectomy (ORP) for patients with clinically localized prostate cancer (PCa) is based on observational retrospective studies.
- The adoption of standardized endpoints is mandatory when evaluating the comparative effectiveness of different surgical approaches for the treatment of PCa.
- The currently available retrospective studies evaluating oncologic and nononcologic outcomes of RARP are limited by selection bias, short follow-up, and the inclusion of patients for the most part treated in high-volume tertiary referral centers.
- Well-designed prospective investigations are needed to comprehensively assess the benefits of RARP compared with other treatment modalities in patients with clinically localized PCa.

INTRODUCTION

PCa is the most common noncutaneous malignancy in the United States and Europe. For the year 2014, 233,000 men are estimated diagnosed with PCa in the United States alone.[1] Radical prostatectomy (RP) represents one of the standard-of-care treatment approaches for patients with clinically localized PCa.[2] Since its description in a landmark study by Walsh and Donker in 1982,[3] ORP has been the most commonly performed approach for the surgical treatment of patients with clinically localized PCa. This surgical technique is associated with excellent cancer control rates, where only 14% of patients treated with ORP experience cancer-specific mortality at long-term follow-up.[4] Long-term side effects, however, such as erectile dysfunction and urinary incontinence, might substantially affect patient health-related quality of life.[5–8] This holds particularly true in young and physically active individuals.

Disclosure Statement: Dr Q-D. Trinh reported having received an honorarium from Intuitive Surgical.
[a] Division of Oncology, Unit of Urology, Urological Research Institute, San Raffaele Scientific Institute, IRCCS Ospedale San Raffaele, Vita-Salute San Raffaele University, Via Olgettina 57, Milan 20132, Italy; [b] Division of Urologic Surgery and Center for Surgery and Public Health, Brigham and Women's Hospital, Dana-Farber Cancer Institute, Harvard Medical School, 45 Francis St, ASB II-3, Boston, MA 02115, USA
* Corresponding author.
E-mail addresses: giorgio.gandaglia@gmail.com; giorgan10@libero.it

Urol Clin N Am 41 (2014) 597–606
http://dx.doi.org/10.1016/j.ucl.2014.07.014
0094-0143/14/$ – see front matter

Over the past 15 years, the introduction of minimally invasive technologies has revolutionized the treatment of clinically localized PCa.[9,10] In particular, the adoption of RARP immediately gathered much enthusiasm in the field. First described in a case report by Abbou and colleagues,[11] Menon's standardization[12–16] of RARP has resulted in the dissemination of robotics in the United States, where a majority of RPs are now done robotically.[10,17]

Robot-assisted surgery offers many hypothetical benefits, such as stereoscopic vision, enhanced visual magnification, and more degrees of freedom for surgical instruments. As such, many investigators hypothesized that this surgical approach would lead to lower rates of short- and long-term side effects, including urinary incontinence and erectile dysfunction, relative to the conventional ORP.[18–22] Additionally, these technical advantages may also result in better oncologic outcomes compared with ORP. For example, several investigators postulated that the adoption of minimally invasive approaches would result in lower rates of positive surgical margins and additional cancer therapies after surgery.[23–26] Conversely, the dissemination of RARP took place in the absence of high-level evidence supporting its efficacy or safety. There are now enough data to suggest that market competition between hospitals and patient demands in response to aggressive marketing strategies were the main drivers of its adoption.[9] The rapid adoption of robotic surgery has had an impact on the costs of PCa care, because RARP is generally more expensive than ORP.[27–33] For example, investigators have estimated that the widespread adoption of minimally invasive surgery is associated with excess expenditures of approximately $2.5 billion per year in the United States alone.[31,33] Given the concerns and the demand for greater value, these considerations highlight the need for a comprehensive evaluation of the safety and efficacy of minimally invasive approaches. Understanding and quantifying the benefits of RARP would allow policymakers to better estimate the true value of this technique to health care systems, providers, and patients. On the basis of these considerations, this study aims to systematically evaluate the models adopted in investigations assessing the comparative effectiveness of RARP versus ORP.

OUTCOMES DEFINITION

There is tremendous variation in the reporting of postoperative complications, functional outcomes, and oncologic results in urologic oncology, regardless of the surgical approach.[5,34–36] Consequently, the implementation of commonly accepted definitions for postoperative endpoints is necessary to compare the results of RARP with ORP. Currently, the lack of such standardized endpoints undermines the validity of studies comparing RARP with ORP. In this context, several efforts have been recently made to standardize the definition of postoperative endpoints.

Short-Term Outcomes

The manner in which perioperative outcomes or complications are reported is a significant confounder when trying to assess differences in complication rates between RARP and ORP.[37] Such confusion has led to efforts to standardize the reporting of complications after surgery. Specifically, Martin and colleagues[38] developed 10 criteria for the evaluation of studies reporting postoperative complications (**Table 1**). These include methods of data accrual, definition of complications, outpatient information, severity grading, procedure-specific complications, length of stay, mortality rates and cause of death, duration of follow-up, and data on preoperative risk factors.[38] These criteria were subsequently modified and adapted for urologic surgery by Donat.[39] Although many notable studies[40–42] have adopted the Martin-Donat criteria for standardized reporting of complications, these criteria are not routinely applied in most settings. For example, a recently published systematic review comparing the perioperative outcomes of RARP and ORP identified only 1 publication that fulfilled all of the 10 Martin criteria.[19,43] Regardless, retrospective comparative assessments critically need to fulfill these criteria to be considered valid and relevant.[19,44]

The cornerstone of the Martin-Donat criteria is using a standardized grading system for complications.[38] The most commonly used grading system is based on the work by Clavien and colleagues.[45] In their pioneering investigation, the investigators systemically categorized postoperative complications into 4 grades according to their severity. In 2004, this grading system was updated by Dindo and colleagues,[46] who modified these criteria to improve their accuracy and applicability to the surgical community.

The current grading system uses the following definitions:

- Grade 0: absence of any complications
- Grade 1: presence of any deviation from the normal postoperative course
- Grade 2: management that includes not more than intravenous blood transfusion
- Grade 3: complications that require surgical, endoscopic, or radiologic intervention

Table 1
Martin criteria for the evaluation of article reporting complications after surgery

Criteria	Requirement
Method of accruing data defined	Prospective or retrospective accrual of data are indicated.
Duration of follow-up indicated	Report clarifies the time period of postoperative accrual of complications, such as 30 d or same hospitalization.
Outpatient information included	Study indicates that complications first identified after discharge are included in the analysis.
Definitions of complications provided	Article defines at least 1 complication with specific inclusion criteria.
Mortality rate and causes of death listed	The number of patients who died in the postoperative period of study are recorded together with cause of death.
Morbidity rate and total complications indicated	The number of patients with any complication and the total number of complications are recorded.
Procedure-specific complications included	Radical prostatectomy: anastomotic leak, lymphocele, urinary retention, obturator nerve injury, etc.
Severity grade used	Any grading system designed to clarify severity of complications, including major and minor, is reported (eg, Clavien and Dindo grading system).
Length-of-stay data	Median or mean length of stay is indicated in the study.
Risk factors included in the analysis	Evidence of risk stratification and method used is indicated by study.

- Grade 4: life-threatening complications requiring intensive care management
- Grade 5: complications that cause the death of the patient

This system is notable for recording any deviation from the regular postoperative course as a complication.[37,45–47] Previous studies showed that this grading system is easily applicable and reproducible in patients treated with RP.[37,44,47] Many comparative assessments between ORP and RARP do not consider blood transfusions as complications but as a separate endpoint. As such, many investigators have argued that if blood transfusions were considered complications, most if not all evidence would show lower complication rates with RARP compared with ORP. Regardless, the adoption of these standardized evaluation tools in more recent publications facilitates the comparison of short-term outcomes of RARP and ORP. For example, Agarwal and colleagues[40] demonstrated the safety of robotic surgery in a large cohort of patients with clinically localized PCa treated at a single referral tertiary center; this report represents one of the first efforts to use the standardized Martin-Donat criteria to examine morbidity and mortality after RARP.

Functional Outcomes

The use of clear definitions for potency and continence recovery is essential for comparing functional outcomes between patients treated with RARP and ORP. Indeed, the adoption of validated questionnaires, such as the International Index of Erectile Function (IIEF), has been widely advocated for the assessment of erectile function after surgery.[6,20,21,36] Briganti and colleagues[36] showed that an erectile function domain of the IIEF greater than or equal to 22 represents a reliable score for defining a satisfactory erectile function after radical prostatectomy. Therefore, such a definition should be applied when assessing the rates of erectile function recovery after ORP and RARP.[36]

Similarly, when evaluating postoperative urinary continence, previous studies have demonstrated that the definition of incontinence substantially affected the rates of continence recovery after surgery.[48–50] In an effort to define more stringent criteria for satisfactory continence, Liss and colleagues[50] recently observed that patients reporting the use of 1 pad or more per day had a significant decrease in postoperative quality of life compared with their counterparts using no pad. Consequently, many investigators have advocated that urinary continence recovery after surgery should be strictly defined as the use of no pad.[50] Additionally, the odds of functional outcomes recovery significantly vary over time; however, improvements in urinary continence and erectile function recovery after 36 months of follow-up are trifling. In consequence, a median follow-up of at least 3 years should be considered compulsory when comparing functional outcomes between open and minimally invasive surgery.

Oncologic Outcomes

When evaluating oncologic outcomes, the short follow-up in series of patients treated with RARP prevents investigators from comprehensively comparing cancer-specific mortality rates between the 2 surgical approaches.[5,25] Given the indolent natural history of clinically localized PCa, a long-term follow-up is needed to assess important postoperative oncologic outcomes, such as metastasis-free survival and cancer-related mortality. In consequence, secondary endpoints have been considered.

Biochemical recurrence (BCR) represents one of the most frequently reported surrogate endpoints. It needs to be taken into consideration, however, that the rates of BCR are conditional to several confounders, such as preoperative and pathologic characteristics, length of follow-up, and use of adjuvant hormonal or radiation therapies.[51–54] The pioneering study by Menon and colleagues[55] was the first to report the 5-year BCR-free survival rates in a large cohort of patients treated with RARP alone (without adjuvant therapies), supporting the safety of this approach.

The presence of positive surgical margins at final pathology has also been proposed as a proxy for cancer control.[23–25,56–58] Again, caution should be used when considering this endpoint. The impact of positive margins on the long-term risk of BCR and cancer-specific mortality remains controversial and is likely dependent on the presence of other adverse pathologic features at RP as well as patient life expectancy.[59–64] Additionally, the rates of positive margins may depend more on surgical expertise[64] and/or surgical technique (ie, aggressiveness of nerve sparing) rather than represent the quality of the approach (RARP vs ORP). The learning curve phenomenon may play a more significant role in patients treated with minimally invasive surgery, given the recent introduction of the robotic technique and the low cumulative case volume of early adopters.[65] Consequently, the use of this endpoint may not be adequate to comprehensively assess the oncologic safety of robot-assisted versus open surgery.[63,66]

Similar limitations apply when comparing the use of postoperative cancer-related therapies between patients treated with RARP or ORP.[23,66,67] The administration of adjuvant radiotherapy and hormonal therapy strongly depends on disease characteristics at final pathology.[66,68] For example, evidence from randomized trials supports the use of adjuvant androgen deprivation therapy after RP in patients with node-positive PCa.[2,53] Because the likelihood of lymph node invasion at RP depends on the extent of the pelvic lymph node dissection performed[2,69,70] and because patients treated with RARP are less likely to receive a lymph node dissection at RP,[65] the use of postoperative cancer therapies may be higher in ORP patients when it really reflects more precise nodal staging. Moreover, given the lack of consensus on the benefits of adjuvant radiotherapy after RP, the selection of patients for adjuvant therapies relies immensely on patient-physician perceptions and preferences.[71–73] Such considerations undermine the validity of this endpoint as a proxy of cancer control after RP.[66]

Costs and Expenditures

In an era of heightened scrutiny for health care spending and resource allocation, treatment-associated expenditures represent an important endpoint when comparing RARP and ORP.[23,27,74] One of the purported disadvantages related to the adoption of minimally invasive surgery is the substantially higher costs associated with the purchase of robotic equipment and the use of disposables.[29,75,76] On the other hand, several investigators have postulated that shorter length of stay and lower rates of transfusions may result in lower costs of RARP compared with ORP in the early postoperative setting.[74] The absence of prospective studies, however, comparing the costs and expenditures associated with RARP and ORP limits the ability to fully grasp these interesting hypotheses.[27,29,74] Moreover, the proposed savings from a shortened length of hospitalization and lower transfusion rates rely on health care provider reimbursement policies, which may vary from one country to another.[31,74] The potential benefits of RARP with regard to lower rates of positive surgical margins and use of additional cancer therapies would also result in substantial savings for the health care system in the long term[23]; however, prospective studies incorporating these endpoints are needed to fully address this.

OBSERVATIONAL STUDIES

Retrospective Studies from Tertiary Referral Centers

Several retrospective studies from high-volume tertiary referral centers showing better short-term postoperative outcomes for patients undergoing RARP fueled the initial enthusiasm for minimally invasive approaches for PCa surgery.[55,56,77–79] These data should be interpreted with caution, however. First, results obtained from high-volume hospitals and surgeons may not be applicable to the broader general population, because most patients are treated at community hospitals.[80] Second, the introduction of a robotics training program at high-volume centers is associated with more stringent patient selection with regard to preoperative disease and patient characteristics.[81,82] Specifically, patients with more favorable disease and health are more likely to be selected to the novel approach (ie, minimally invasive surgery).[81] Such selection bias may result in better short- and long-term outcomes for patients treated with minimally invasive approaches compared with their open counterparts. Some of these selection biases are often unrecorded in retrospective observational studies, thus may undermine the validity of retrospective comparative investigations, because these unmeasured confounders may exert strong influence on the outcomes, to an extent that any statistical adjustment would not appropriately mitigate.[83]

Several systematic reviews and meta-analyses based on these retrospective data from high-volume centers showed significant benefits for RARP with regard to perioperative outcomes, functional results, and oncologic endpoints.[19–21,25,84] Unfortunately, the aforementioned limitations apply also to these investigations, in addition to the usual publication bias for positive studies.[85] Consequently, despite the high number of patients evaluated, these meta-analyses do not provide a definitive and compelling answer to the question, Which surgical approach is best for the treatment of patients with clinically localized PCa? If it is assumed that adjustment for case mix is appropriately performed (which is not a given), the best interpretation of these data may be that the outcomes of the best RARP series (or surgeons) are better than those of the best ORP series (or surgeons).

Population-Based Studies

As discussed previously, data from high-volume referral centers may not be generalizable to the overall population. In the absence of randomized controlled trials, several investigators give credence to population-based analyses evaluating the comparative effectiveness of RARP versus ORP in large contemporary cohorts of patients with clinically localized PCa.[8,18,23,29,86] Such studies allow for comparison of competing therapies across a broad range of health care settings.[86]

Results obtained from these data differ somewhat from those originating from high-volume referral centers.[8,27,65,67,86] In their assessment of a large population-based cohort of patients within the Nationwide Inpatient Sample, Trinh and colleagues[18] were able to demonstrate superiority of RARP over ORP for virtually all perioperative outcomes. In a landmark investigation by Hu and colleagues,[86] however, no differences were observed between ORP and RARP with regard to perioperative outcomes and long-term functional results when evaluating a population aged 65 years or older enrolled in Medicare. Gandaglia and colleagues[17] examined postoperative complications and use of additional cancer treatments in a more contemporary cohort of Medicare beneficiaries and corroborated the results of the Hu and colleagues' study. Similarly, Barry and colleagues[8] compared the odds of problems with continence and sexual function after RARP and ORP in Medicare beneficiaries treated between 2008 and 2009 using rigorous survey instruments and validated questionnaires. They observed that robotic surgery was associated with a nonsignificant trend toward greater problems with urinary continence. Additionally, the adoption of RARP was not associated with better erectile function recovery rates at a median follow-up of 14 months.[8]

The reasons for such discrepancy may reside in preoperative case mix, where individuals included in these population-based studies may be older and sicker compared with their counterparts treated in referral centers. Many of these studies originate from Medicare enrollees, who are by definition older than 65 years of age. This may also explain why Trinh and colleagues'[18] study showed a benefit for RARP with regard to perioperative outcomes, whereas the other studies did not. Additionally, the learning curve phenomenon may be more influential at a population-based level. From a practical prospective, when results of institutional series conflict with large population-based studies, these findings highlight the importance of the surgeon rather than the surgical approach.[9,87] For example, relying on Nationwide Inpatient Sample data that showed that RARP was associated on average with better perioperative outcomes than ORP,[18] Sammon and colleagues[87] nevertheless observed that ORP performed at high-volume hospitals had better outcomes than RARP performed at low-volume hospitals.

Statistical Methodology Applied in Retrospective Studies Comparing the Two Techniques

Several efforts have been made to limit the effect of selection bias in retrospective observational studies comparing RARP with ORP. Several advanced statistical tools have been applied to minimize the effect of confounders. For example, propensity score matching represents a commonly used approach in observational retrospective investigations. This method allows the selection of control subjects matched with treated subjects for readily available covariates, which, if unaccounted for, lead to biased estimates of treatment effects.[88] When matching is performed, the covariates in the control and treatment groups are balanced after the matching process.[88] Thus, analyses performed on the postpropensity score–matched population should lead to theoretically unbiased comparisons between postoperative outcomes of the 2 surgical techniques. Many investigators think, however, that although the effect of measured confounders is minimized with propensity score matching, the effect of unmeasured confounders may be amplified.[89]

Another statistical method gaining traction in the field is the instrumental variable analysis. This approach claims to perform pseudorandomization by accounting for both measured and unmeasured confounders.[90] By definition, an instrumental variable should be associated with the odds of receiving the treatment of interest (eg, RARP) but should not be associated with the analyzed endpoint (eg, cancer-specific survival) except through the choice of treatment. Examples of instrumental variables that could be used to compare RARP with ORP are the density of RARP cases performed in a given area, the distance to the closest hospital performing RARP, or even physician-level preference for RARP. These instruments are conceptually sound; however, the quality of the instrument must always be verified using statistical calculations, such as the F-statistic.[91,92] For example, the density of RARPs performed in a given area are expected to influence the choice of treatment; however, that variable is not expected to affect the endpoint (for example, postoperative complications) except through the choice of treatment (RARP vs ORP). The instrumental variable is subsequently used for pseudorandomization, thereby allowing estimation of the effect of a certain treatment on the marginal population (eg, individuals for whom the likelihood of undergoing the treatment is based on the instrumental variable).[93]

Although these statistical tools may limit the effect of selection bias when applied correctly, data from observational studies will never be as compelling as evidence from well-designed prospective randomized trials.

PROSPECTIVE RANDOMIZED TRIALS

To the best of the authors' knowledge, there is no published randomized trial comparing the outcomes of RARP with those of ORP. Two randomized trials have been accruing patients, however, and results are expected in the short term.[94,95] Gardiner and colleagues[94] are recruiting 200 patients per treatment arm (RARP vs ORP) at a major public hospital clinic in Queensland, Australia. One surgeon is performing all RARPs whereas another surgeon is performing all ORPs. The endpoints considered are both oncologic (positive surgical margins, BCR, and need for further treatments) and nononcologic (pain, physical and mental functioning, fatigue, urinary continence, erectile function recovery, and quality of life). Cost modeling for each approach, as well as a full economic appraisal, will also be performed.[94] The second trial is currently recruiting participants at the Mayo Clinic, and the preliminary results are expected by May 2016.[95] The primary endpoint is trifecta status (ie, free of BCR, potency, and continence, at 2-year follow-up).

Finally, results from 2 randomized controlled trials comparing RARP with pure laparoscopic RP have recently been published.[96,97] Asimakopoulos and colleagues[96] randomized 128 patients with clinically localized PCa in 2 groups: RARP and laparoscopic RP. The primary endpoints were erectile function and urinary continence recovery, postoperative complications, and pathologic results.[96] The study showed that patients treated with RARP had higher erectile function recovery rates compared with their laparoscopic counterparts. No differences were found, however, between the 2 surgical approaches when evaluating the other endpoints. Recently, Porpiglia and colleagues[97] presented the results of their prospective randomized trial comparing RARP and laparoscopic RP. The investigators included 120 patients with clinically localized PCa, who were randomly assigned to RARP or laparoscopic RP. The same surgeon performed all cases. The investigators did not find any differences between the 2 surgical approaches with regard to postoperative complications and pathologic results; however, RARP provided better recovery of functional outcomes (ie, urinary continence and erectile function) at 12-month follow-up.[97] The small number of patients included limits the generalizability of these prospective trials. Ultimately, critics can argue that these studies do not constitute a randomized trial of 2 surgical techniques but rather a randomized trial of a single surgeon's ability to perform RARP versus laparoscopic RP.

SUMMARY

Several methodological aspects should be considered when evaluating the effectiveness of robotic surgery in patients with clinically localized PCa. First, the adoption of standardized endpoints is needed to compare these 2 techniques. Second, the level of evidence supporting the superiority of one approach over the other (RARP vs ORP) depends on the type of study design. Currently, the comparative effectiveness of RARP and ORP has been exclusively evaluated through retrospective observational studies. Selection bias and short follow-up undermine the findings obtained in this setting. Therefore, prospective randomized trials are needed to comprehensively assess the superiority or inferiority of RARP compared with other surgical approaches for the treatment of PCa.

REFERENCES

1. Siegel R, Ma J, Zou Z, et al. Cancer statistics, 2014. CA Cancer J Clin 2014;64(1):9–29.
2. Heidenreich A, Bastian PJ, Bellmunt J, et al. EAU guidelines on prostate cancer. part 1: screening, diagnosis, and local treatment with curative intent-update 2013. Eur Urol 2014;65(1):124–37.
3. Walsh PC, Donker PJ. Impotence following radical prostatectomy: insight into etiology and prevention. J Urol 1982;128(3):492–7.
4. Mullins JK, Feng Z, Trock BJ, et al. The impact of anatomical radical retropubic prostatectomy on cancer control: the 30-year anniversary. J Urol 2012;188(6):2219–24.
5. Boorjian SA, Eastham JA, Graefen M, et al. A critical analysis of the long-term impact of radical prostatectomy on cancer control and function outcomes. Eur Urol 2012;61(4):664–75.
6. Gandaglia G, Suardi N, Gallina A, et al. Preoperative erectile function represents a significant predictor of postoperative urinary continence recovery in patients treated with bilateral nerve sparing radical prostatectomy. J Urol 2012;187(2):569–74.
7. Suardi N, Moschini M, Gallina A, et al. Nerve-sparing approach during radical prostatectomy is strongly associated with the rate of postoperative urinary continence recovery. BJU Int 2013;111(5):717–22.
8. Barry MJ, Gallagher PM, Skinner JS, et al. Adverse effects of robotic-assisted laparoscopic versus open retropubic radical prostatectomy among a nationwide random sample of medicare-age men. J Clin Oncol 2012;30(5):513–8.
9. Trinh QD, Ghani KR, Menon M. Robot-assisted radical prostatectomy: ready to be counted? Eur Urol 2012;62(1):16–8 [discussion: 18–9].
10. Lowrance WT, Eastham JA, Savage C, et al. Contemporary open and robotic radical prostatectomy practice patterns among urologists in the United States. J Urol 2012;187(6):2087–92.
11. Abbou CC, Hoznek A, Salomon L, et al. Laparoscopic radical prostatectomy with a remote controlled robot. J Urol 2001;165(6 Pt 1):1964–6.
12. Menon M, Shrivastava A, Tewari A, et al. Laparoscopic and robot assisted radical prostatectomy: establishment of a structured program and preliminary analysis of outcomes. J Urol 2002;168(3):945–9.
13. Tewari A, Peabody J, Sarle R, et al. Technique of da Vinci robot-assisted anatomic radical prostatectomy. Urology 2002;60(4):569–72.
14. Menon M, Tewari A, Peabody JO, et al. Vattikuti Institute prostatectomy, a technique of robotic radical prostatectomy for management of localized carcinoma of the prostate: experience of over 1100 cases. Urol Clin North Am 2004;31(4):701–17.
15. Menon M, Hemal AK, Tewari A, et al. The technique of apical dissection of the prostate and urethrovesical anastomosis in robotic radical prostatectomy. BJU Int 2004;93(6):715–9.
16. Menon M, Tewari A, Peabody J, et al. Vattikuti Institute prostatectomy: technique. J Urol 2003;169(6): 2289–92.
17. Gandaglia G, Sammon JD, Chang SL, et al. Comparative effectiveness of robot-assisted and open radical prostatectomy in the postdissemination era. J Clin Oncol 2014;32(14):1419–26.
18. Trinh QD, Sammon J, Sun M, et al. Perioperative outcomes of robot-assisted radical prostatectomy compared with open radical prostatectomy: results from the nationwide inpatient sample. Eur Urol 2012;61(4):679–85.
19. Novara G, Ficarra V, Rosen RC, et al. Systematic review and meta-analysis of perioperative outcomes and complications after robot-assisted radical prostatectomy. Eur Urol 2012;62(3):431–52.
20. Ficarra V, Novara G, Rosen RC, et al. Systematic review and meta-analysis of studies reporting urinary continence recovery after robot-assisted radical prostatectomy. Eur Urol 2012;62(3):405–17.
21. Ficarra V, Novara G, Ahlering TE, et al. Systematic review and meta-analysis of studies reporting potency rates after robot-assisted radical prostatectomy. Eur Urol 2012;62(3):418–30.
22. Gandaglia G, Suardi N, Gallina A, et al. How to optimize patient selection for robot-assisted radical prostatectomy: functional outcome analyses from a Tertiary Referral Center. J Endourol 2014;28(7): 792–800.
23. Hu JC, Gandaglia G, Karakiewicz PI, et al. Comparative effectiveness of robot-assisted versus open

radical prostatectomy cancer control. Eur Urol 2014. [Epub ahead of print].
24. Sooriakumaran P, Srivastava A, Shariat SF, et al. A multinational, multi-institutional study comparing positive surgical margin rates among 22393 open, laparoscopic, and robot-assisted radical prostatectomy patients. Eur Urol 2013. [Epub ahead of print].
25. Novara G, Ficarra V, Mocellin S, et al. Systematic review and meta-analysis of studies reporting oncologic outcome after robot-assisted radical prostatectomy. Eur Urol 2012;62(3):382–404.
26. Suardi N, Ficarra V, Willemsen P, et al. Long-term biochemical recurrence rates after robot-assisted radical prostatectomy: analysis of a single-center series of patients with a minimum follow-up of 5 years. Urology 2012;79(1):133–8.
27. Close A, Robertson C, Rushton S, et al. Comparative cost-effectiveness of robot-assisted and standard laparoscopic prostatectomy as alternatives to open radical prostatectomy for treatment of men with localised prostate cancer: a health technology assessment from the perspective of the UK National Health Service. Eur Urol 2013;64(3): 361–9.
28. Bjartell AS, Steineck G, Haglind E. Modeling costs for prostate surgery: are we close to reality? Eur Urol 2013;64(3):370–1.
29. Kim SP, Shah ND, Karnes RJ, et al. Hospitalization costs for radical prostatectomy attributable to robotic surgery. Eur Urol 2013;64(1):11–6.
30. Sleeper J, Lotan Y. Cost-effectiveness of robotic-assisted laparoscopic procedures in urologic surgery in the USA. Expert Rev Med Devices 2011; 8(1):97–103.
31. Nguyen PL, Gu X, Lipsitz SR, et al. Cost implications of the rapid adoption of newer technologies for treating prostate cancer. J Clin Oncol 2011; 29(12):1517–24.
32. Lowrance WT, Eastham JA, Yee DS, et al. Costs of medical care after open or minimally invasive prostate cancer surgery: a population-based analysis. Cancer 2012;118(12):3079–86.
33. Barbash GI, Glied SA. New technology and health care costs–the case of robot-assisted surgery. N Engl J Med 2010;363(8):701–4.
34. Cookson MS, Aus G, Burnett AL, et al. Variation in the definition of biochemical recurrence in patients treated for localized prostate cancer: the American Urological Association Prostate Guidelines for Localized Prostate Cancer Update Panel report and recommendations for a standard in the reporting of surgical outcomes. J Urol 2007;177(2):540–5.
35. Mir MC, Li J, Klink JC, et al. Optimal definition of biochemical recurrence after radical prostatectomy depends on pathologic risk factors: identifying candidates for early salvage therapy. Eur Urol 2013. [Epub ahead of print].
36. Briganti A, Gallina A, Suardi N, et al. What is the definition of a satisfactory erectile function after bilateral nerve sparing radical prostatectomy? J Sex Med 2011;8(4):1210–7.
37. Graefen M. The modified Clavien system: a plea for a standardized reporting system for surgical complications. Eur Urol 2010;57(3):387–9.
38. Martin RC 2nd, Brennan MF, Jaques DP. Quality of complication reporting in the surgical literature. Ann Surg 2002;235(6):803–13.
39. Donat SM. Standards for surgical complication reporting in urologic oncology: time for a change. Urology 2007;69(2):221–5.
40. Agarwal PK, Sammon J, Bhandari A, et al. Safety profile of robot-assisted radical prostatectomy: a standardized report of complications in 3317 patients. Eur Urol 2011;59(5):684–98.
41. Ghazi A, Scosyrev E, Patel H, et al. Complications associated with extraperitoneal robot-assisted radical prostatectomy using the standardized Martin classification. Urology 2013;81(2):324–31.
42. Jhaveri JK, Penna FJ, Diaz-Insua M, et al. Ureteral injuries sustained during robot-assisted radical prostatectomy. J Endourol 2014;28(3):318–24.
43. Novara G, Ficarra V, D'Elia C, et al. Prospective evaluation with standardised criteria for postoperative complications after robotic-assisted laparoscopic radical prostatectomy. Eur Urol 2010;57(3):363–70.
44. Hakimi AA, Faleck DM, Sobey S, et al. Assessment of complication and functional outcome reporting in the minimally invasive prostatectomy literature from 2006 to the present. BJU Int 2012;109(1): 26–30 [discussion: 30].
45. Clavien PA, Sanabria JR, Strasberg SM. Proposed classification of complications of surgery with examples of utility in cholecystectomy. Surgery 1992;111(5):518–26.
46. Dindo D, Demartines N, Clavien PA. Classification of surgical complications: a new proposal with evaluation in a cohort of 6336 patients and results of a survey. Ann Surg 2004;240(2):205–13.
47. Loppenberg B, Noldus J, Holz A, et al. Reporting complications after open radical retropubic prostatectomy using the Martin criteria. J Urol 2010; 184(3):944–8.
48. Wei JT, Dunn RL, Marcovich R, et al. Prospective assessment of patient reported urinary continence after radical prostatectomy. J Urol 2000;164(3 Pt 1): 744–8.
49. Wei JT, Montie JE. Comparison of patients' and physicians' rating of urinary incontinence following radical prostatectomy. Semin Urol Oncol 2000; 18(1):76–80.
50. Liss MA, Osann K, Canvasser N, et al. Continence definition after radical prostatectomy using urinary quality of life: evaluation of patient reported validated questionnaires. J Urol 2010;183(4):1464–8.

51. Bolla M, van Poppel H, Tombal B, et al. Postoperative radiotherapy after radical prostatectomy for high-risk prostate cancer: long-term results of a randomised controlled trial (EORTC trial 22911). Lancet 2012;380(9858):2018–27.
52. Briganti A, Joniau S, Gandaglia G, et al. Patterns and predictors of early biochemical recurrence after radical prostatectomy and adjuvant radiation therapy in men with pT3N0 prostate cancer: implications for multimodal therapies. Int J Radiat Oncol Biol Phys 2013;87(5):960–7.
53. Messing EM, Manola J, Sarosdy M, et al. Immediate hormonal therapy compared with observation after radical prostatectomy and pelvic lymphadenectomy in men with node-positive prostate cancer. N Engl J Med 1999;341(24):1781–8.
54. Punnen S, Cooperberg MR, D'Amico AV, et al. Management of biochemical recurrence after primary treatment of prostate cancer: a systematic review of the literature. Eur Urol 2013;64(6):905–15.
55. Menon M, Bhandari M, Gupta N, et al. Biochemical recurrence following robot-assisted radical prostatectomy: analysis of 1384 patients with a median 5-year follow-up. Eur Urol 2010;58(6):838–46.
56. Masterson TA, Cheng L, Boris RS, et al. Open vs. robotic-assisted radical prostatectomy: a single surgeon and pathologist comparison of pathologic and oncologic outcomes. Urol Oncol 2013;31(7): 1043–8.
57. Jayram G, Decastro GJ, Large MC, et al. Robotic radical prostatectomy in patients with high-risk disease: a review of short-term outcomes from a high-volume center. J Endourol 2011;25(3):455–7.
58. Magheli A, Gonzalgo ML, Su LM, et al. Impact of surgical technique (open vs laparoscopic vs robotic-assisted) on pathological and biochemical outcomes following radical prostatectomy: an analysis using propensity score matching. BJU Int 2011;107(12):1956–62.
59. Ploussard G, Drouin SJ, Rode J, et al. Location, extent, and multifocality of positive surgical margins for biochemical recurrence prediction after radical prostatectomy. World J Urol 2014. [Epub ahead of print].
60. Choo MS, Cho SY, Ko K, et al. Impact of positive surgical margins and their locations after radical prostatectomy: comparison of biochemical recurrence according to risk stratification and surgical modality. World J Urol 2013. [Epub ahead of print].
61. Briganti A, Karnes RJ, Joniau S, et al. Prediction of outcome following early salvage radiotherapy among patients with biochemical recurrence after radical prostatectomy. Eur Urol 2013. [Epub ahead of print].
62. Stephenson AJ, Eggener SE, Hernandez AV, et al. Do margins matter? The influence of positive surgical margins on prostate cancer-specific mortality. Eur Urol 2014;65(4):675–80.
63. Yossepowitch O, Briganti A, Eastham JA, et al. Positive surgical margins after radical prostatectomy: a systematic review and contemporary update. Eur Urol 2014;65(2):303–13.
64. Vickers A, Bianco F, Cronin A, et al. The learning curve for surgical margins after open radical prostatectomy: implications for margin status as an oncological end point. J Urol 2010;183(4):1360–5.
65. Gandaglia G, Trinh QD, Hu JC, et al. The impact of robot-assisted radical prostatectomy on the use and extent of pelvic lymph node dissection in the "post-dissemination" period. Eur J Surg Oncol 2014;40(9):1080–6.
66. Karnes RJ, Joniau S, Blute ML, et al. Caveat Emptor. Eur Urol 2014. [Epub ahead of print].
67. Gandaglia G, Abdollah F, Hu J, et al. Is robot-assisted radical prostatectomy safe in men with high-risk prostate cancer? Assessment of perioperative outcomes, positive surgical margins, and use of additional cancer treatments. J Endourol 2014; 28(7):784–91.
68. Abdollah F, Suardi N, Cozzarini C, et al. Selecting the optimal candidate for adjuvant radiotherapy after radical prostatectomy for prostate cancer: a long-term survival analysis. Eur Urol 2013;63(6): 998–1008.
69. Abdollah F, Sun M, Thuret R, et al. Decreasing rate and extent of lymph node staging in patients undergoing radical prostatectomy may undermine the rate of diagnosis of lymph node metastases in prostate cancer. Eur Urol 2010;58(6):882–92.
70. Briganti A, Larcher A, Abdollah F, et al. Updated nomogram predicting lymph node invasion in patients with prostate cancer undergoing extended pelvic lymph node dissection: the essential importance of percentage of positive cores. Eur Urol 2012;61(3):480–7.
71. Pfister D, Bolla M, Briganti A, et al. Early salvage radiotherapy following radical prostatectomy. Eur Urol 2014;65(6):1034–43.
72. Briganti A, Wiegel T, Joniau S, et al. Early salvage radiation therapy does not compromise cancer control in patients with pT3N0 prostate cancer after radical prostatectomy: results of a match-controlled multi-institutional analysis. Eur Urol 2012;62(3):472–87.
73. Thompson IM, Valicenti RK, Albertsen P, et al. Adjuvant and salvage radiotherapy after prostatectomy: AUA/ASTRO Guideline. J Urol 2013;190(2):441–9.
74. Bolenz C, Freedland SJ, Hollenbeck BK, et al. Costs of radical prostatectomy for prostate cancer: a systematic review. Eur Urol 2014;65(2):316–24.
75. Tomaszewski JJ, Matchett JC, Davies BJ, et al. Comparative hospital cost-analysis of open and robotic-assisted radical prostatectomy. Urology 2012;80(1):126–9.
76. Yu HY, Hevelone ND, Lipsitz SR, et al. Use, costs and comparative effectiveness of robotic assisted,

laparoscopic and open urological surgery. J Urol 2012;187(4):1392–8.
77. Menon M, Tewari A, Baize B, et al. Prospective comparison of radical retropubic prostatectomy and robot-assisted anatomic prostatectomy: the Vattikuti Urology Institute experience. Urology 2002;60(5): 864–8.
78. Ahlering TE, Woo D, Eichel L, et al. Robot-assisted versus open radical prostatectomy: a comparison of one surgeon's outcomes. Urology 2004;63(5):819–22.
79. Rocco B, Matei DV, Melegari S, et al. Robotic vs open prostatectomy in a laparoscopically naive centre: a matched-pair analysis. BJU Int 2009;104(7):991–5.
80. Schmitges J, Trinh QD, Bianchi M, et al. The effect of annual surgical caseload on the rates of in-hospital pneumonia and other in-hospital outcomes after radical prostatectomy. Int Urol Nephrol 2012; 44(3):799–806.
81. Briganti A, Bianchi M, Sun M, et al. Impact of the introduction of a robotic training programme on prostate cancer stage migration at a single tertiary referral centre. BJU Int 2013;111(8):1222–30.
82. Jacobs BL, Zhang Y, Schroeck FR, et al. Use of advanced treatment technologies among men at low risk of dying from prostate cancer. JAMA 2013;309(24):2587–95.
83. Giordano SH, Kuo YF, Duan Z, et al. Limits of observational data in determining outcomes from cancer therapy. Cancer 2008;112(11):2456–66.
84. Moran PS, O'Neill M, Teljeur C, et al. Robot-assisted radical prostatectomy compared with open and laparoscopic approaches: a systematic review and meta-analysis. Int J Urol 2013;20(3):312–21.
85. Thornton A, Lee P. Publication bias in meta-analysis: its causes and consequences. J Clin Epidemiol 2000;53(2):207–16.
86. Hu JC, Gu X, Lipsitz SR, et al. Comparative effectiveness of minimally invasive vs open radical prostatectomy. JAMA 2009;302(14):1557–64.
87. Sammon JD, Karakiewicz PI, Sun M, et al. Robot-assisted versus open radical prostatectomy: the differential effect of regionalization, procedure volume and operative approach. J Urol 2013;189(4): 1289–94.
88. D'Agostino RB Jr. Propensity score methods for bias reduction in the comparison of a treatment to a non-randomized control group. Stat Med 1998; 17(19):2265–81.
89. Brooks JM, Ohsfeldt RL. Squeezing the balloon: propensity scores and unmeasured covariate balance. Health Serv Res 2013;48(4):1487–507.
90. Korn EL, Freidlin B. Methodology for comparative effectiveness research: potential and limitations. J Clin Oncol 2012;30(34):4185–7.
91. Newhouse JP, McClellan M. Econometrics in outcomes research: the use of instrumental variables. Annu Rev Public Health 1998;19:17–34.
92. Lu-Yao GL, Albertsen PC, Moore DF, et al. Survival following primary androgen deprivation therapy among men with localized prostate cancer. JAMA 2008;300(2):173–81.
93. Stukel TA, Fisher ES, Wennberg DE, et al. Analysis of observational studies in the presence of treatment selection bias: effects of invasive cardiac management on AMI survival using propensity score and instrumental variable methods. JAMA 2007;297(3): 278–85.
94. Gardiner RA, Yaxley J, Coughlin G, et al. A randomised trial of robotic and open prostatectomy in men with localised prostate cancer. BMC Cancer 2012;12:189.
95. Thompson RH, Tollefson MK. Available at: http://clinicaltrials.gov/show/NCT01365143. Accessed March 26, 2014.
96. Asimakopoulos AD, Pereira Fraga CT, Annino F, et al. Randomized comparison between laparoscopic and robot-assisted nerve-sparing radical prostatectomy. J Sex Med 2011;8(5):1503–12.
97. Porpiglia F, Morra I, Lucci Chiarissi M, et al. Randomised controlled trial comparing laparoscopic and robot-assisted radical prostatectomy. Eur Urol 2013;63(4):606–14.

Index

Note: Page numbers of article titles are in **boldface** type.

Urol Clin N Am 41 (2014) 607–612
http://dx.doi.org/10.1016/S0094-0143(14)00093-7

O

P

R

S

T

U

United States Postal Service

Statement of Ownership, Management, and Circulation
(All Periodicals Publications Except Requestor Publications)

1. Publication Title	2. Publication Number	3. Filing Date
Urologic Clinics of North America	0 0 0 - 7 1 1	9/14/14

4. Issue Frequency	5. Number of Issues Published Annually	6. Annual Subscription Price
Feb, May, Aug, Nov	4	$355.00

7. Complete Mailing Address of Known Office of Publication (*Not printer*) (*Street, city, county, state, and ZIP+4®*)

Elsevier Inc.
360 Park Avenue South
New York, NY 10010-1710

Contact Person: Stephen R. Bushing
Telephone (Include area code): 215-239-3688

8. Complete Mailing Address of Headquarters or General Business Office of Publisher (*Not printer*)

Elsevier Inc., 360 Park Avenue South, New York, NY 10010-1710

9. Full Names and Complete Mailing Addresses of Publisher, Editor, and Managing Editor (*Do not leave blank*)

Publisher (*Name and complete mailing address*)

Linda Belfus, Elsevier, Inc., 1600 John F. Kennedy Blvd. Suite 1800, Philadelphia, PA 19103-2899

Editor (*Name and complete mailing address*)

Kerry Holland, Elsevier, Inc., 1600 John F. Kennedy Blvd. Suite 1800, Philadelphia, PA 19103-2899

Managing Editor (*Name and complete mailing address*)

Adrianne Brigido, Elsevier, Inc., 1600 John F. Kennedy Blvd. Suite 1800, Philadelphia, PA 19103-2899

10. Owner (*Do not leave blank. If the publication is owned by a corporation, give the name and address of the corporation immediately followed by the names and addresses of all stockholders owning or holding 1 percent or more of the total amount of stock. If not owned by a corporation, give the names and addresses of the individual owners. If owned by a partnership or other unincorporated firm, give its name and address as well as those of each individual owner. If the publication is published by a nonprofit organization, give its name and address.*)

Full Name	Complete Mailing Address
Wholly owned subsidiary of	1600 John F. Kennedy Blvd, Ste. 1800
Reed/Elsevier, US holdings	Philadelphia, PA 19103-2899

11. Known Bondholders, Mortgagees, and Other Security Holders Owning or Holding 1 Percent or More of Total Amount of Bonds, Mortgages, or Other Securities. If none, check box → ☐ None

Full Name	Complete Mailing Address
N/A	

12. Tax Status (*For completion by nonprofit organizations authorized to mail at nonprofit rates*) (*Check one*)
The purpose, function, and nonprofit status of this organization and the exempt status for federal income tax purposes:
☐ Has Not Changed During Preceding 12 Months
☐ Has Changed During Preceding 12 Months (*Publisher must submit explanation of change with this statement*)

PS Form 3526, August 2012 (Page 1 of 3 (Instructions Page 3)) PSN 7530-01-000-9931 **PRIVACY NOTICE**: See our Privacy policy in www.usps.com

13. Publication Title: Urologic Clinics of North America
14. Issue Date for Circulation Data Below: August 2014

15. Extent and Nature of Circulation		Average No. Copies Each Issue During Preceding 12 Months	No. Copies of Single Issue Published Nearest to Filing Date
a. Total Number of Copies (*Net press run*)		1,296	1,060
b. Paid Circulation (By Mail and Outside the Mail)	(1) Mailed Outside-County Paid Subscriptions Stated on PS Form 3541. (*Include paid distribution above nominal rate, advertiser's proof copies, and exchange copies*)	625	437
	(2) Mailed In-County Paid Subscriptions Stated on PS Form 3541 (*Include paid distribution above nominal rate, advertiser's proof copies, and exchange copies*)		
	(3) Paid Distribution Outside the Mails Including Sales Through Dealers and Carriers, Street Vendors, Counter Sales, and Other Paid Distribution Outside USPS®	316	342
	(4) Paid Distribution by Other Classes Mailed Through the USPS (e.g. First-Class Mail®)		
c. Total Paid Distribution (*Sum of 15b (1), (2), (3), and (4)*)		941	779
d. Free or Nominal Rate Distribution (By Mail and Outside the Mail)	(1) Free or Nominal Rate Outside-County Copies Included on PS Form 3541	105	131
	(2) Free or Nominal Rate In-County Copies Included on PS Form 3541		
	(3) Free or Nominal Rate Copies Mailed at Other Classes Through the USPS (e.g. First-Class Mail)		
	(4) Free or Nominal Rate Distribution Outside the Mail (Carriers or other means)		
e. Total Free or Nominal Rate Distribution (Sum of 15d (1), (2), (3) and (4))		105	131
f. Total Distribution (Sum of 15c and 15e)		1,046	910
g. Copies not Distributed (See instructions to publishers #4 (page #3))		250	150
h. Total (Sum of 15f and g)		1,296	1,060
i. Percent Paid (15c divided by 15f times 100)		89.96%	85.60%
16. Total circulation includes electronic copies. Report circulation on PS Form 3526-X worksheet.			

17. Publication of Statement of Ownership
If the publication is a general publication, publication of this statement is required. Will be printed in the November 2014 issue of this publication.

18. Signature and Title of Editor, Publisher, Business Manager, or Owner

Stephen R. Bushing – Inventory Distribution Coordinator

Date: September 14, 2014

I certify that all information furnished on this form is true and complete. I understand that anyone who furnishes false or misleading information on this form or who omits material or information requested on the form may be subject to criminal sanctions (including fines and imprisonment) and/or civil sanctions (including civil penalties).

PS Form 3526, August 2012 (Page 2 of 3)

Printed and bound by CPI Group (UK) Ltd, Croydon, CR0 4YY
03/10/2024
01040376-0015